Table of Contents

Praise for
The Sensitive Patient's Healing Guide

"Have you ever walked out of a doctor's office and said to yourself *This doctor thinks I'm crazy. All my tests are 'normal,' but then why am I so exhausted, so sore, and always in a fog? To make matters worse, just a whiff of someone's cologne, a too-bright light, a sudden loud noise, even a strong electrical field, will send me into a tailspin.*

"No, you're not crazy. *The Sensitive Patient's Healing Guide* clearly explains what's going on and why, how to diagnose it, and how to treat it. Created by Dr. Neil Nathan, acclaimed author of the book *Toxic,* who has supplemented his own chapters with a masterfully curated list of celebrated contributing authors, this book collectively serves as a reference work not just for the sensitive patient but also for their loved ones, colleagues, and yes, even their physicians. An invaluable resource for the sensitive patient, the guide offers a roadmap for moving on from a life with a 'mystery illness' to one with a future of hope, recovery and health."

—Joseph Burrascano, M.D., pioneer in the treatment of Lyme Disease

"As a specialist in mold problems in buildings, I found Dr. Neil Nathan's *Sensitive Patient's Healing Guide* an enlightening read, especially regarding the complexities of mold exposure and its interactions with other health conditions. Dr. Nathan's emphasis that sensitive patients cannot truly heal while continuously exposed to toxic and water-damaged buildings with unresolved mold and other microbial issues resonates deeply with my work and underscores the indispensable connection between our surroundings and our health.

What sets this book apart is its practical approach, blending Dr. Nathan's fifty years of medical experience with contributions from twenty specialists in their respective fields. This collaborative effort, is an invaluable guide to working with people with sensitivities.

Having known Dr. Nathan for over a decade, I've always been impressed by his depth of understanding and compassion for those suffering from chronic illnesses. *The Sensitive Patient's Healing Guide* is more than a medical book; it's a testament to the power of collaborative knowledge and the importance of environmental awareness in the healing journey. It has reinforced and expanded my understanding of the vital interplay between our internal and external environments, an insight I believe will resonate with a diverse range of readers.

—John C. Banta, CIH, coauthor of *Prescriptions for a Healthy House:*
A Practical Guide for Architects, Builders, and Homeowners

"Now, more than ever, we need a medical manual for the highly sensitive patient (HSP). Dr. Neil Nathan has created a powerful guide for all who suffer from unexplained chronic complex and debilitating illness, and has given us a template for healing. Being a highly sensitive patient myself, I recommend this book to anyone who has felt frustrated by the fact that they are extra-sensitive and have struggled with traditional medical treatments and protocols that do not take into account their exquisitely delicate nature."

—**Jill Carnahan, MD, best-selling author of** *Unexpected:*
Finding Resilience through Functional Medicine, Science, and Faith

"Clinicians, if you want to know how to help patients with chemical and environmental sensitives, this is the book for you! Dr. Nathan provides a comprehensive guide to the sensitive patient, and brings to light the suffering of individuals whose conditions are poorly understood and often dismissed as psychological. The book unites a group of experts who offer a wealth of knowledge and provide models for treatment. Each chapter presents a unique perspective on the initiation and persistence of sensitivity. The book offers a comprehensive look at a complex health issue, and gives hope to thousands of individuals who suffer debilitating conditions. It's a must-read for any professional who works with patients with multiple sensitives. I highly recommend it."

—**Carolyn Torkelson MD, Adjunct Associate Professor, U of Minn.,**
author of *Beyond Menopause: New Pathways to Holistic Health*

"Dr. Nathan has created a magnificent resource for both patients and providers seeking solutions to the most elusive health problems. A gift to the future of healthcare, *The Sensitive Patient's Healing Guide* is a much-needed beacon that will lead generations forward into a new field of knowledge."

—**Hilary Crowley,** author of *The Power of Energy Medicine:*
Your Natural Prescription for Resilient Health

"With an informed and compassionate voice, Dr. Nathan speaks on the often-neglected topic of patients who are ill for reasons that are very difficult to elucidate but turn out to be sensitivity to factors in the environment or in the diet. This book is immensely comforting to patients because it establishes that their illness is legitimate, something in which the medical profession is commonly remiss. I hope health-care professionals will listen more carefully to patients after reading it, and will think more deeply about their problems. *The Sensitive Patient's Healing Guide* is well researched and well written, and will be helpful to patients and informative to providers."

—**Kirk Heriot, MD, PhD,** author of *Practical Surgical Pathology: Morphology & Molecular Pathology* and *The Prophet Returns: Calm Words for Troubled Times*

The Sensitive Patient's Healing Guide:

Top Experts Offer New Insights and Treatments for Environmental Toxins, Lyme Disease, and EMFs

Neil Nathan, MD

Cypress House
Fort Bragg, California

Cypress House
155 Cypress Street
Fort Bragg, CA 95437
800 773-7782
www.cypresshouse.com

Book Design and Production by Cypress House
Cover Design by Allegra Pescatore
Cranial Nerve Pairs with Anatomical Sensory Functions iStock.com / VectorMine
Cranial Nerves iStock.com / ttsz
Diaphragm iStock.com / madigraphics
Oxalate Crystals iStock.com / Md Babul Hosen
Sympathetic and Parasympathetic Nervous System iStock.com / ttsz
Vagus Nerve iStock.com / ttsz

Publishers Cataloguing-inPublication Data
Names: Nathan, Neil, author.
Title: The sensitive patient's healing guide : top experts offer new insights and treatments for environmental toxins, Lyme disease, and EMFs / Neil Nathan, MD.
Description: First edition. | Fort Bragg, CA : Cypress House, [2024] | Includes bibliographical references and index.
Identifiers: ISBN: 979-8-9854086-4-5 (print) | 979-8-9854086-5-2 (ebook)
Subjects: LCSH: Environmentally induced diseases. | Multiple chemical sensitivity. | Sick building syndrome. | Lyme disease. | Electromagnetic fields--Health aspects. | Molds (Fungi)-- Toxicology. | Food intolerance. | Environmental toxicology. | Allergy. | BISAC: MEDICAL / Toxicology.
Classification: LCC: RB152.5 .N38 2024 | DDC: 616.9/8--dc23
Library of Congress Control Number 2023920194

Printed in the USA

2 4 6 8 9 7 5 3

First edition

Dedication

We dedicate this book to the millions of struggling patients who have, through no fault of their own, become unusually sensitive to the normal stimuli of light, sound, touch, food, chemicals, and EMF, such that they can no longer tolerate those stimuli without significant suffering.

For many years, health-care practitioners have dismissed their experience as trivial or psychological, which has added to their suffering.

Having had the privilege of providing healthcare for thousands of these patients, I want to thank them for their patience with me, and with medical science, for taking so long to bring them answers.

It is our hope that this book will bring them the reward for that patience—a new understanding of the neurology, physiology and biochemistry of what creates this kind of sensitivity, and the medical conditions that are most likely to set it off. Even more important, we want to share with them the many new approaches to reducing and curing these sensitivities, based on our newly obtained knowledge.

We invite those individuals and their families and physicians to soak up this information with a realistic hope for restoration of their normal faculties.

Foreword

This book really needed to be written. An increasing number of patients are being discounted, discarded, and disheartened by the conventional model of medicine. Because their symptoms and body reactions don't fit into the current medical paradigm, these people are told, "It's all in your head," or "You're too sensitive," even though their lives are greatly impacted.

Despite new research and information about the physiology, neurology, physics, chemistry, and genetics behind what makes a person become "sensitive," the patients' experiences are discounted as purely psychological. In addition, despite innovative treatments based upon this new research and information, the medical system has still not adopted these therapies, leaving these patients without adequate care.

Medicine needs to move out of the Dark Ages and catch up, and this book provides us the necessary catch-up. By inviting some of the finest experts in the field to contribute a chapter on their expertise, each covering a different aspect, Dr. Nathan has created the most comprehensive resource imaginable for patients who have slipped through the cracks, and those caring for them. We have the opportunity to learn from an array of top-notch researchers and practitioners, encompassing clinically useful information for both professional clinicians and people identified as sensitive.

Truly, there's no one more suited to author this book than Dr. Nathan—a seeker, collaborator, and seasoned physician, whose fifty-year medical career has been focused on treating the most ill patients. Rather than discounting these people, he became increasingly curious about them, honoring their lived experience, and digging to get to the bottom of their conditions. Through his long career, he's developed collaborative relationships with top experts in the field, many of whom have contributed to this book, resulting in a tour de force lineup of authors.

Through this vital work, Dr. Nathan is setting the record straight. In other words, this is not "all in your head." If a medical practitioner has labeled you as sensitive, you can bet that you have a very real medical condition whose cause has not yet been discovered and whose treatment may lie within the pages of this comprehensive book.

I will never forget the first time I saw Dr. Nathan teach. It was in 2008, at a conference on Lyme disease. The room was packed with people, some sitting on the floor and many standing, for there were no seats left. The subject? Chronic Inflammatory Response Syndrome, more commonly known as CIRS—one of the many illnesses addressed in this book that conventional medicine has missed, leaving those who suffer from it without help or hope. CIRS patients are often labeled as sensitive, and Dr. Nathan has been working with them for a very long time.

My lasting impression from that lecture was that this man was a seeker. He had studied with one of the experts in the field of CIRS, but then skillfully took what worked according to his extensive patient experience and translated it marvelously for those of us in the room to take back to our practices as actionable information.

Dr. Nathan is not only a seeker, he's a true collaborator. He developed one of the first integrative practices in the country, though no one called it that at the time. My belief is that his passion to help as many patients as possible fuels his unending curiosity and drive to collaborate. It's this collaborative nature that inspired the format of this book.

As Dr. Nathan is known to do when he reads a book or listens to a scientific presentation that expands his understanding, he picks up the phone and calls the author to learn more. This is how we met. I was so lucky as to receive one of those life-changing phone calls. What you'll find in this book is a fabulous collection of writings from others who've received such a call. They represent various areas of expertise such as neurology, biochemistry, physics, physiology, and genetics. I can't imagine a more impressive panel of experts, including Dr. Nathan.

While he himself could have written on each topic area, having studied them thoroughly and put most of the principles to work in his own practice, he chose instead to allow each expert the opportunity to write on his or her own subject matter in his or her own way. The result is as definitive a book as possible for those struggling with extreme sensitivities.

I'm incredibly grateful that Dr. Nathan heard the call and made it happen. It's in line with what I understand his passion to be—to teach, mentor, and share what he's learned with as many people as possible in order to offer healing. May it help you heal and bring you hope.

Jill Crista, ND
Author of *Break the Mold* and *A Light in the Dark for PANDAS & PANS*

Preface

The following description is a composite of hundreds of patients whom I've had the privilege of working with for the past thirty years. At first, it may sound a bit excessive, but I assure you that variations of this story are more common than you might suspect.

Imagine that you were once a very healthy young person, just completing graduate school and starting your dream job. You're in great shape; after running cross-country in high school and playing on the soccer team, you recently completed your second marathon. You have a flourishing relationship with a bright, kind, lovely person, and marriage seems just around the corner. You feel really good about your life and what you have accomplished, and you're excited to see what lies ahead.

Then you move into an older home, hoping to fix it up and make it a great place for your spouse and perhaps a child or two. There's a mild smell of mildew in the basement, but it's probably nothing, so you ignore it as an unimportant detail in your world.

As you train for your third marathon, however, you find yourself inexplicably short of breath by the fifth mile, which is both surprising and annoying, as is the unusual feeling of sore and achy muscles and fatigue that lasts into the next day, which has never happened before.

Initially, you don't pay much attention to this; everyone has an off day from time to time, so you take a day off to rest up. When you run again the next day you find yourself tired, achy, and short of breath by the third mile, and it takes two days to recover. This is weird—what's going on? Ahh, probably just a hiccup, maybe a bug of some kind, and it will go away soon.

At work, usually able to multitask easily with a sharp and active mind, you find yourself having trouble focusing on the tasks at hand; you forget a client's name midsentence, and can't seem to get motivated to complete your assigned workload. You find yourself making excuses to avoid some social outings with your partner because, honestly, you're too tired to enjoy them. Your partner notices, and feels a little frustrated, but this is going to go away soon, right?

Over the next few weeks, running becomes even more difficult. You become a bit short of breath even climbing the stairs. You come home from work exhausted, knowing you haven't been able to complete your work in a timely fashion. You find yourself ordering food in, since you don't have the energy to cook. Even with your increasingly poor appetite, you have gained several pounds—but maybe that's just because you haven't been as active as usual.

Getting to sleep has become increasingly difficult, and you wake up feeling unrefreshed and not at all ready to face the day. It's too hard to even think about going for a short run, which is odd because you loved being active and how great it felt while you were running.

You're starting to feel a bit depressed about how work and other activities are losing their meaning—it's become a chore to just get up and shower and get through work. For no reason you can discern, you are becoming more and more anxious about everything. You become more moody; you get angry and irritable when you know you shouldn't. All sorts of worries begin to intrude into your thoughts: Perhaps you'll get fired because you aren't performing up to snuff. Perhaps your partner will get frustrated with how you're interacting and leave you. The slightest stress makes you unusually antsy, and at night you sometimes wake up with your heart beating hard and fast, sweating—your first panic attack of many yet to come.

Finally, you admit to yourself (your partner has been nagging you about this for a while) that something is wrong, so you see your family physician who examines you briefly and does some basic tests (blood count, thyroid, chemistries), which turn out "normal." Your physician recommends an antidepressant like Lexapro for both the anxiety and depression, and suggests that perhaps you've been under more stress than you realized.

You took the medication and felt a little better for a while, but the fatigue got worse, you gained a bit more weight, and on reflection, the antidepressant just didn't seem to help much. The vitamins and supplements you've taken for years didn't do much either and now you notice, with increasing concern, that you can't take them without getting nauseated or having a headache. What on earth is going on here?! You are falling apart! Going out into the daylight on a sunny day seems way too bright. You even have to wear sunglasses inside your home to keep from squinting or having blurred vision. It's harder to read; the words just don't string together in a logical pattern, and you have to read whole sentences over and over again to understand them. Innocuous sounds, like children at play, have become odious and intolerable. You jump when you hear a car horn or the dishwasher comes on. Your sense of smell has become more acute—the aromas of cooking foods you used to enjoy are now off-putting, and that smell from the basement is awful!

Spending time on your computer becomes increasingly difficult. After fifteen minutes of sitting in front of the computer, your brain feels like it will stop working and it takes too much of an effort to continue. This is particularly annoying since your work requires quite a bit of screentime, and this is one more area of enjoyment that's being taken away from you.

Your physician is stumped. He doesn't know what is wrong, so he refers you to a rheumatologist for your sore joints and muscles, to a pulmonologist for your shortness of breath, to an ophthalmologist for your eye symptoms, and to a psychiatrist for your anxiety and depression. It takes a few months before all of these visits can be scheduled, and disappointment after disappointment follows when all of these specialists shake their heads and don't know what to do to help you. The message from all of your doctors is clear: this is so complicated that it must be in your head. Your partner and your parents have accompanied you to some of these visits and they too hear this message. They become less and less supportive and understanding of the reality of your condition, and they too begin to tell you that it's all in your head. Your partner is increasingly frustrated with your inability to make plans and keep them—you keep bailing on social outings because you never know when you will be able to muster the energy to go out without becoming exhausted afterward, or have to stop and turn back because you don't have the energy to proceed.

Just when you thought it couldn't get any worse, you notice that after eating many of your meals, you immediately begin to itch all over, or have heart palpitations, or an increase in brain fog and fatigue, or bloating and abdominal pain.

This scenario is recounted in my office over and over again, with only slight variations. If you are lucky, you'll finally make your way into the office of a medical practitioner who specializes in integrative medicine. For the first time, you may feel truly listened to and heard. They will nod and tell you that no, you are not going crazy, but that you are suffering from a medical condition (not a psychological one) that goes by many names, some of which include: Multiple Chemical Sensitivity (MCS), Chronic Fatigue Syndrome (CFS), Fibromyalgia, Mast Cell Activation, Mitochondrial Dysfunction, and/or Post Exertional Malaise (PEM).

Ah, finally a diagnosis! But wait a second—we're not quite there yet, because all of these named conditions are triggered or caused by other, more specific, agents: mold toxicity, Lyme disease (with its coinfections), chronic viral infections, other infectious diseases (Chlamydia, Mycoplasma), dental diseases, and more. This may sound like a lot, and it is, but here's the good news—all of these conditions can be diagnosed and treated. There is real hope that we can get to the bottom of your illness and get you back on the road to healing—and this goes for all our patients!

That is what this book is about. For so many patients who have been marginalized, disrespected, ignored, and left with no hope or future, isolated from their spouses, families, and communities, the ones who have slowly become so sensitive and reactive to their environment that they have become severely limited in their connection to the world they used to love, there is a way to make a clear diagnosis of what you have, what caused it, and how to treat it! This is realistic, true hope. I, and my colleagues who have contributed to the writing of this book, have treated thousands of patients like you, and have helped the vast majority to a complete restoration of health and resumption of a meaningful life.

We will describe to you, in detail, how the body slowly but inexorably becomes sensitized to light, sound, touch, smell, chemicals, foods, and EMFs (Electromagnetic Frequencies). This is *not* a psychological condition (though most patients become anxious and depressed when they have not been given a diagnosis and the treatments offered haven't worked). It is a neurological condition triggered initially by environmental toxins, infections, and/or stress.

In the past twenty-five years, MCS has gone from a rare diagnosis to a common one, but the medical profession has not kept pace with the knowledge that has accumulated to treat this condition. I am delighted that the medical practitioners who've joined with me in putting together this volume are all experts in understanding this condition and have helped to create the treatments that we know will work for the vast majority of patients and enable them to recover their health. There is a wealth of information here, and it is our hope that it will lead you into a brighter future filled with hope and meaning.

Introduction

Here is one of the most important things I have learned during my fifty years of medical practice: Human beings are complicated. Your immediate reaction to this is likely to be a sarcastic "Yeah, that's a revelation, tell me more."

What I mean by this is not the obvious, but that we are all biochemically, structurally, and genetically very different. The reason that this is worthy of note is that it has to do with how the same medical condition can manifest in so many different ways in different individuals. Again, while that might sound obvious, surprisingly, many medical practitioners don't see it that way—and there's the rub.

Most physicians were taught in medical school that each named disease has a predictable set of symptoms attached to it. This makes it easier for medical students to assimilate the knowledge they are striving for, but the price of that oversimplification leads to a life-long craving for that same simplicity in all the patients they will see.

Unfortunately, life is just not like that. Medicine is just not like that. The same named disease, or diagnosis, such as, say, psoriatic arthritis, may show up in some people as the classical form, a severe arthritis associated with the skin plaques of psoriasis. In others, however, those symptoms may be minimal, but they may have fatigue, digestive symptoms, conjunctivitis, or other eye symptoms that predominate. As rheumatologists are well aware, these same patients might present with classic blood-test results that confirm the diagnosis, or they might have the disease without those tests being positive, which is referred to as seronegative arthritis.

We find, therefore, that the simple approach learned in medical school to making the diagnosis of psoriatic arthritis must be viewed in the light of the complicated fashion in which patients actually experience their disease. This means that a good physician must be aware of *all* the symptoms a patient is experiencing to gain the most comprehensive overview of what might be causing the patient's illness to make the most accurate diagnosis, without which effective treatment is not possible.

This is not a theoretical discussion; I have seen quite a few patients who were diagnosed by their rheumatologist with "psoriatic arthritis" and treated for years—unsuccessfully—with medications that affect the immune system. When a careful review of the entire gamut of symptoms was made, these patients were actually found to have Lyme disease, and when treated for that, they recovered completely, with no sign of residual "psoriatic arthritis."

This is a somewhat long-winded way of telling you that no matter what symptoms a patient has, the diagnosis must truly fit those symptoms, and we must get to the root cause of those symptoms to have any chance of treating them properly.

Over the past thirty years, it has been disheartening to me to find that the practice of medicine has changed so much that physicians, well-intentioned as they are, usually don't have the time or energy to embrace this basic principle of medical practice, and too many patients are treated in a kind of knee-jerk way, just to keep the work from piling up to an unmanageable extent.

What does this have to do with patients who have become increasingly sensitive to their medications, supplements, chemicals, smells, light, sound, touch, food, or EMFs? Everything. As you'll see in this comprehensive volume, with chapters written by some of the finest experts in this field, the emergence of these sensitivities is a gradual, insidious process, created to some degree by a lack of understanding of how missed, partial, or incorrect diagnoses can trigger a series of neurological, biochemical, and hormonal events that produce an individual who has become so overly sensitive and reactive. In fact, despite a wealth of research and new information about how this process evolves and how to treat it, a large percentage of physicians still believe that this sensitivity is mostly or entirely psychological on the patient's part, and that it cannot be successfully treated but merely ameliorated with the use of antidepressant and anti-anxiety medications.

This has led to the travesty of leaving these unfortunate people, who are already suffering from their very real medical conditions, without a diagnosis, and the medical label "This is all in your head." This unfairly adds another layer of stress to an already struggling patient, and tends to alienate their families and friends who accept the incorrect medical dismissal. But this is rare, right? Every system will have a few outliers, no?

Rare? Reports from around the world show that all people, regardless of age or race, now appear to be moving in that direction. A national US study found that 11.2% of respondents reported an increased sensitivity to common chemicals. This would mean that in the United States alone, perhaps 30 million people are experiencing some form of chemical sensitivity to some degree—and the research shows that this has been increasing geometrically for many years!

Let me share with you how this has manifested in my own experience. When I began practice in the 1970s, I rarely encountered anyone with chemical or other sensitivities. Admittedly, neither was I attuned to the existence of such sensitivities, as it was not taught in medical school. With each passing decade, more and more of my patients showed up with these sensitivities to the point that in the past ten to fifteen years, I can say that I've treated over a thousand patients with these issues. I admit that part of my increasing awareness of these sensitivities is that my practice has evolved over the years to specializing in treating patients with chronic fatigue syndrome, fibromyalgia, mold toxicity, and Lyme disease. It turns out that those conditions are major triggers for the creation of sensitivities. You might not be aware that these conditions are no longer rarely encountered. It's estimated that up to 10 million people have some degree of mold toxicity. In 2018, the CDC (Centers for Disease Control) recognized publicly that there are 400,000 new cases of Lyme disease every year. It is estimated that 5–10 million people have chronic fatigue or fibromyalgia. Rare? More accurately, seriously underdiagnosed!

Unfortunately, my profession has not yet realized that these epidemics have already arrived, and I'm embarrassed that there continues to be ongoing debate about the existence of all these medical conditions. For example, until the medication Lyrica was released fifteen years ago, fibromyalgia was considered a psychological condition—until a medication was found that could impact it and the medical field began to accept fibromyalgia as a valid diagnosis. Until that time, like everything else we're discussing, it was considered a psychological issue.

Another example: The IDSA (Infectious Disease Society of America), a national group of infectious disease specialists, has long doubted the existence of chronic Lyme disease, and those patients are told they have "post-Lyme syndrome." You might think this is merely semantics (it is), but the consequence of this terminology is that those unfortunate patients are then told by many specialists that nothing can be done for them—that their condition is untreatable. A separate group of physicians, ILADS (the International Lyme and Associated Diseases Society), has long recognized the reality of chronic Lyme disease and has pioneered its treatment. The tragedy here is that a large group of specialists, with a great deal of clout (the insurance industry has been very happy to agree with their point of view), has discouraged patients from seeking help with a serious medical disease and has attempted to make those physicians, who are trying to help their patients, look like quacks. This has placed both physicians on the front lines (who are not sure whom to follow) and their patients in a compromised position, and those patients are more often than not left untreated and suffering with little hope in sight.

So, when a sensitive patient presents to a health-care provider with a description of their symptoms, unless they are lucky, or do their research, they are likely to have their condition dismissed as psychological and be sent away with a prescription for a medication that will not even come close to dealing with the root cause of their problem. I am embarrassed that my profession has treated these folks so dismissively—it flies against everything that I believe constitutes the compassionate intention that should be the essence of good medical practice.

Here is the good news. In this book, a group of experts will communicate to you that there's a great deal of new information about the causes of these sensitivities, and especially important, new and effective treatments. To embrace this information, which will do a great service to the millions of affected individuals, we urge you to disregard the older "It's all in your head" model, which has left so many patients disrespected and allowed to suffer with no hope.

Yes, a patient who is extremely sensitive is likely to become anxious and/or depressed about their situation. If you were walking down the street, or passing down the aisle in the grocery store, and you suddenly passed someone wearing perfume or cologne (or who washed their clothes in a scented detergent), and you dropped to the ground, unable to think, or even having odd twitching or seizure-like activity, and, embarrassed and frightened, had to be helped out to your car—can you imagine what that would feel like? This happens to countless people daily. You would know that you could never feel safe, never know when something like this could happen again. Understandably, you'd become increasingly vigilant simply to survive your daily activities, or severely curtail them to prevent these events. How could this not engender anxiety and/or depression?

What's crucial to understand is that anxiety and depression are consequences of sensitivity, not the cause. They add another element to an already difficult situation. Because taking antidepressants can't cure this presentation (you could think of it as a band-aid), we must find the cause of these reactions so we can address them.

The astute reader might recognize that the first few chapters of this book reflect my previous book, *Toxic*, in which I began to broach this major subject. *Toxic* contains a great deal of information about the sensitive patient, and can be viewed as preparatory for this book. These reworked introductory chapters are followed by a comprehensive discussion of the science behind what creates sensitization, its most common triggers, and most important, what we've learned about how to treat it successfully.

This book is written for two main audiences: Those who suffer from excessive sensitivities (and their families and friends), and the medical professionals who've been searching for an understanding of how to help those patients. Accordingly, some of these chapters will be a bit more academic than others, and readers are encouraged to gravitate to those chapters that resonate most strongly for them. If you do chose to read this book cover to cover, it's organized in such a way as to provide a comprehensive approach to this subject.

Throughout the book, we will discuss an overview of this process, with an effort to clarify how these stimuli (smells, sound, light, foods, chemicals, or EMFs) trigger such distressing reactions. We will delve into the biochemistry, neurology, and genetics that contribute to creating the perfect storm by which these symptoms manifest. We'll discuss the underlying medical conditions that set the stage for these reactions to evolve. Spoiler alert: mold toxicity and Lyme disease are key players in the process.

Above all, this is a book of hope—for those who have been told, often repeatedly, that they have to "live with it" and have had to isolate themselves from the world in order to survive. We, the authors, have helped thousands of patients recover their health and rejoin their families and communities with a new sense of purpose and meaning. If you are struggling with medical conditions that have left you in this position, we are hoping you will join them.

An Overview of
the Sensitive Patient

During my many years of medical practice, I found myself treating patients whose illnesses were increasingly complicated. I began my career as a family physician and gradually became more interested in those folks who were not responding to conventional medical approaches. Initially, many of these patients were experiencing chronic pain of various types. My first partners included a chiropractor and a massage therapist; our practice grew to include acupuncturists and body workers of every sort, and we shared our information to work on individuals who were struggling. I studied with all of my colleagues, and expanded my studies to learn about osteopathic manipulation, homeopathy, energy medicine, Reichian therapy, injection techniques, prolotherapy, and hypnosis. It soon became clear that there was no single treatment that worked for all patients; rather, each new field that I studied added to my "toolbox" and enabled me to help more and more patients.

Over many years, my colleagues learned of my interest in patients who were floundering with traditional treatments that weren't working, and they referred more and more of their challenging patients to me. I helped many, but was always aware that there was much more to learn to help more of them. By the early 1990s we saw a dramatic increase in our knowledge of the biochemistry of chronic illnesses, and I added each new piece to my ability to help these patients.

There is no name for the field of medicine that has evolved here, and I (and many others) have come to call it Complex Medical Problem Solving. Many of the health-care providers who have entered this field call it integrative medicine or functional medicine. The bottom line is that the patients who seek our help have developed illnesses that escape the notice of conventional medicine, and those unfortunate individuals are left with the impression that there is no hope for them, or that the experiences they describe are "in your head," or both.

Here is the good news: For those of you who have not received a diagnosis or treatment that has helped you, there is realistic hope that this help is near. This volume, a collection of knowledge accumulated over the past twenty years, will help you to understand not only why you are sick but also what you can do about it.

Because patients who have become unusually sensitive have received so little attention and so much dismissal by my profession (for which I apologize profusely), they are the focus of this book. Keep in mind that this sensitivity is usually associated with, or accompanied by, many other common symptoms, including fatigue, cognitive impairment, pain of various sorts, breathing difficulties, cardiovascular issues, allergies and/ or autoimmunity, headaches, anxiety and depression, and more, so please don't confine your interest to sensitivity alone, as many of the chapters in this book will probably speak to you as well. Let's quickly get one important subject out of the way: the sensitivity we are talking about is *not* emotional sensitivity to language or to the behavior of others and how it affects us. If you were hoping for some pointers about dealing with your reactions to the nasty, mean, or insensitive comments of those around you, such as

- "You're fat."
- "You're ugly."
- "You're stupid."
- "Who gave you that awful haircut?"
- "Did you really just buy that hideous couch?"
- "Whatever would have motivated you to _____?"
- "Are you *still* going out with *him?*"
- Any number of disapproving looks, gestures, or suggestions,

then you're going to be disappointed, because that's not what we explore here, and this book won't help you in that regard. A sensitivity to language or actions is *psychologically* induced and quite different from *neurological* and *biochemical* sensitivity, which is the focus of our discussions. The detailed information we present here can be summarized as concerning our patients' increasing sensitivity to specific stimuli that our nervous systems monitor constantly and carefully, including the five basic senses of light, sound, smell, touch, and taste, as well as the newly recognized effects of electromagnetic frequencies (EMFs). To clarify, when we speak about chemical sensitivity, we're not referring to a mere dislike of being around strong perfumes but to a significant and immediate reaction to any number of scents, including perfumes, of headache, fatigue, cognitive dysfunction, and even certain types of seizures. Reaction to sound is not just avoiding certain kinds of music but startling noticeably at certain noises. Reaction to light is not squinting when first coming out of a movie theater, but needing to wear sunglasses indoors. Reactions to EMFs include intense fatigue, headache, or cognitive impairment within minutes of using a computer.

This, as you will discover, is no small subject, and I'm happy to report that we've learned a tremendous amount about it in the past fifteen years. Ultimately, we intend this as a book of hope, so that those who have been affected by increasing sensitivity and the many symptoms that accompany it (which differ according to what is causing it) will be able to understand the possible contributing causes to their sensitivities, and will realize that there are many new techniques and treatments that can help them to heal.

To bring this discussion into immediate focus, I present the case of Lisa (the names of all of our patients have been changed to protect their privacy, but the medical details are entirely accurate.)

Lisa's Story

Lisa first came to see me in October 2010, at age forty-seven. She had been essentially healthy until January 2008 when she returned home from a hike with her dogs and discovered that they were covered with small seed ticks. Lisa doesn't recall receiving a tick bite, but two weeks later she came down with a flulike illness that involved fatigue and intense pain in her neck, spine, and foot. She was fortunate because her family physician realized that the issue could be Lyme disease (an unusually quick diagnosis), but when treated with antibiotics, Lisa experienced severe gastrointestinal symptoms and got progressively worse. By August she had become weaker and more fatigued and required a walker to move about. Within a few months, she developed an extreme sensitivity to scents; mere exposure to perfumes or certain detergents would cause immediate collapse and a brief loss of consciousness. Sometimes she would twitch or shake uncontrollably or writhe about (movements technically called dyskinesias). Her doctor continued to treat her for Lyme disease and gave her intravenous fluids, which did help a bit. By March 2009, however, Lisa required the use of a wheelchair. Her sensitivities (multiple chemical sensitivities, or MCS) had escalated to include exposure to fluorescent lights, and she had developed intense anxiety with panic attacks and depression, none of which she had ever had before.

A complete neurological evaluation that included an MRI was done to rule out MS (multiple sclerosis) or any other clear cause of Lisa's debilitating symptoms. Two physicians continued to treat her with antibiotics aimed primarily at Lyme disease (caused by the bacteria *Borrelia burgdorferi*) and *babesiosis,* a common co-infection of Lyme disease caused by a parasite similar to the one that causes malaria. Despite receiving expert care, her condition continued to deteriorate, and by May 2010, the spasmodic twitching and jerking motions had become even more prominent and incapacitating. Lisa lost the use of her right hand and was unable to read or walk.

Shortly thereafter, she came into my office for the first time. My overriding question during that visit was, as always, "What are we missing?" While her testing and current diagnosis gave clear indication of Lyme disease and *Babesia,* Lisa's symptoms—chemical sensitivity, anxiety, depression, and unusual neurological presentation with intense fatigue and cognitive impairment—pointed to other important possibilities, namely, mold toxicity and *Bartonella,* another co-infection of Lyme disease, which had not yet been specifically addressed.

Recognizing Lisa's extreme sensitivity, I started her on one drop of A-Bart, once a day (an herbal tincture specific for treatment of *Bartonella*), and very slowly increased her dosage to one drop once a day, then twice a day, which was as much as she could comfortably take. Any higher dosing triggered a severe Herx reaction, which is a worsening of her underlying symptoms, and as you might expect, quite unpleasant. As she slowly stabilized, I was able to add a small dose of the herbal supplement *Houttynia* and a small amount of hydrosol silver in the form of argentyn 23. It took several months to achieve even these tiny doses, but we were encouraged by her slow, steady improvements. I then added a tiny dose of Bactrim, an antibiotic sulfa drug which tends to work well for *Bartonella,* in August; it took until November to double that small dose. Lisa was still improving and getting stronger, and we were able to start LENS (low-energy neurobiofeedback systems) treatment, which helped so much with her dyskinesias that she was no longer in a wheelchair, but she still could not leave her home without the risk of chemical exposure that would cause her to crumple in her church or a grocery store. I witnessed several of these episodes at our clinic, when I watched Lisa walk fairly well down our hallway, pass a woman who had washed her clothes in Tide, and fall to the floor writhing.

Typically, the treatment for *Bartonella* requires several antibiotics given concurrently, and we were slowly able to add several others after trial-and-error efforts showed which ones Lisa could tolerate to any degree. She continued to make slow but steady progress, and we were able to start LDA (low-dose antigen) treatments (see chapter 25) to begin to quiet the extreme reactivity that was so limiting for her.

I was encouraged by Lisa's improvements, but felt that something else was contributing to her illness, so by August we began to look into the possibility of mold toxicity, a condition that can elicit similar symptoms. At that time, the urine mycotoxin tests we now use routinely were not yet commercially available, so we used the crude visual contrast test (VCS), which was clearly abnormal, suggesting mold as a possible diagnosis. It was not until December that Lisa was able to test her home for the presence of mold, and it turned out that she was indeed being exposed to a significant degree there. Starting with tiny amounts of intravenous phosphatidyl choline (1cc) we were slowly able to increase that dose to 5cc, then 10cc, which are more normal dosages. Lisa tolerated her LDA treatments well.

By March 2012, Lisa was finally able to tolerate some of the binders for mold toxicity that we typically use, including Welchol (colesevalam).

She continued to be able to be more active after remediating the mold in her home, but chemical exposures still limited her going to church or to the grocery store. By June 2013, she could drive short distances and resumed bicycling. She then started Annie Hopper's Dynamic Neural Retraining System (DNRS), which I had just learned about, and she made more rapid improvements (see chapter 1). As she improved, she became aware of some old, repressed memories of traumatic experiences that a therapist helped her to work through, and with these additions to her treatment, she was able to stop all antibiotics and start working part-time. By December 2014, Lisa was able to fully resume her life; she was even able to fly to another city and stay in a hotel for her daughter's wedding.

I have followed Lisa ever since, and as of early 2022 she was working as a health coach and donating funds to help other patients who had struggled as she had and needed the extra help. Her life was full, and she was excited about all that her current vibrant state of health enabled her to give back.

Lisa's story is fairly typical of patients from my practice. That may seem extreme to some readers, but alas, it's more common than you might realize. Of course, there are millions of individuals out there who have some of these symptoms, though to a lesser extent.

As I reviewed Lisa's story, it dawned on me that I was not only describing her journey but my own as well. It reflects the process by which I began to acquire more and more information about the causes of patients' sensitivities and tools for their treatment. You can plainly see that Lisa's progress was linked to the growth of my own knowledge and experience. When we started in 2010, discovering the missing diagnosis of *Bartonella*, we made slow but limited progress. Adding our knowledge of mold toxicity and LDA, we made further progress, and with the addition of limbic retraining with DNRS in 2013, Lisa was able to move forward toward complete health.

Definitions of Sensitivity

In the next chapter, we'll examine the important distinctions between sensitivity, toxicity, and reactivity, but first, let's try to get a definition of what *sensitivity* means. We'll start with MCS (multiple chemical sensitivity), which, though recognized as quite common, is the only aspect of sensitivity that medical authorities have even *tried* to define. For sensitivities to light, sound, food, touch, and EMFs, while recognized, only limited attempts at definition have been made.

Unfortunately, the medical profession won't be very helpful to us here. For many years, MCS was considered a purely psychological condition, which as we know is not useful and actually incorrect. More recently, medical authorities have proposed that MCS is *both* a medical condition and a psychological one. Though closer to reality, their new explanation still does our patients an injustice. This is reflected in the 1996 expert panel at the WHO (World Health Organization), which accepted the existence of "a disease of unclear pathogenesis" but rejected the claim that MCS was caused by chemical exposure. WHO provided three diagnostic requirements for this illness, which they renamed "idiopathic environmental intolerances." These requirements are:

1. The disease was acquired (not present from birth) and must produce multiple relapsing symptoms.
2. The symptoms must be closely related to "multiple environmental influences, which are well tolerated by the majority of the population."
3. These symptoms cannot be explained by any other medical conditions.

Well, this was a start. Remember: It was 1996, and a great deal of newer information is now available that has not yet been assimilated into medical science. In 2017 a Canadian task force reported that there was very little peer-reviewed research in this field, but admitted that "some peer-reviewed clinical research has emerged from centers in Italy, Denmark and Japan suggesting that there are fundamental neurobiologic, metabolic and genetic susceptibility factors that underlie ES/MCS" (ES is environmental sensitivity).

Where has this left our patients? Generally, holding the short end of the stick. When government agencies can't agree on a definition, or even the cause, it leaves medical practitioners and their patients out on a limb. In 2014, OSHA (the United States Occupational Safety and Health Administration) continued this thread by noting that MCS is highly controversial and that there is insufficient science to explain its possible causes, listing "allergy, dysfunction of the immune system, neurobiological sensitization, and various psychological theories" as potential causes.

We have to start somewhere. I propose something simple: that we honor and respect our patients' observations and experiences. What they tell us, consistently, is that when they are exposed to certain chemicals (often scented products, plastics, smoke, petroleum products, paint fumes, and outgassing products) or to strong light, different sounds, touch of various degrees, the medications and supplements they take, and EMFs, they react quickly (usually within minutes) upon exposure to these stimuli, with predictable symptomatology. To me, that seems pretty straightforward: you are exposed to something, then you react.

How the patient reacts varies, depending on the amount of their exposure, under-lying medical conditions, biochemistry, genetics, and stress levels—all of which we discuss in this book. The "how" seems to have baffled many researchers and observ-ers because they came to the table looking for absolute consistency, expecting that the same stimulus would have an identical effect on multiple individuals complaining of sensitivity.

Not finding this consistency, they have doubted the observations of the patients reporting these experiences and have concluded that this must not be a real phenome-non. To me, and many others, that is an unreasonable assumption, but it seems, for rea-sons that still baffle me, to have stymied the acceptance of the reality of this condition.

Let's keep it simple: patients get exposed to a stimulus and then react to that stimu-lus in a way that creates a variety of symptoms that range from uncomfortable to fright-ening. This is as real as it gets.

While there are, understandably, psychological consequences to these experiences, these are not primarily psychological in origin. I hope that by the time you finish this book you will have a much better grasp of the entire sensitization process, which will in turn help you understand the many effective treatments that are now available.

Sensitive vs. Toxic

At the risk of offending the membrane physiologists and toxicologists who might read this chapter, I'm going to simplify a very complicated subject so as to give you an understanding of what I, and our authors, mean when we use terms such as *sensitivity, toxicity,* and *reactivity.* I often see references to articles that discuss sensitivity and toxicity in a general sense, but I hope you will ask the important question: *"Sensitive (or toxic, or reactive) to what, exactly?"* The *time* it takes between exposure to a substance and how quickly the body reacts is equally important. These questions are very useful from both a diagnostic and therapeutic standpoint.

What Is Sensitivity?

Sensitivity refers to a nervous system that has become overexcited or hyperreactive in response to a wide variety of stimuli. These include sound, light, touch, food, chemicals, smells, and EMFs. A sensitive patient can have one, several, or all of these. Although we briefly touched on this kind of sensitivity, it's so essential to our discussion that some of that bears repeating.

You might, for example, be so sensitive to light that you need to wear sunglasses in indoor settings or spend most of your day in a darkened room. You might be unusually responsive to noises, jumping at unexpected sounds that others don't even notice. You might develop food sensitivities that can include true food allergies or mast-cell activation. Mast cells are immune cells that coordinate how your immune system and nervous system respond to infectious and toxic threats. An "activated" mast cell reacts quickly and intensely and seemingly at random (depending on how activated it is at that moment) to a spectrum of stimuli, especially food coming down the alimentary canal, by releasing large amounts of histamine and other biochemical mediators that create an immediate onset of symptoms such as flushing, sweating, palpitations, abdominal pain, and/or diarrhea (see chapter 4).

You might develop multiple chemical sensitivities (MCS) such that even the slightest exposure to certain odors, such as perfume, gasoline, or cigarette smoke, can within seconds cause profound fatigue, cognitive impairment, or headache. In especially sensitive individuals, we see more dramatic reactions, such as pseudoseizures and dyskinesias (spasmodic twitching and jerking motions) that look like seizures but without the usual accompanying EEG changes. In An Overview of the Sensitive Patient, I told the story of Lisa, who had some of these unusual neurological presentations.

Some patients become unusually sensitive to EMF exposure and find they can no longer work around computers or other electronic devices. I've worked with several patients who could not tolerate Wi-Fi exposure, which is ubiquitous, and when exposed to Wi-Fi experienced fatigue, cognitive impairment, and/or other neurological symptoms, which made it difficult for these patients to find a safe environment that they could live in. Several years ago, when the state of California mandated the use of smart meters, my office saw new cases of severe EMF reactivity in people who had been apparently healthy prior to the installation of those meters. Several of my patients were so profoundly affected that they had to leave the Bay Area and move to rural settings so they could get away from EMF exposure in order to function. With the introduction of 5G, this has become even more prevalent (see chapter 9).

Often, people who are not sensitive can't fathom this level of sensitivity and might think these reactions must be psychosomatic. *They are not!* Though the medical profession has considered this possibility for many years, we are talking about as many as 30 million Americans who could be wrestling with some form of increased sensitivity to some degree, so it's nowhere near as rare as many suppose.

This marked increase in the reactivity of the nervous system is a serious problem for many of my patients. It's hard enough for them to try to work through these difficulties without having to face skepticism and ridicule from those who don't believe them. I've seen these dynamics tear families apart, as patients' family members struggle to understand what is happening and assume attitudes that undermine communication, caring, and healing.

Here it is in a nutshell: *Sensitivity* is created by a hyperreactive or hypersensitive nervous system. You could think of it as a hypervigilant nervous system that is not convinced that it's "safe." In actuality, it's *not* safe, so the parts of the brain, specifically the limbic system (see chapters 4 and 5) and the vagal nerve system (involving the ventral branch of the tenth cranial nerve (the vagus nerve) and the associated cranial nerves (see chapter 3) that monitor the body's internal and external stimuli for safety move from a protective mode into an overprotective mode and question every arriving stimulus.

When a sensitive individual walks down the street and passes someone wearing cologne or perfume, and then suddenly drops to the sidewalk twitching and writing—they know they are not safe. At any given moment, someone or something could enter their world and bring it crashing down around them, so they really are not safe. This is a correct neurological perception, and it leads to serious consequences. It is not psychological in origin, but rather becomes more so with each frightening, unexpected reaction.

What I'll stress throughout this book is that we must not only accept the reality of this sensitivity but *look for the root cause(s)*.

We will delve into these causes in detail, but I will emphasize that toxins, especially mold toxicity, and infections, particularly Lyme disease and the coinfection *Bartonella*, are the most common causes I've found. Most important, once found, they are treatable.

Sarah's story will clarify what sensitivity looks like.

Sarah's Story

Sarah was referred to me in 2010 by a colleague who had seen her for chronic fatigue syndrome, which he felt was caused by Lyme disease and possibly *Bartonella* and *Babesia* as well. He also suspected a viral component to her illness, and treated her with multiple antibiotics for all of those potential causes.

I discovered that Sarah also had a degree of adrenal fatigue (a deficiency of adrenal hormones created by prolonged stress), and incorporated adrenal support into her treatment program. Though she appeared to improve initially, it became clear over time that she continued to struggle with extreme fatigue, which was accompanied by exercise intolerance (often referred to as post-exertional malaise (PEM), headaches, and cognitive impairments that included brain fog and difficulties with focus, memory, and concentration.

By 2014, seeing little improvement, I evaluated Sarah for mold toxicity, despite having no clear evidence of current mold exposure ("But I grew up in a moldy basement," she later recalled). The newly available urine mycotoxin test showed a significant elevation of trichothecenes (over three times the upper limit of "normal"), so I began treating her for mold toxicity. This proved more difficult than I'd anticipated, because Sarah became more and more sensitive to every treatment we tried. She could only take a few drops of the tinctures I prescribed, or the nasal sprays we provided—far less than the usual dosing amounts. By April 2015, she reported, "I'm reacting to pretty much everything." In addition to a worsening of her symptoms, she became depressed and physically weaker. She described a severe exacerbation of her condition when she took even one sixth of a drop of cilantro (used for detoxification), and she noted an immediate onset of symptoms after eating a variety of foods, which suggested that she had now developed mast-cell activation syndrome.

Despite her best efforts, Sarah could barely tolerate the treatments for mast cell activation, and by early 2017 she had become very frustrated with her worsening condition.

We then started Annie Hopper's DNRS (Dynamic Neural Retraining System (see chapter 1), and Sarah's extremely sensitive body finally began to quiet down. She responded beautifully to this form of limbic retraining. Within several months she was able to not only start tolerating the treatments for mast-cell activation (which could now help her a great deal) but was finally able to take the binders and antifungal treatments for her underlying mold toxicity and respond to them. Over the course of that year, she got progressively stronger and healthier. She reported a marked decrease in her depression and sensitivities, an improvement in energy and cognitive abilities, and she was able to exercise for the first time in years. Sarah was able to fully resume all her life activities, including full-time work, and was delighted by her return to complete health.

As I review the chronology of Sarah's story, I can't help but reflect on my own journey in understanding the evolution of sensitivity and what we've learned about how to treat it. For difficulties that first presented in 2010, we were unable to nail down the diagnosis of mold toxicity until 2014, when urine mycotoxin testing became available. Despite this, we did not make progress (even when we identified mast-cell activation) until 2017 when we instituted Annie Hopper's DNRS program, which set the healing wheels in motion. Readers who have struggled for many years can now see that hope, in the form of improved diagnosis (causes) and effective treatments are now available.

What is Toxicity?

In her lectures to medical audiences, Patricia Kane, PhD, a pioneer in the understanding and treatment of cell membrane disorders, projects slides that show electron microphotographs of cells from toxin-laden individuals. In these close-ups, you can see cell membranes that are chock-full of toxin. Some cells are so loaded that you can see molecules of toxin precariously attached to the outer membrane, ready to be dislodged at the slightest provocation. This visual can be helpful for showing how easily the tiniest insult or stressor—a shower that's a little too hot or too cold, a barometric weather change, or exposure to a certain food, chemical, or scent—will knock loose those toxic molecules and send them into the bloodstream, exacerbating that person's symptoms.

That the cell membranes are so clogged up with toxin is an obvious (but easily overlooked) problem: There is no room on the membrane for it to function properly by allowing substances in or out, which is the membrane's fundamental job. As toxins accumulate, that membrane cannot get rid of those additional toxins because it is literally stuck. Once toxins have begun to saturate the cell membranes, the toxins, which can include mycotoxins (mold), heavy metals (e.g., mercury or lead), and pesticides and herbicides (such as glyphosate), poison the body's systems of excretion and elimination, preventing those systems from doing their jobs.

Being poisoned prevents the body from doing what it needs to do—namely, eliminate that poison. The body cannot rid itself of what is making it sick. This is a vicious cycle: the more toxic one becomes the more difficulty one has with detoxification. This has profound implications for both diagnosis and treatment, as you will see in chapter 7, which discusses mold toxicity in more detail.

Some mold toxins are *ionophores*. An ionophore is a small molecule that has a fat-soluble part of its structure (technically called *lipophilic*, meaning "lipid-loving" or "fat-loving") on one end, and a water-soluble part of its structure (called *hydrophilic* or "water-loving") on the other end. The importance of this is that these molecules can attach to, or blend in with, the fatty materials that constitute every membrane in the body, or dissolve into watery solutions that make up the liquids that bathe all of our cells and tissues.

The body typically prevents unwanted substances, like toxins, from entering cells by using a complicated system of membrane physiology. A foreign substance is not allowed to enter the cell unless it binds to specific receptors of the cell membrane. Ionophores, by their unique structure, can bypass these normal membrane defenses and go anywhere they please, meaning they can enter any cell and travel through the bloodstream, and our bodies have very few defenses against them.

So, how does the body get rid of these toxins? In the case of mold toxins, if a person has the proper genetic makeup (which exists in 75% of the human population), they can make antibodies to these toxins that will help to bind those toxins in such a way that the immune system can neutralize them and get rid of them. For the 25% of the population that is not genetically engineered to make these antibodies, the only way to deal with these toxic molecules is to bring them to the liver, our major organ of detoxification, to be processed. Other systems of elimination, including the skin, gastrointestinal tract, kidneys, lymphatic system, and lungs, can also help remove these toxins from our bodies.

If these systems are poisoned, they may not be able to do their jobs, and toxins can accumulate. This is the state of affairs for many of my sickest patients. Even if we can figure out what is making them toxic—whether a mold toxin or mercury, for example,—we may have to address this shutdown of the organs of elimination before we can even begin to consider treatment. If we plunge into treatment with the intention of healing a patient *before we've addressed the patient's ability to detoxify,* there's very good chance that the patient's condition will get worse. Unlike sensitivity, which primarily involves an increased reactivity of the nervous system, toxicity represents the direct action of a toxin on body tissues. Robert's story will help clarify what toxicity looks like.

Robert's Story

Robert was a forty-four-year-old man who came to see me several years ago after having been ill four years prior. He described increasing fatigue, insomnia, frontal headaches, nausea (occasionally with vomiting), brain fog, anxiety, and depression. Of particular concern was an intense sensation of tingling and numbness around his mouth (technically called *perioral paresthesia*). Another physician had diagnosed him with Lyme disease, but antibiotics produced what Robert called a "huge Herx." (A Herx reaction— short for Herxheimer, the name of the physician who first described it—is a two-to-three-day exacerbation of symptoms caused by the sudden release of toxins produced by killing a bacteria such as Lyme (*Borrelia*) or *Bartonella*. With treatment for his Lyme disease, Robert became progressively worse. As he researched his condition, he discovered the possibility of mold toxicity. Upon considering this diagnosis, he realized that a shower in his weekend home, which he visited regularly, had developed a leak, and he himself had been involved in the repair process by which mold was uncovered and removed. Upon further reflection, Robert recalled other instances of possible exposure to mold at work and in previous homes. He also reported that he'd begun to notice increasing sensitivity to light, sound, and smells.

Robert persuaded his physician to do a RealTime urine mycotoxin test, which showed an ochratoxin level of 3.10 (normal is less than 1.8) and a gliotoxin level of 1.76 (normal is less than 0.5). (See chapter 7 for a detailed discussion of these tests.) With a clear diagnosis of mold toxicity based on his symptoms, history of exposure, and laboratory testing, we started treatment with the binders that are best for those two categories of mold toxin, namely, bentonite clay, *Saccharomyces boulardii*, N-acetyl cysteine (NAC), activated charcoal, and the prescription medication cholestyramine. (Binders are natural or pharmaceutical materials that have the ability to attach loosely to a specific mycotoxin and carry it out of the gastrointestinal system and out of the body).

One month after beginning this treatment, Robert reported marked general improvement, noting, "My strength is coming back." The perioral paresthesia that had been so bothersome to him was greatly reduced, and Robert was able to resume swimming for the first time in a long time. His sensitivities to light, sound, and smells had also decreased.

Here is a clear example of toxic exposure to mold. Over time, Robert's classic mold toxicity symptoms, untreated while he was focused on Lyme, slowly amplified until specific treatment was provided. I'm happy to report that he continued to improve as we fine-tuned his treatment program. Simply put, toxin exposure had made Robert ill. Treating that exposure began the process of helping him get well. Notice, too, that while Robert did have toxicity, he also had a certain degree of sensitivity, so you can see how they often coexist. In fact, the longer toxicity continues untreated the more likely a patient is to develop sensitivity, which will get worse and worse unless its cause is addressed.

What Is Reactivity?

Reactivity is a more generic term than either toxicity or sensitivity. Simply put, it is a reaction, or response of the body to a stimulus of any kind. This means that toxicity and sensitivity both fall into the category of reactivity, but are far more specific as to what could be causing that reaction. From this perspective, it is correct to describe these symptoms in our patients as representing "reactivity," but the more specific terms "sensitivity" and "toxicity" can be far more precise about what's causing what we're seeing.

The Difficulty in Distinguishing Toxicity from Sensitivity

I've tried to distinguish sensitivity from toxicity because they are not the same thing, even though clinically they sometimes look alike. Reactivity is an even more general term, and though it's frequently used interchangeably with the other terms, I think you can see that it's less specific.

When a patient experiences an increase in toxicity, their *symptoms* can appear identical to those of patients who experience reactions to stimuli they are sensitive to. This has led many clinicians to lump toxicity and sensitivity together, frustrated by the difficulties of clarifying *causation* in a complex situation. If, however, we make the effort to separate them, we realize that they need to be understood and treated differently, and this is of overriding importance.

Patients dealing with sensitivity, for example, are often unable to tolerate the treatment for toxicity. A sensitive patient will often have a severe reaction to even tiny doses of the supplements and medications provided to remove toxins from the body. Therefore, not recognizing the difference between toxicity and sensitivity can inadvertently lead to worsening the patient's condition.

What makes this a little more complicated is that many patients are both toxic and sensitive. Worse yet, the presence of toxicity predisposes, even triggers, a person to become more sensitive, and that increase in sensitivity predisposes that person to have an increased reactivity to the toxins he or she is exposed to. Thus it can be quite difficult to tease these phenomena apart with any precision. Often, physicians must use a process of trial and error to figure out the right approach to each patient who presents with unique issues shaped by his or her own specific biochemistry and genetics.

The Current Epidemic of Increasing Toxicity and Sensitivity

I emphasize that the increase in sensitivity and toxicity we are seeing is largely unacknowledged by the medical community. As I write these words, I don't feel that I'm being overly dramatic. I began treating chronically ill patients in the mid-1980s, and I can't recall a single patient who presented with these symptoms. Perhaps they were there and I was simply not picking up on them (and neither were most of my colleagues). By the late 1990s, when I was treating a large number of patients with CFS/ME and fibromyalgia, I had begun to see more and more individuals who were reacting to substances that I thought of as so benign that I sometimes questioned the validity of those reactions. Rare patients would complain that probiotics made them feel worse; others reported reactions to vitamin B-12; still others complained about miniscule doses of homeopathic remedies. Having never seen this kind of reactivity before, I was baffled. These were not neurotic patients, but credible citizens from whom I did not expect "weird" reactions. I didn't know what to do with those reactions, and unfortunately I had little to offer, either as explanation or treatment. I apologize to those patients if I conveyed any sense of disbelief or disrespect in my reactions to their complaints. I have always strived to be respectful, but I fear that my disbelief may have inadvertently slipped out, and for that I am deeply sorry.

In just a few years, these reports became more common, and I realized that I had to take them more seriously. I still didn't understand what was happening to these patients, but I was beyond the point of questioning their descriptions. I was convinced that what they were telling me was accurate; I just didn't know what to do about it.

Empirically, using trial and error, I found several types of treatments that could help to quiet their hyperreactive systems. (At that time I had no grasp at all that there was a difference between toxicity and sensitivity). Osteopathic cranial manipulation, frequency specific microcurrent (FSM), and low-dose antigen therapy (LDA) were of some help to quite a few patients. I began to see a pattern emerge: Almost all of these patients had been exposed to mold or had Lyme disease and its coinfections. When we were able to successfully remove the mold toxin from their bodies and treat the infections, their reactivity slowly dissipated, and the patients eventually recovered their health. In the ensuing years, several other components of sensitivity came to light, notably mast cell activation syndrome and porphyria (see chapters 4 and 23).

Along with these causes, or triggers, of sensitivity, I also began to learn about the role of limbic dysfunction and vagal nerve dysfunction as central to the presence of sensitivity (see chapters 1, 2 and 3). The pioneering work of Annie Hopper's Dynamic Neural Retraining System (DNRS, see chapter 1) and Ashok Gupta's Amygdala Retraining (see chapter 2) made major contributions to the effectiveness of treatment.

Prior to my retirement from clinical practice after five decades of patient care, these patients made up the majority of my practice. I would estimate that at least 70% exhibited this debilitating reactivity. As we have slowly recognized the epidemic nature of Lyme disease (the CDC recognizes 400,000 new cases every year) and have just begun to realize the same for mold toxicity (some experts estimate 10 million Americans have a degree of mold toxicity), it should come as no surprise that what was once rare is now quite common.

I have the privilege of mentoring over 150 physicians, all of whom are seeing the same thing that see. These physicians are on the cutting edge of medicine and are finding the same successes I do with diagnosis and treatment. Unfortunately, many other physicians, who deny the existence of these illnesses or who have no awareness of them, do not "see" these patients at all. Rather, baffled by the unusual presentation of symptoms in their patients, these physicians assume that the symptoms are psychological in origin and refer their patients for psychotherapy. Alas,, as we have learned, psychotherapy does not usually help, as it completely misses the diagnoses that are triggering these conditions.

I hope that the information we are acquiring will somehow reach my colleagues, because given the state of toxicity of the world we live in, I can assure them that they'll be seeing more and more of these patients in the near future.

Why Now?

While the formal "scientific proof" that the medical community insists upon might not be as overwhelming as it needs to be, increasing information and a growing number of physicians agree with me that these phenomena are triggered by a significant increase in the toxicities of the world we live in. We are currently exposed to tens of thousands of chemicals that simply did not exist fifty years ago, the vast majority of which have never been tested for safety in humans (see chapter 11). We are also exposed to massive amounts of electromagnetic fields (EMF) that did not exist fifty years ago. Worse, we hold them in our hands, in our laps, to our ears, and on our bodies all day long. Commercials bombard us with the joy that 5G (a vastly more powerful EMF exposure than 4G) can bring us electronic information even faster now, with no mention of the growing body of information that suggests that these represent a serious health hazard (see chapters 9 and 10). We are continuously exposed to all kinds of heavy metals (such as mercury and lead) and other environmental pollutants and radiation (see chapter 11). The long-term effects of the Fukushima Daiichi nuclear disaster have not yet been studied, and concerns about genetically modified organisms (GMOs) and food additives abound. There is increasing concern about the long-term effects of the vaccines provided for COVID (see chapter 24).

We are exposing our bodies to chemicals and radiation in amounts and varieties never before encountered in the history of humankind. Without complete or adequate knowledge, we are messing around with our environment in ways that we're just beginning to understand, and unless we start doing something about it right now, the future won't be all that bright. I fear that if we don't devote ourselves to fully understanding what we are doing, and limit these exposures now, we will suffer damage that cannot be undone.

Canaries In the Coal Mines

Quite a few contemporary writers have alluded to what I am describing. It is not a new idea, but sadly, one that our politicians and captains of industry have not embraced.

Long ago, when coal miners explored a new vein of ore, they brought caged canaries down into the mines with them. Canaries are more sensitive to toxic gases than humans are, so when the birds keeled over in their cages without warning, it was a clear signal to get out of the mine immediately. I cannot help but view the epidemic increase in chronic fatigue, fibromyalgia, mold toxicity, multiple chemical sensitivities, autism, Lyme disease, and cancer as a manifestation of the growing toxicity of our modern world.

You could view these chronically ill patients as unlucky, and in a sense, they are. Their unique biochemistry, genetics, and exposures due to being at the wrong place at the wrong time do predispose them to one or more of these illnesses, but take care, because they are just the tip of the iceberg, the canaries in the coal mine, if you will. We are right behind them, as are our children and grandchildren, who will inherit this world we have unwittingly polluted.

How Do I Know If I'm Sensitive – And To What?

While many of you have already had the experience of sharing your symptoms with others (physicians, family, or friends) and find yourself not being believed, it may be helpful to know that there are well-validated methods of knowing that you are indeed sensitive, and even methods for knowing what may have triggered, or be continuing to trigger, your symptoms. Not only that, but this method, developed by Claudia Miller, MD, is an excellent way to follow your progress with treatment.

I hope you'll want to take these questionnaires before you receive treatment, and then repeat them following your treatments. If you would be so kind as to send them on to me, once treatments have been completed, at www.neilnathanmd.com, we can use your information to not only help you but to help countless others who are suffering with sensitivities and not receiving the medical help they need.

Three Simple Questions

The BREESI: Brief Environmental Exposure and Sensitivity Inventory

Let's start with three simple questions developed by Dr. Miller and validated by medical publications.

1. Do you feel sick (headache, brain fog, weakness, dizziness, shortness of breath, or stomach upset) when exposed to tobacco smoke, cleaning supplies, nail polish, gasoline, fresh tar, asphalt, new carpets, furnishings, air "fresheners," pesticides, etc.?
2. Are you unable to tolerate or have you had adverse reactions to antibiotics, painkillers, anesthetics, contrast dyes, oral contraceptives, vaccines, or medical prostheses and other such devices?
3. Are you unable to tolerate or do you react to dairy, corn, wheat, eggs, soy, alcohol, caffeine, or food additives (MSG, food dyes)?

If you answered yes to all three questions, it is *very suggestive* that you have a 90% likelihood of meeting the criteria for chemical intolerance (MCS). If you answered yes to 2 of the 3 questions, it suggests that you'd have a 70% likelihood for this diagnosis.

Most of my patients would answer yes to all three questions. Here is the beginning of validating your experiences. No, this is not in your head—your experiences are very real and need to be honored.

Additional Validation

The QEESI: Quick Environmental Exposure and Sensitivity Inventory

Dr. Miller developed the QEESI as a screening questionnaire for multiple chemical intolerances (MCI, which some of our authors refer to as MCS). This instrument has 4 scales: Symptom Sensitivity; Chemical Intolerances; Other Intolerances, and Life Impact. Each scale contains 10 items, scored from 0 = "not a problem" to 10 = "severe or disabling problem." A 10-item Masking Index gauges ongoing exposures that may affect an individual's awareness of their intolerances as well as the intensity of their responses to environmental exposures.

Individuals whose symptoms began or intensified following a particular exposure can fill out the QEESI using two different ink colors, one showing how they were before the event, and the second how they've been since the event. Below is a "Symptom Star," which provides a graphical representation of patients' responses to this test.

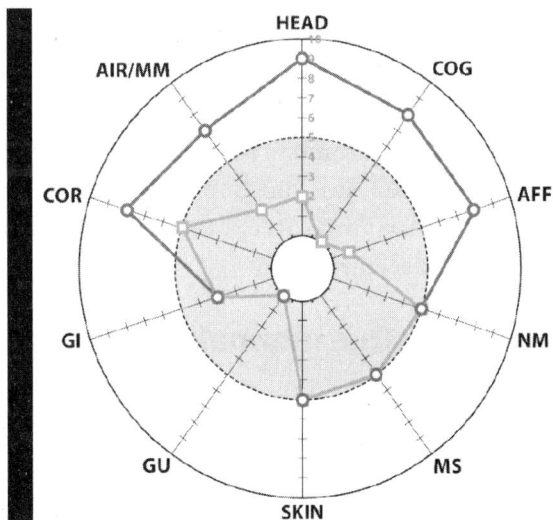

Symptom Star

HEAD = Head-related symptoms
COG = Cognitive symptoms
AFF = Affective symptoms
NM = Neuromuscular symptoms
MS = Musculoskeletal symptoms
SKIN = Skin-related symptoms
GU = Genitourinary symptoms
GI = Gastrointestinal symptoms
COR = Heart/chest-related symptoms
AIR/MM = Airway or mucous membrane symptoms

□————□ Before exposure event

○————○ After exposure event

We are unable to provide the full QEESI here, but you can go to Dr. Miller's website and take this questionnaire for free. Just google UT Health San Antonio/Hoffman Tilt Program and these questionnaires will become immediately available for you.

This test has been validated by the experiences of over 10,000 patients, and this result has been published in the medical literature. As you complete your questionnaire, the further out from the center of the star the more symptoms you have and the greater the likelihood that you are suffering from chemical intolerance.

You now have in hand proof that this is very real, that what you're experiencing can be measured, and that as you receive helpful treatments this will be validated by an improvement in your scores.

Dr. Miller's research, which spans many decades (see chapter 14 for more details), has demonstrated, from their completed QEESIs, that nearly half of those who were chemically intolerant reported one or more initiating events.

Of those, mold was the most common initiator in 14%, followed by remodeling (or new construction) in 13.2%, medical procedure in 13.2%, pesticides in 11.8%, combustion products in 6.9%, and implants (breast or others) 2.6%.

I readily admit that we have high hopes for this book. First and foremost, we envision that the thousands—perhaps millions—of patients currently impaired by their severe sensitivities will be able to both understand how they have become so sensitive and also use the blueprint we provide to recover their health and live normal lives again.

This is also an opportunity for patients to help us and the medical profession to document just how successful these treatments can be, by completing some online questionnaires before they begin treatment and repeating the questionnaires once they've completed their treatments. By collecting this important data, we can continue our efforts to refine and improve our approach and at the same time demonstrate to the larger medical community that our understanding is not only useful but can be statistically validated. It is our hope that this will provide additional impetus to move the medical profession to accept the reality our sensitive patients live in, and to realize that they can indeed help them.

Inventory Questionnaire for Sensitive Patients

Evaluation: QEESI Pre- and Post-Test

Treatments

Mold: ☐ Binders
☐ Antifungals
☐ Remediation
☐ Moving Location

Lyme: ☐ Antibiotics
☐ Herbal Treatments

Mast Cell Treatments: ☐ H1 blocker
☐ H2 Blocker
☐ Ketotifen
☐ Singulair
☐ Cromolyn Sodium
☐ Other Pharmaceuticals
☐ Quercetin
☐ NeuroProtek
☐ Perimine
☐ AllQlear
☐ DAO
☐ PEA
☐ Others

Other Environmental Strategies: ☐ Natural Gas Removal
☐ Personal Health Items
☐ Glyphosate
☐ Sauna/Hot Tub
☐ Ionic Foot Baths
☐ Epsom Salt Baths
☐ Oil Pulling
☐ Dry Brushing
☐ Other

Thiamine: ☐ Thiamine Hydrochloride
☐ Benfotiamin
☐ TTFD

LDI: ☐ Antigen(s):
☐ **Effective Dosages:**

NAET: ☐

EMF Exposure: ☐ Testing Home Devices
☐ Testing Dirty Electricity
☐ Shielding Devices
☐ Home

Physical Structure: ☐ Osteopathy
☐ Chiropractic
☐ TMJ
☐ Other

Limbic System: ☐ DNRS
☐ Amygdala Retraining
☐ Other

Vagal System: ☐ Rosenberg Exercises
☐ Osteopathic Cranial Work
☐ FSM
☐ Emotional Freedom Technique
☐ Brain Tap
☐ Vagal Nerve Stimulator
☐ Safe & Sound Program
☐ Gargling, singing, gagging
☐ Other

Ketamine: ☐ Intravenous
☐ Other

Food Allergy Testing: ☐ **Laboratory and Findings**
Oxalates: ☐ **Evaluation and Treatment**
Salicylates: ☐ **Evaluation and Treatment**
Benzodiazepine Withdrawal ☐
SSRI Withdrawal ☐

Avoidance(s):
Food ☐ Gluten
☐ Dairy
☐ Other

Environmental: ☐ VOCs
☐ Tobacco
☐ Alcohol
☐ Natural gas
☐ Wildfires
☐ Solvents
☐ Cleaning agents
☐ Pesticides
☐ Other

Which treatments do *you* feel have been most beneficial?

Which treatments do *you* feel have not helped?

References

1. Validation of a Brief Screening Instrument for Chemical Intolerance in a Large U.S. National Sample. Palmer RF, Walker T, Kattari D, Rincon R, Perales RB, Jaén CR, Grimes C, Sundblad DR, Miller CS. *Int J Environ Res Public Health.* 2021 Aug 18;18(16):8714. doi: 10.3390/ijerph18168714.PMID: 34444461.
2. The Environmental Exposure and Sensitivity Inventory (EESI): a standardized approach for measuring chemical intolerance for research and clinical applications. Miller, CS, Prihoda, TJ, *Toxicology and Industrial Health* 15: 370-385 (1999).
3. A controlled comparison of symptoms and chemical intolerance reported by Gulf War Veterans, implant recipients and persons and multiple chemical sensitivity, Miller, CS, Prihoda, TJ., *Toxicology and Industrial Health,* 15: 386-397 (1999).

Part I

The Neurology, Biochemistry, and Physiology of Sensitivity

What Creates Sensitivity?

This section will give you an understanding of the origin of sensitization—the what, how, and why of it, which is of the utmost importance to grasp how the body initiates the process of sensitization, using primary elements of neurophysiology and biochemistry to do so. For a clinician trying to learn how to help their patient, exploring these areas is essential, as they provide a roadmap of how to reverse the sensitization process. For a patient, this is the starting point for your healing journey.

It's crucial to realize that all of these systems come into play to protect you, not to harm you—it's all about *safety*. If your body doesn't feel safe, or has any hint of danger, it will do everything in its power to protect you by warning you of what it perceives as a threat.

The three most important components of the perception of safety are the limbic system, the vagal nerve system (sometimes referred to as polyvagal theory), and Mast Cell Activation Syndrome (MCAS), and for all three, inflammation is the underlying causative physiology. In virtually all patients who become sensitized, the limbic system and vagus nerve are key, neurologically, to that process. This should come as no surprise, since the limbic system is the part of the brain responsible for monitoring and evaluating all the stimuli we are exposed to from the perspective of safety, and thus is key to the development of sensitivity. While the vagus nerve is anatomically separate from the limbic system, physiologically it works together with the limbic system to monitor our stimuli for *safety*. If either system suspects that any given stimulus (light, sound, touch, food, chemicals, or EMFs) is unsafe, it will alert us by finding a way to get our attention. That can include the sudden and immediate onset of fatigue, brain fog, headache, pain, or even severe neurological conditions such as pseudoseizures (seizure-like activities that don't show up on EEGs but are still categorized by neurologists as true seizures) or dyskinesias (writhing, twisting, spasmodic movements of the limbs). *Limbic and vagal issues are clearly neurological, not psychological.* It's important to keep in mind that these are attempts at protection, though often it might not seem that way.

For most patients who develop these sensitivities, as their triggers, or causes, persist untreated, they will gradually develop Mast Cell Activation Syndrome. This is a cellular process, as opposed to a neurological process. It meshes with, and integrates with, limbic and vagal physiology to provide yet another way of monitoring our environment for safety. Mast cells are found in every tissue of our bodies, but particularly in parts that closely interface with the outside world: our gastrointestinal tract and sinuses. Mast cells are designed to react to a variety of stimuli, and when activated, they do so with gusto, releasing hundreds of biological mediators into our bodies that have profound and immediate effects.

As I do throughout this book, I reiterate that these three systems are central to understanding and treating sensitivity. Underlying these systems, as the basis for triggering their emergence, is a persistent inflammatory response to either a toxin or an infection. It is especially important to understand that inflammation is at the root of these difficulties and to appreciate that *inflammation does not usually create damage* but rather is amenable to treatment so that its effects can resolve. I emphasize this because so many of our patients are worried that their illness has damaged them to the point that recovery may not be possible. I want to reassure them that the vast majority of our patients have recovered completely. The effects of inflammation on the brain, which can be evaluated with a version of an MRI called a Neuroquant, show that in the throes of an inflammatory response from a toxin or an infection, certain brain areas become enlarged and others shrink. When they receive the report of this test, many patients are terrified that they won't be able to improve. We've discovered that when we treat the toxins (such as mold) or the infections (such as Lyme disease), these brain changes resolve completely and our patients' symptoms resolve as well. Irreparable damage is very rare, since the inflammation can be treated.

The next chapters focus on these subjects so you can understand the underlying mechanisms of sensitivity. We can then explore the triggers that evoke sensitivity reactions in these systems, which will lead us directly into effective treatments.

The limbic system is so essential to these discussions that I invited the two people who have understood and treated limbic dysfunction for the longest time—Annie Hopper and Ashok Gupta—to share their perspectives on how to view and work with the limbic system. Both Annie and Ashok have found that Long Haul COVID can trigger a limbic issue and that using their methods, many patients with Long COVID have recovered.

In chapter 1, Annie discusses her grasp of the limbic system and how her method, Dynamic Neural Retraining System (DNRS), has helped so many patients to heal.

In chapter 2, Ashok discusses his view of the limbic system and how his process, Amygdala (another name for limbic) Retraining Program (ARP), has also helped so many patients to heal.

Chapter 3 is written by Stephen Porges, the brilliant researcher who essentially put our understanding of vagal nerve physiology on the map, and by me. Stephen goes into detail about what the vagus nerve does and how this impacts sensitization.

In chapter 4, Beth O'Hara offers a thorough discussion of mast cell activation—what it is, what causes it, and how to treat it.

Chapter 5 presents a cutting-edge concept developed by Andrew Maxwell and Deborah Wardly that ties together some seemingly disparate ideas into a cohesive discussion about how mast cell activation and inflammation trigger a sequence of events that lead to illness and sensitization, and with that, how to approach treatment from different perspectives.

In chapter 6, Kurt Woeller adds another dimension to our understanding of these processes by examining the immune system and how immune function is biochemically related to sensitivity. Here we learn the fundamentals of inflammation as a central component of these physiological processes.

These six chapters not only give us a great starting point for understanding the most important components of sensitization but also provide models for treatment.

Chapter 1: The Limbic System, Part 1

Annie Hopper

Introduction by Dr. Nathan

Given that we have discovered that limbic dysfunction, vagal nerve dysfunction, and mast cell activation are key elements in the development of sensitivity, we begin with the limbic system. We are honored to have Annie Hopper, a pioneer in the understanding and treatment of limbic issues, present to us her understanding of this important subject. Annie will utilize her own story as a way of personally connecting her journey of debilitating illness to her discoveries about how, exactly, one can reboot this aspect of neurological dysfunction. Knowing Annie well, it is hard to imagine that this vital, vibrant teacher that I work with was once barely able to function, but I also know that her illness was the motivating force for these discoveries. Having been seriously ill myself, on two occasions, I understand how precious it is to recover completely and get one's life back.

✿ ✿ ✿

Exploring The Limbic System and the Sensitivities Involved in Long COVID

When discussing sensitivities involved in Long COVID or any complex, chronic health condition, it is imperative that we look at how limbic-system impairment and a nervous system stuck in a "fight, flight, or freeze" trauma response may be involved.

The limbic system is a complex set of structures in the midbrain that is associated with emotion, learning, memory, threat evaluation, the body's stress response, and sense of smell. Under stress or during trauma (viral, emotional, physical, or toxic exposure), the brain can get stuck in a protective trauma response. The brain and body may remain on high alert, even if the initial threat or trauma is no longer present. This is called limbic-system impairment (also known as central sensitization).

This impairment can be caused by a single trauma or more often from a combination of stressors and traumas over time. For many, it is at the very root of their ongoing suffering, especially for those wrestling with debilitating sensitivities. If the brain remains in a high-alert state, the body will chronically release stress hormones that affect the autonomic nervous system (automatic body functions), the immune system (protection against disease), and the endocrine system (hormone production). It also affects the ability to rest and digest, the accuracy of messages being sent by the brain regarding threat evaluation, sensory perception, and overall health and well-being. Symptoms may include chronic inflammation, poor memory, brain fog, digestive issues, lowered energy levels, numerous sensitivities, chronic pain, and sleep issues, as well as many other symptoms. Bodily functions such as detoxification, absorption of nutrients, and cellular communication can also become compromised. Limbic-system impairment also has a direct impact on thoughts, emotions, and behaviors. Dysfunction of the limbic system is central to the process of sensitization.

Simply said, the brain remains on high alert and never gets the "all clear" signal. An easy analogy is a home alarm system gone awry. Imagine installing an alarm system to alert you when an intruder enters. All is calm until one day the alarm goes off. You suddenly become fearful and adrenaline surges through your body, but when you check to see if there are any intruders, you don't see anyone. Day after day the alarm goes off—first, the cat trips the alarm; then a tree branch scraping the side of your window sets it off; then a leaf falling off the tree sets it off. Unbeknown to you, the alarm system has a software bug. Each day it grows more sensitive. Your alarm system has become hypersensitive and is sending false messages of impending threats.

This is similar to what happens in limbic-system impairment. The brain begins to send the body false alarm signals. The brain can misinterpret information and send a message that danger is present when it is not or when the danger has passed.

If you have experienced trauma (viral, emotional, physical, or toxic exposure) and have tried various treatments but still find yourself suffering in a cycle of illness, your limbic system may be stuck in this protective state, and you would likely benefit from retraining your brain. It doesn't matter whether your condition is mild or severe, if you have the same symptoms as someone else, or how long you've been suffering—the common denominator in many cases is limbic-system impairment.

Here are the common conditions and symptoms related to limbic-system impairment: Multiple chemical sensitivities, chronic fatigue syndrome, neurological disorders, fibromyalgia, chronic Lyme disease, food allergies or sensitivities, anxiety disorders, post-acute COVID-19 syndrome (COVID Long Haulers), posttraumatic stress disorder, depressive mood disorder, postural orthostatic tachycardia syndrome, irritable bowel syndrome, chronic pain, migraines or general headaches, electric hypersensitivity syndrome, mast cell activation disorder, chronic inflammatory response syndrome or mold illness, sensory sensitivities, adrenal insufficiency, dysautonomia, and more.

I have good news and bad news: The good news is that retraining your brain to provide the "all clear" signal can be done from the comfort of your own home through a self-paced online program. The bad news is that there is no magic pill, and it's going to take focus, energy, and consistent effort. Don't let that scare you—it doesn't take more energy or time than current coping mechanisms such as avoidance behaviors, special diets, or coping strategies to manage energy expenditure. The challenge with rewiring the limbic system is that it's an experiential process, not an intellectual one.

The Dynamic Neural Retraining system (DNRS) program that I developed is a drug-free, self-directed, neural rehabilitation program. It uses principles of neuroplasticity to help reverse limbic-system impairment and regulate autonomic nervous-system function. While I can share with you the basic overview of the steps involved, you will need to take the time to learn how to retrain your limbic system and practice daily for a minimum of six months. The DNRS online instructional video program will show you exactly what you need to do and how to do it. Six months might sound like a long time but is a small sacrifice when this can be the missing key to healing.

It is certain that millions have developed limbic-system impairment due to the trauma involved in the pandemic, triggering a tsunami of chronic health conditions. Let's take a closer look at the pandemic in general and how it has affected limbic-system function. We have been focusing on the threat of COVID, the undeniable loss involved, and the hardships that we have endured for a very long time. The direct impact on the limbic system from the virus, or a reaction to the vaccine, along with the generalized fear, stress, and fallout from the pandemic, have affected us all on some level. Some may have had health challenges prior to the pandemic that have gotten worse, while millions of others are dealing with chronic health issues for the first time. And yet, even during these challenging times, there are people who have been able to recover from chronic health issues by rewiring their limbic system through self-directed neuroplasticity.

Regardless of whether you are suffering from disabling sensitivities, Long COVID, autonomic nervous-system dysfunction, anxiety, depression, chronic fatigue, chronic pain, or are just in the beginning stages of developing several sensitivities, if you suspect that you have limbic-system impairment, it is imperative to address brain function sooner rather than later. The faster you address brain function, the less time you'll spend suffering.

While other treatments are helpful for some, they may not have
a positive or lasting impact until a neurological reset takes place.

How do I know this? I once suffered from severe limbic-system impairment that rendered me disabled and homeless. Let me explain. My perfect storm for developing limbic-system impairment might sound familiar to you. I was exposed to heavy wildfire smoke, involved in a motor vehicle accident, and was exposed to toxic mold and industrial chemical cleaners within a six-month period. Combined with childhood distress, this created a host of traumas and changed the structure and function of my brain. My limbic system became stuck in a "fight, flight, or freeze" trauma response.

The tipping point was the exposure to toxic mold and industrial chemical cleaners in my workplace where I had a very busy counseling practice. My symptoms started with headaches, muscle and joint pain, insomnia, and unexplained anxiety. Over time, I developed an increase in sensitivity to scented products like perfumes, cleaning products, detergents, and any amount of mold. It felt like I was literally being poisoned by everything around me, and I was also in chronic pain. I spent thousands of dollars on various treatments with well-intended health-care practitioners and various specialists. I was an obedient patient and tried everything that was recommended. I detoxed my way to Mars and back, tried desensitization treatments, took a ton of supplements, and was on a restricted diet, but any positive effects were short-lived. I ended up sling-shotting back into a state of chronic illness, often worse than before. It got to the point that the mere whiff of perfume or walking by dryer exhaust could send me into neurological convulsions. My cognitive abilities were also affected, and often I could not string words together to make a coherent sentence. My memory declined, I would lose my voice with each exposure, and I felt like a dumbed-down, sick, and depressed version of my former self.

As a writer, and someone who depended on communication for a living, this was more than deeply disturbing. It would take me days to recover from the smallest exposure, and as you can imagine, it became increasingly difficult to navigate the world. The only answer I could see was to avoid anything that seemed to be causing the symptoms. I thought that scented products were the enemy. They felt like kryptonite to me. I couldn't believe that other people could not detect what I could. Perfumes that used to smell inviting now smelled like toxic bug spray. Due to the severity of reactions to common exposures, I had to completely overhaul my life and live a life of isolation and loneliness. I could no longer work, and rarely left my home except for medical appointments, which were very difficult to manage. No more going out and no more being involved in my community or being around my friends. If anyone came to visit, they would have to jump through hoops to make it "safe" for me. Eventually, my circle of friends dissolved to none—except for my loving partner James.

My complete focus was on my health and trying to find an answer to my increasing nosedive into poor health and a life of science fiction. I knew that my brain was no longer filtering information in a healthy way, and started to research how it might be involved.

Then things went from bad to worse. Overnight, I developed electric hypersensitivity syndrome and could no longer tolerate electromagnetic fields that were being emitted from things like WIFI or electronics of any sort. If I was talking on my phone or typing on the computer, I would lose my voice and would experience the same symptoms as I did with scented chemical products. That's when I became homeless, or more accurately, I could not find a home to live in that didn't cause a reaction. My brain's protective response was stuck in emergency mode, and the resulting increased sensory distortions and illness made it impossible to live in a "normal" environment.

In my exhaustive search for answers, I came across the book *The Brain That Changes Itself* by Dr. Norman Doidge. This was a huge source of inspiration and for realizing that my situation was most likely not a life sentence after all. From what I could gather, if I could rewire my limbic system, it was quite likely that all my symptoms of illness would disappear. I matched the theories in the book about neuroplasticity with everything I was studying about the limbic system, which happened to be the area of the brain responsible for the sense of smell. Studying that part of the brain seemed like the logical place to start.

It finally made sense to me that despite my exhaustive search for answers, the treatments I had tried in the past were largely ineffective because my nervous system was stuck on high alert, and it was impossible to make lasting gains until my brain function was addressed. Combining the theory that neuroplasticity was involved in the development of illness, and that applying neuroplasticity could be the way out, I was able to retrain my brain's response to perceived threat—and my symptoms started to fade. It was this new understanding of the brain and retraining my brain that led me to developing the DNRS program.

Understanding how neuroplasticity was involved with my illness turned out to be the missing link. I achieved full recovery by implementing my own daily program of brain-based rehabilitation, which focused on retraining my brain's unconscious conditioned response and rewiring faulty neural pathways in the brain. Fortunately, my nervous system regulated, my sensory perception returned to normal, the chronic pain and other symptoms eventually disappeared, and my immune system went back to regular function. Within six months I went from being disabled to a vivacious, driven woman on fire to liberate millions from suffering.

When I was sick, I promised myself that if I recovered, I would spend my life liberating those who were still suffering. Since 2008, the DNRS program has helped thousands of people worldwide find relief from a growing list of chronic and hard-to-treat conditions, allowing them to reverse often disabling symptoms of illness. The intention is to move your brain and body out of a state of survival and chronic stress response into a state of growth and repair, where true healing can take place.

If you would like to know more about my personal history and the development of the program, I encourage you to read my book, *Wired for Healing: Remapping the Brain to Recover from Chronic and Mysterious Illnesses.* If you want to learn how to rewire your limbic system, I encourage you to implement the program as taught in the DNRS Instructional Video Program available on our website: www.RetrainingTheBrain.com.

How Do Sensitivities Relate to Long COVID?

Like many other chronic and complex health conditions related to limbic-system impairment, the brain never gets the "all clear" message and gets stuck on high alert. This alarm state sends inaccurate messages about levels of safety to all systems of the body and can result in myriad symptoms in multiple body systems. For example, elevated stress hormones can lead to an increase in histamine release and overactive immune responses. This can also negatively affect vagus nerve function (your ability to rest, digest, and connect with others) and your ability to use energy resources to complete the healing cycle.

While loss of smell and taste is a hallmark symptom of COVID in its acute form, this loss can last well into a chronic stage, and patients can also develop other sensory distortions and multisystem issues. Some people will go on to develop sensory sensitivities and become sensitive to stimuli that they used to tolerate very well. They might develop light, sound, and food sensitivities, or suffer chronic pain, or experience gastrointestinal and digestive issues. When their sense of smell returns, some people become overly sensitive to smells and develop a condition known as multiple chemical sensitivity. Others may be diagnosed with conditions such as dysautonomia or postural orthostatic tachycardia syndrome or chronic fatigue syndrome and more. Regardless of the diagnosis, rewiring the limbic system can set the stage for healing to take place.

Patients with Long COVID usually recognize that brain function is involved in the condition because of neurological issues such as cognitive decline and brain fog, but for most, symptoms are multisystemic, and some symptoms seem to wax and wane, leaving most medical teams perplexed. Additional symptoms commonly include sensory distortions, headaches, fatigue, food sensitivities, gut problems, rapid heart rate, low blood pressure, depression, and anxiety.

These symptoms, which are related to limbic-system impairment, can remain long after the COVID infection or other viral or bacterial infections are no longer present. The virus has affected the limbic system of the brain. It's not your fault. The symptoms are not in your head, but, ironically, brain function is involved. The COVID infection was a trauma your brain and body attempted to defend against. Your limbic system, through no fault of its own, got stuck in defense mode. Depending on the injuries you sustained from the virus, implementing the DNRS program can resolve a vast majority of the long-hauler symptoms you just can't seem to shake.

While implementing the program can't repair organ damage to the lungs, heart, or kidneys, it can interrupt the chronic fight, flight, or freeze response. Through daily implementation of the program, you'll find that your limbic-system function will regulate and help you find your way back to health.

In a research study published in *Nature* medical journal in 2022, UK researchers studied the brain scans of 401 people with Long COVID and found changes in the limbic portion of the brain. The study found reduced gray matter in several regions associated with olfaction (sense of smell). They also found abnormalities in structures in the limbic system important for producing behavioral and emotional responses. The hypothesis is that the virus directly impacted the portion of the brain responsible for the sense of smell, and that other changes in brain structure may be the consequence of an overactive immune response occurring throughout the brain.

Research: Douaud, G. et al. (2022) SARS-CoV-2 is associated with changes in brain structure in UK Biobank. Nature https://doi.org/10.1038/s41586-022-04569-5

DNRS addresses the brain directly and assists in the recovery process through retraining limbic function. The program focuses on the five pillars of recovery. Consistent application of all five pillars can bring about changes in brain function that result in greater health on the physical, mental, and emotional levels. Symptoms can wax and wane during the rehabilitation process but will eventually abate. Each pillar is unique and is thoroughly explained in the online instructional video program available at www. RetrainingTheBrain.com.

The Five Pillars of Recovery with DNRS

Pillar 1: Recognize the Link Between Your Brain and Your Condition. This mindset introduces a new way of thinking about how brain function may be involved in your condition.

Pillar 2: Interrupt and Redirect Your Pathways of the Past (POPs). This pillar focuses on how to interrupt old neural pathways that keep the brain in a state of survival, and learn to redirect our thoughts, emotions, and behaviors to create new, positive neural pathways.

Pillar 3: Practice Full Rounds of DNRS Retraining Steps. The steps utilize a variety of methods that involve speech, movement, visualization, and thought and emotional restructuring. The intention of this step is to decrease firing of threat centers in the brain by flooding the brain with neurotransmitters and hormones related to a state of growth and repair. The limbic-system retraining steps are not about immediate symptom relief, though sometimes an immediate change in symptoms may be noticed. The goal is to rewire the limbic system and regulate the stress response.

Pillar 4: Apply Incremental Training. This pillar involves changing trauma associations and graduated exposure therapy (imaginary and real) to desensitize the brain, change fear associations and strengthen positive neural pathways that lead to optimal health.

Pillar 5: Elevate Your Emotional State: Elevating your emotional state helps to provide a cue of safety to the brain, allowing for the brain to move out of survival-related emotions and pave the way for positive neuroplastic changes.

In some ways rewiring your limbic system is like learning how to drive a car or ride a bike. At first, it might seem very complex to remember all the steps involved when merging onto the highway or finding your sense of balance on a bicycle for the first time, but like all learned skills, rewiring your limbic system gets easier with practice.

How Can Implementing the Program Change Sensitivities and the Symptoms of Long COVID?

Let's look at Sandra's case, for example. We will explore the perfect storm for developing limbic-system impairment, her experience with Long COVID, and her recovery journey.

Sandra contracted COVID-19 in March 2020. Prior to that, Sandra describes herself as a healthy person, though as a child she was very prone to catching infections, had chronic skin issues with eczema, and had an overactive immune response to mosquito bites. In her teens she had developed temporary sensitivities to mold and EMFs that coincided with emotional trauma. The sensitivities resolved over time. During Sandra's university years she was very healthy. As a young adult, while traveling in Indonesia for doctoral field work, she suffered a severe case of malaria that took her three years to recover from. Following this infection, she once again became prone to other infections and catching colds.

In the acute stage of the COVID-19 infection, she displayed a full spectrum of symptoms—high fever, chills, loss of sense of smell and taste, persistent cough, fatigue, brain fog, rapid pulse, headache, aches and pains, gastrointestinal issues, and difficulty breathing and swallowing. She also developed sensitivities to light and sound, insomnia, and numbness in her hands and face.

After resting for a few weeks, Sandra felt worse instead of better. After a month, she developed severe lung pain and neurological symptoms. No longer able to care for her four-year-old daughter, Sandra and her daughter moved in with Sandra's parents. She felt like the signals from her brain were not reaching her legs, and she was losing control of the movement in her legs. Similarly, she could no longer write or print with a pen as the signals from her brain were not reaching her hands properly. She was also experiencing difficulty balancing and at times was too weak to stand up. Sandra was in a wheelchair most of the time or walked slowly with support. She also developed excruciating chronic pain. Her pulse was very high, her blood pressure had gone haywire, and her oxygen saturation levels became unstable.

As the neurological symptoms increased, her arms and hands trembled as if she had Parkinson's disease. Sandra had been to the emergency Covid Clinic in Sweden a number of times, but her medical team could not provide any concrete answers as to what was happening.

Sandra was one of the first Long COVID patients in Sweden to try an alternative antiviral treatment, and within two weeks she could walk again and did not have to wear sunglasses all the time. Unfortunately, after two months she had to stop the treatment due to the onset of severe hypersensitivities. She developed a rash and had difficulty swallowing. It became difficult to pinpoint the source of her reactions, as she grew more and more sensitive.

Her tongue would suddenly become swollen, and she began to have acute breathing difficulties after eating. When the sensitivities worsened, Sandra started to restrict her diet in the hope of decreasing the reactions, but soon realized that the list of sensitivities was growing, not getting better. At this point she also developed severe chemical sensitivities and was reacting to all products that contained artificial scent. Her smell sensitivities escalated to include some natural smells as well—like the smell of food cooking. Sandra moved into a home close to her parents where she could be alone and manage her exposures. Her sensitivities increased, however, and exposures would leave her disabled. All the symptoms that had improved with the antiviral treatment were coming back. Along with severe neurological symptoms, Sandra lost her voice and also suffered from chronic elevated mucus production. She was also losing control of her left eye, and color input had become distorted.

Sandra was very active in long-haul COVID groups on social media. A doctor from the Karolinska Institute who was familiar with the DNRS program contacted her and suggested she try neuroplasticity training to reset her limbic system. Sandra immediately resonated with the whole concept because she was already familiar with neuroplasticity from her research studies, After learning about the limbic system and how it can affect the body, Sandra said, "It made sense that I was stuck in a fight-or-flight response because of the trauma my body had gone through with the COVID-19 infection and that my brain was reacting as if the event were still happening."

It was easy for Sandra to commit to the DNRS program, and she started to notice an immediate change. "On the very first day I started doing the DNRS program, I got an explosion of the sense of taste in my mouth without even eating anything," she said. "I hadn't been able to feel the sensation of taste for a year."

After a couple of days, her voice returned, and she was able to remove her allergy mask. Then Sandra felt that she had the energy to start moving again. "In the first week I started moving again and going for walks, first in the neighborhood and then venturing farther away. This was only days after I started the program. Prior to that, I had just been inside the house, hardly getting out of bed," she said.

After one month she was able to return to work part-time, and within four months she was back at work full-time. In the fifth month Sandra stated, "Today I lead a very active life. I go for walks every day. I go jogging, I play with my daughter, I can cook every day and take care of all the household chores. I can do everything that I couldn't do before."

Sandra could not have imagined that she would be doing so well in such a short time after having been so ill. She can eat whatever she wants and do whatever she wants. She feels healthy and resilient, and happily says, "I'm just so grateful to have my life back and to be the mother my daughter deserves."

Sandra kept in touch with a handful of people experiencing Long Covid symptoms who also started to implement the DNRS program, and she reports that all of them were experiencing a positive change.

When I asked Sandra what she would say to people who experience Long Covid symptoms, she said, "Give neuroplasticity training a go. It might be difficult to comprehend the basic concept behind neuroplasticity training, but then again, it doesn't really matter why or how it works. It works, and it can make you feel better. I recommend trying this non-invasive, easy-to-follow program. It might take you longer to see results, and that's okay. It can give you your life back!"

The acronym "IMAGINE" describes the neuroplasticity principles involved in the program.

I: Intention – The immediate intention is not to decrease symptoms, though at times this can happen; the goal is to bring your attention inward and use self-directed neuroplasticity to change your brain. If the focus is on the immediate reduction of symptoms, or if a temporary increase in symptoms occurs, you may become frustrated and feel that the program is not effective. Implemented appropriately, however, the program has a cumulative effect on the brain that will in turn have a gradual positive impact on your symptoms.

M: Motivation – Motivation does not require extra energy but can simply be viewed as changing old habits for new ones. Your willingness and desire to become an active participant in the healing process will help you greatly. Motivation often improves with experiencing signs of progress and using our ongoing support services.

A: Awareness – An important part of the rewiring process is stepping into the state of a "curious observer" to develop awareness of the subconscious neural patterns associated with limbic-system impairment. What is challenging about this step is to recognize that coping behaviors and beliefs about the condition that seemed to help with managing symptoms are not necessarily helpful in the neural rehabilitation process. Many people manage their illness through avoidance and isolation and have been forced to adapt their lives to illness. This makes sense from a survival perspective. Understandably, no one wants to experience symptoms or discomfort if they can avoid it. That reasoning, however, is built on the premise that symptoms are a direct reflection of one's experience of safety or well-being. This is not to say that the symptoms are not real. Limbic-system impairment negatively impacts the immune system, endocrine system, and the autonomic nervous system. Conversely, rebalancing the limbic system can reverse the effects and act on these systems in a positive way.

Bringing awareness to symptoms of limbic-system impairment is the first step to rewiring the brain. The goal is to question the exaggerated messages the brain is sending and create a reverse effect on the brain in that moment. Overriding the distorted messages of an impaired limbic system through top-down regulation can move your brain and body from a state of survival into a state of growth and repair, where healing can take place.

G: Gains – While undergoing limbic-system rehabilitation, it is important to consciously focus on your gains, no matter how big or small. This will include improvements on physical, psychological, or emotional levels. While physical symptoms seem to be the most apparent with limbic-system impairment, psychological and emotional processes are often affected. One of the most common shifts recognized early on is a change in emotional state. As structural changes in the brain begin to occur, one's emotional capacity and thought patterns are greatly affected. Alongside these structural and functional changes, a sense of hope replaces a feeling of despair, and the very common cloud of depression begins to lift.

I: Incremental Training – Incremental Training is a form of neural shaping that may involve graduated exposure therapy in a safe, healthy, and informed way. During incremental training, one mildly activates symptoms to create a heightened neuroplastic state. Practicing the DNRS limbic-retraining steps when the brain is in a heightened state facilitates the process of redesignating the neural networks associated with an overactivated limbic response. Incremental training can be imaginary and work up to a real-life situation. In short, rewiring the limbic system is not necessarily a comfortable process, but it shouldn't be debilitating either. Whenever one becomes aware of a limbic response, it's a perfect time to interject and redirect brain patterns. In doing so, a "symptom" of illness is turned into a direct opportunity to act back on the brain.

Note that not every challenge requires incremental training. Every instance of incremental training helps recalibrate overall limbic-system function and can influence responses to other triggers, even if those triggers are unknown.

N: Neurological and Emotional Rehearsal – Rewiring the limbic system involves the conscious use of emotion as a tool to alter brain structure and function. Emotions strengthen neural connections, and we can use this understanding to our advantage. While ruminating on past trauma can strengthen the neurological pathways involved in the impairment, cultivating a positive emotional state can provide a safety cue for the brain that assists in the rewiring process. This is not about denial or repression of emotions, but rather understanding the brain's involvement in emotional responses.

Part of the process of rewiring the limbic system with DNRS involves describing positive past memories and positive future events in great detail by using your senses and imagining yourself in a state of optimal health. If you have difficulty remembering positive memories, you can create imaginary ones, as the brain does not distinguish between what is real and what is imagined. We capitalize on brain function by neurologically and emotionally rehearsing positive scenarios that bypass any trauma-related associations and create a context of safety. Like a professional athlete who uses mental rehearsal as part of their training, as we recall a positive memory, the brain uses the same neural pathways that are associated with that event.

The hormones and neurotransmitters that are generated with a positive emotion (i.e., dopamine and oxytocin) cool off the threat centers in the limbic system and increase function in the prefrontal cortex (the area for higher learning and executive function).

Research: Speer, M. E., Bhanji, J. P., and Delgado, M. R. (2014). Savoring the past: positive memories evoke value representations in the striatum. Neuron 84, 1–10. doi: 10.1016/j.neuron.2014.09.028

People who have limbic-system impairment are likely to be inexperienced at remembering positive memories and may feel challenged to cultivate positive emotions. From a brain perspective, this makes perfect sense. Typically, emotions like worry, fear, and hopelessness go hand in hand with limbic-system impairment. In addition, magnification of the brain's innate negativity bias is also involved. It's common for people with limbic-system impairment, who were once optimistic, happy, and easygoing, to become negative, withdrawn, and depressed. While this can be normal given the decrease in quality of life, it is important to recognize that this can also be a symptom of limbic-system impairment. As a pattern recognition organ, when your brain recalls past positive memories with associated emotions, you will naturally start to remember more. This gets easier with practice, and people often report that it feels like a floodgate has opened when they suddenly gain access to several positive memories.

E: Environmental Awareness – For many people, toxic trauma is part of their developing limbic-system impairment; e.g., toxic mold exposure or chemical exposure. Therefore, it makes common sense that we become proactive in creating a healthy home or office environment and become curious about what we put on and in our bodies.

Limbic-system rehabilitation does not replace common sense. Developing environmental awareness, eating nutritious food, exercising regularly, establishing balance in our lives, strengthening our social connections, and managing stress are essential to promote and maintain good health.

While other factors beyond rewiring the limbic system may also need to be addressed, there are times when rewiring limbic-system function is enough. For instance, though vagus-nerve function can be negatively affected, it can also be regulated through limbic-system retraining. The vagus nerve plays a role in the production of acetylcholine, a primary neurotransmitter and natural anti-inflammatory involved in the parasympathetic response. It is also involved in detoxification pathways and in protective responses related to the freeze response. Rewiring limbic-system function provides a cue of safety for the vagus nerve to resume normal function. This cue of safety will help regulate an overactive immune response, prevent the inappropriate release of histamine (an immune response that is often combined with sensitivities), and stop overstimulation of the amygdala (a structure in the limbic system associated with fear), thus breaking the histamine-cortisol cycle and negative feedback loop. With rewiring limbic function, this "all clear" signal also allows for cells to complete their healing cycle and move out of a cell danger response.

Keep in mind that the DNRS program and limbic-system rehabilitation is experiential and accumulative in nature. With repetition, the new neural patterns will make themselves apparent, and symptoms of illness will decrease. It does take dedication and effort, but this is nothing when compared to the energy and time it takes to manage and cope with symptoms. It's important to realize that with limbic-system impairment, you can no longer rely on your brain to be the conveyer of truth. This means you cannot always believe every thought you have, every emotion you experience, or every message your body sends you. This isn't denial, but rather a recognition that the messenger can be impaired.

Recovery times vary from person to person. Every brain is different. Most often, recovery happens gradually. Some people will start to notice changes very soon, while for others it will take more time. Regardless of whether symptoms change immediately or not, strengthening new neural pathways is like planting a seed in the garden. The root system must develop below the surface before the plant starts to sprout. Our recommendation is to practice all aspects of the program daily for a minimum of six months.

Suffering from limbic-system impairment and chronic complex health conditions can be a very harrowing and isolating experience; however, you are not alone in your recovery process. We offer several ongoing support services to provide guidance, connection, and community during your recovery journey.

After you have completed the online instructional video program, we highly encourage you to take advantage of the ongoing support services we offer, including:

DNRS Global Community Forum – The forum is a moderated online resource for all DNRS participants. A lifetime basic membership to the Global Community Forum is included with the DNRS instructional video program. This extensive resource is filled with invaluable information applicable to implementing the DNRS program. With over

13,000 members on our global community forum, many have traveled this journey, and their words of encouragement and experiential accounts of their recovery journey will give you hope and added insight into the program. This community of compassionate people will become your number one cheerleader and celebrate every victory along the way.

DNRS 12-week Support Sessions (Living DNRS) – This optional support service provides professional guidance and group support with implementing the DNRS program into daily life.

DNRS Individual Coaching – Individualized coaching with a Certified DNRS Coach is available for purchase to provide personalized guidance with implementing the program for your unique situation. Our certified DNRS Coaches have all recovered from limbic system impairment and related chronic illnesses through DNRS. They are extensively trained in the program and its applications and are leaders in applied neuroplasticity as it relates to limbic system rehabilitation.

When I was suffering, hope sometimes felt like a luxury I could not afford, because time after time I felt disappointed when treatment efforts failed, not to mention the expense of trying so many treatments. The key to effective recovery is early diagnosis and resetting the limbic system to provide the environment for healing to take place.

If you are suffering from limbic-system impairment, my heart goes out to you. Please do not lose hope. There is an answer, and there is a way to regain your health.

Navigating limbic-system trauma can be challenging as it alters one's ability to think, to be objective, and to feel safe in the world. It alters the brain's normal filtering process, which increases its vulnerability and keeps it in a cycle of trauma. To truly grasp that recovery is possible, one needs to embrace the idea that brain function plays a key role in optimal health. This does not mean that the illness is "all in your head," but rather that recovery, through neuroplasticity, requires that the brain be involved in the rehabilitation process.

Limbic-system rehabilitation through self-directed neuroplasticity represents a new paradigm in treating chronic and complex health conditions. Your story of transformation can and will positively affect people in ways beyond your imagination.

Just like Sandra and the thousands of others who have recovered, you have the power to retrain your brain, regain your health, and reclaim your life!

Ongoing Research

"Neuroplasticity-based treatment for fibromyalgia, chronic fatigue and multiple chemical sensitivity: feasibility and outcomes" Guenter D, et al. (2019). Research findings suggest that quality of life and function improved dramatically while implementing the DNRS program over a period of twelve months. People who enrolled in the study reported suffering from numerous—and often overlapping—conditions. Among these were: anxiety, chronic fatigue syndrome (ME/CFS), chronic pain, depression, fibromyalgia, food allergies/sensitivities, irritable bowel syndrome (IBS), Lyme disease, migraines/headaches, multiple chemical sensitivity (MCS), neurological disorders, and posttraumatic stress disorder (PTSD).

Early research findings from a feasibility study in Sweden suggest that the DNRS program is very effective for people suffering from Long COVID, POTS (Postural Orthostatic Tachycardia Syndrome), and many other limbic system impairment-related conditions. Dr. Söderberg reports, "So far, we have observed great to astonishing full recovery from severe post-acute COVID-19 disease (PACS)/autonomic dysfunction/ postural orthostatic tachycardia syndrome (POTS), chronic inflammatory response syndrome (CIRS), and hyper-reactivity to food, mold, and chemicals, in many patients undergoing DNRS training."

The DNRS Online Instructional Video program and Ongoing Support Services can be found at www.RetrainingTheBrain.com

Annie Hopper is a limbic-system rehabilitation specialist and founder of the Dynamic Neural Retraining System (DNRS), a neuroplasticity-based treatment method to regulate limbic-system function.

Author of *Wired for Healing: Remapping the Brain to Recover from Chronic and Mysterious Illnesses*, Annie is featured regularly in print, online, and in broadcast media. As a speaker, she delivers a unique and riveting message. Her speaking engagements include the Canadian Brain Injury Association, the American Academy of Environmental Medicine, the Canadian Counseling and Psychotherapy Association, the Institute for Functional Medicine, McMaster Teaching Hospital, the International Society for Environmentally Acquired Illnesses, the Finnish Institute for Occupational Health, and the Parliament House, Helsinki, Finland.

Chapter 2: The Limbic System, Part 2

Ashok Gupta and Frances Goodall

Introduction by Dr. Nathan

Ashok Gupta is another pioneer in the development of methods to successfully treat the limbic system. Like Annie, he too began his journey by needing to find a method to treat his own chemical sensitivities, and we are grateful that the answers he found have helped countless patients to recover. Ashok presents a somewhat different explanation of limbic dysfunction, which beautifully compliments those from our last chapter.

☼ ☼ ☼

In patients who react to their environment in ways that affect health and well-being, their brain has become unusually sensitized and conditioned to respond to what would've previously been experienced as inert or neutral stimuli. The good news is that with the tools and support we have developed, the brain can be retrained to no longer respond to triggers in this way. The ability of the brain to heal, or rewire itself, is called neuroplasticity—the idea being that the brain circuitry is not necessarily fixed but can be rewired to regain function.

Thousands of patients with conditions like multiple chemical sensitivity, mold toxicity, electrical sensitivities, food sensitivities, and Mast Cell Activation Syndrome (MCAS), in addition to ME/CFS, fibromyalgia, and Long COVID, have made a recovery using these tools.

In this chapter we shall go through the background hypothesis as to what may be causing these sensitivity reactions. Then we shall look at brain retraining and neuroplasticity, and how you can regain your health.

What Causes Sensitivity Illnesses Such as Mold Illness?

We always like to start with asking the biggest question of all—Why are we here? We are here because over millions of years of evolution, this body that we have inherited was designed to protect us from our environment and ensure survival so we can pass our genes on to the next generation.

Survival is our number one priority. Our physical and emotional well-being comes second. Additionally, in that pursuit of survival, the brain can often make mistakes and overprotect us, which is our first clue as to how sensitivity conditions can start.

Let's now explore how the brain may become hypersensitive and learn to overprotect at the start of a medical condition. There are three unique factors that might trigger a sensitivity condition:

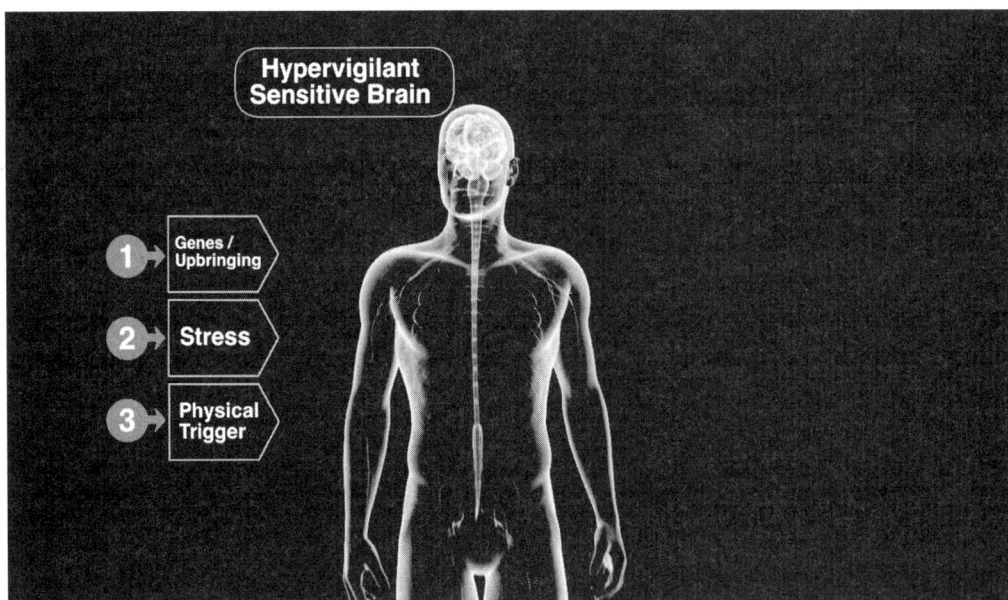

First, we may have inherited some genes from our parents that might be a risk factor. Other risk factors for sensitization may include our childhood experiences, some of which may have been traumatic or frightening. This can affect how we respond to illness and to stress, as we are conditioned to become overly vigilant by our lifelong experiences and genetic predisposition.

Secondly, at the beginning of a medical condition, most people report experiencing acute stress in the buildup to that illness, which can then become chronic stress. Prior to the onset of their illness, many people were working very long hours, or perhaps there was a bereavement or some other source of stress. When we are stressed, our immune system does not function at its full potential, making it more likely that our bodies may not handle what we are being exposed to in an optimal fashion.

Thirdly, in the buildup to the condition, most patients experience a physical trigger, which can be some kind of exposure to a chemical, toxin or mold, or an infection. With IBS and food sensitivities, that trigger tends to be food poisoning or eating a food that creates a sudden sensitivity reaction. In electrical hypersensitivity syndrome (EHS), there may have been exposure to intense electromagnetic fields.

At step 4, the combination of these three factors then may lead to a "rewiring event" in the brain, which is likely to be in two brain structures called the amygdala and the insula, in combination with the hippocampus. The amygdala is the center of our defensive nervous system mechanisms, including emotional reactions, and it sits within the limbic-system part of the brain. The insula has been shown to be where our previous immune system reactions can be stored, ready to deal with future exposures.

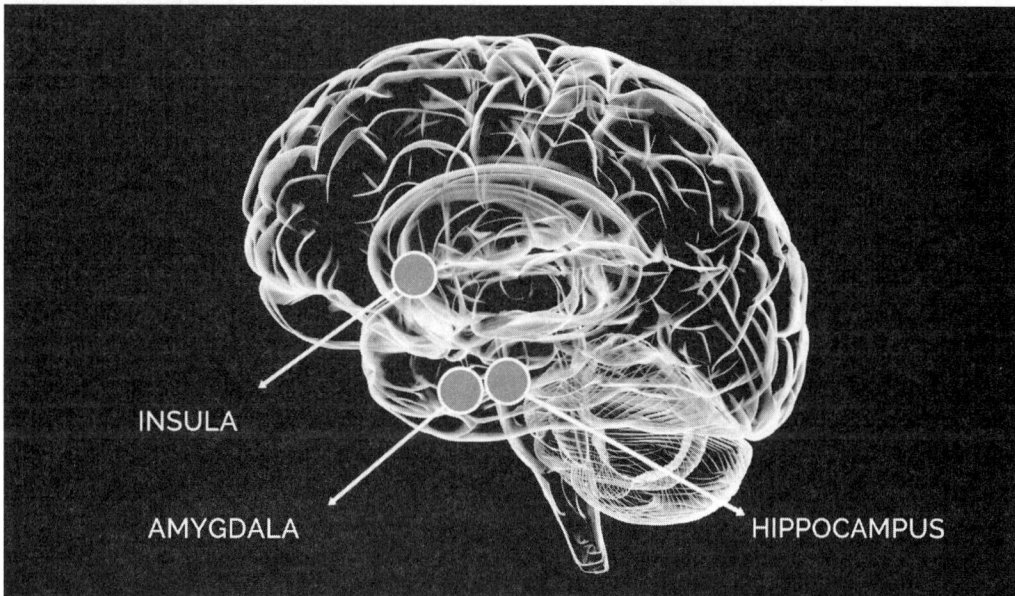

INSULA

AMYGDALA

HIPPOCAMPUS

When I say, "rewiring event," I don't necessarily mean physical damage to these parts of the brain. I simply mean that, neurologically, these brain structures learn to become hyper-defensive—they easily trigger many aspects of the immune system, including mast cell activation, and those systems have become somewhat traumatized as a result of the three factors we spoke about. They retrigger these responses to err on the side of caution, just to ensure survival.

From an evolutionary perspective, it makes sense for our brain to make sure we survive by overprotecting if necessary. This is called "neurological learning" or conditioning—basically our brain has learned to over-defend.

Why does the brain get rewired so easily as a response to a trigger in some people but not in others? Remember, we said that the brain's number one responsibility is to ensure survival. If someone is feeling really stressed and weak, then their immune system will be less effective, so the brain thinks *"Oh, no, we're not going to be able to fight off this mold or infection or chemical or food! This is dangerous. Let's over-trigger our defense responses to make sure we survive!"*

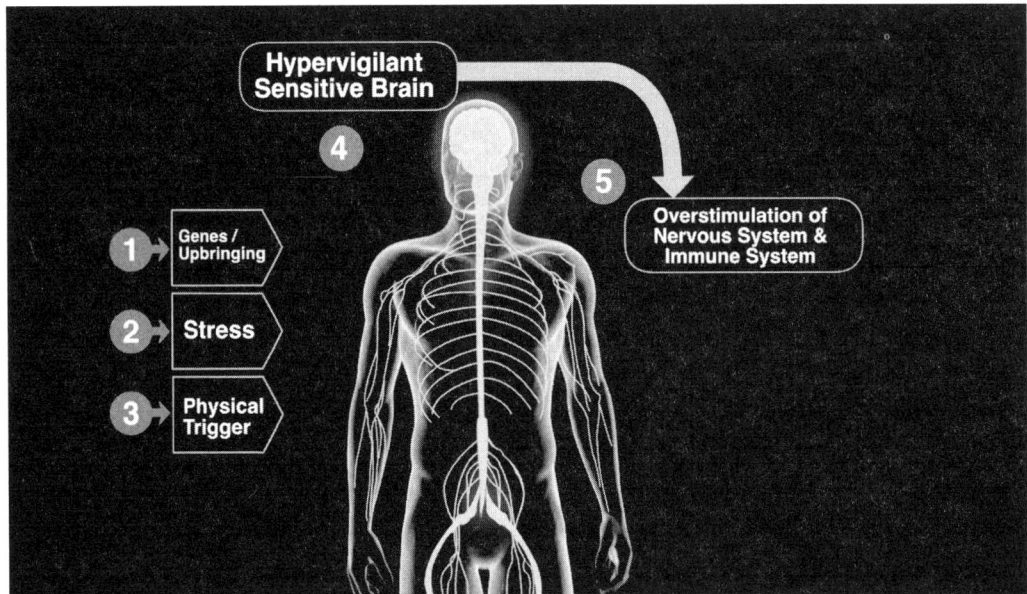

What do you think causes these symptoms? It might not be just the trigger itself! While the trigger may still be present (or it may be long gone) and need to be addressed, usually the first order of treatment is to decrease this overprotective process so the body can accept other treatments it needs. In most cases, a patient's symptoms are caused by the immune system and aspects of the nervous system being triggered, and not solely by the trigger itself. When we over-trigger these systems continually, it makes us have lots of symptoms and uses up our energy and our resources really quickly.

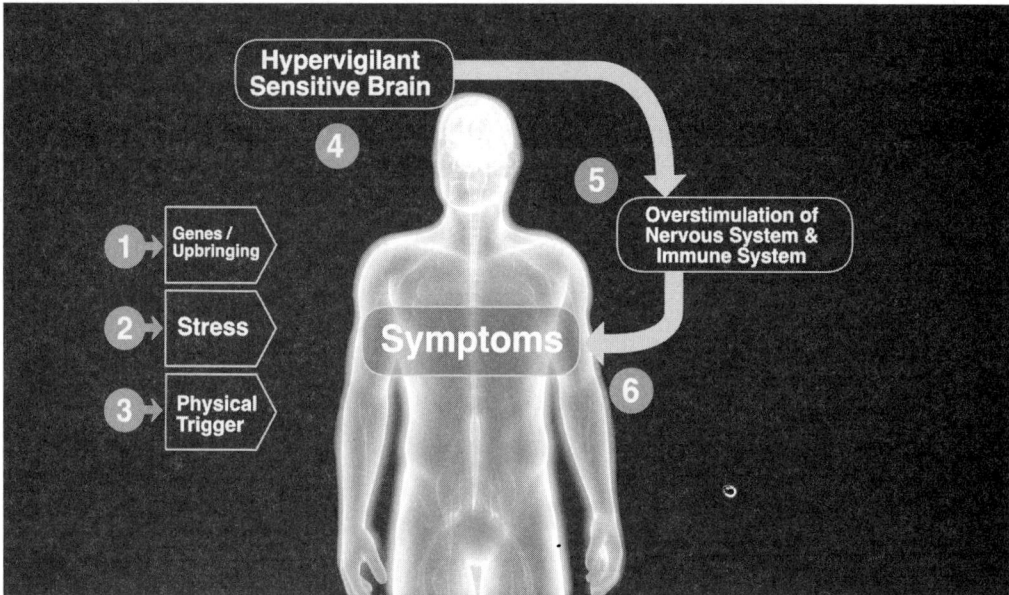

From an evolutionary perspective, this is exactly the right thing to do! The issue arises when this hypervigilant response becomes chronic. When it does, the brain gets stuck in that mode and has to be retrained to get back to balance.

Re-reaction to Triggers

In this diagram we can see the words "External Stress."

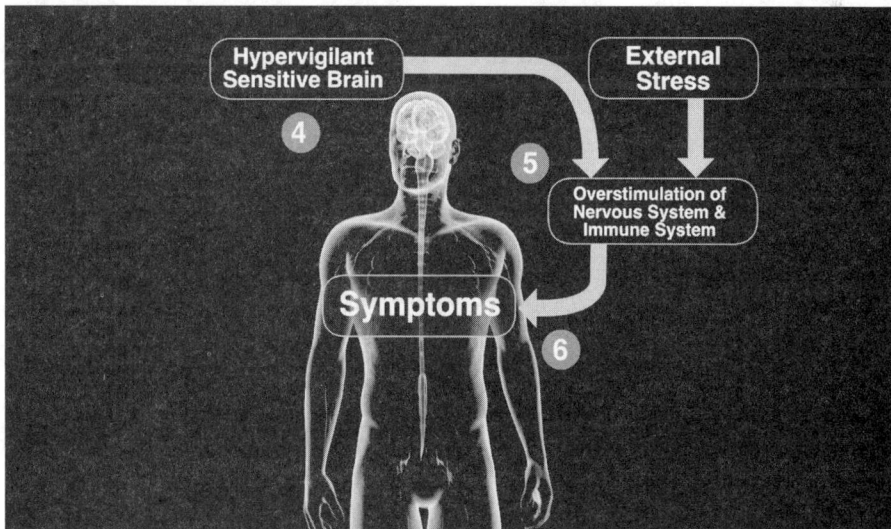

The external stress here can be re-exposure to that initial trigger. Let's say someone was exposed to a high level of mold at the beginning of their condition. Let's call this 100% exposure, which causes a strong sensitivity response measured at 100%. Because the brain has learned to be hypersensitive to this trigger, and errs on the side of caution, just 5% of the original exposure has the ability to cause a 100% sensitivity response in the future. In brain neurology, this is called "differential activation."

This is how one intense exposure has the ability to make the brain hypersensitive to an otherwise neutral trigger. From that moment onwards, a person may have an ongoing strong sensitivity reaction to very small exposures that other people have no response to. Animal studies support the idea that the conditioning of the immune system occurs in the insula part of the brain, and the conditioning of the nervous system occurs in the amygdala.

The Symptoms

At step 5, we can see what systems have been overstimulated. Our fight-or-flight response is hyperstimulated, which is regulated by the sympathetic nervous system. Aspects of the nervous system are over-triggered, and this sympathetic overarousal means that in our body we have an excess or a deficiency of stress hormones such as cortisol and adrenaline.

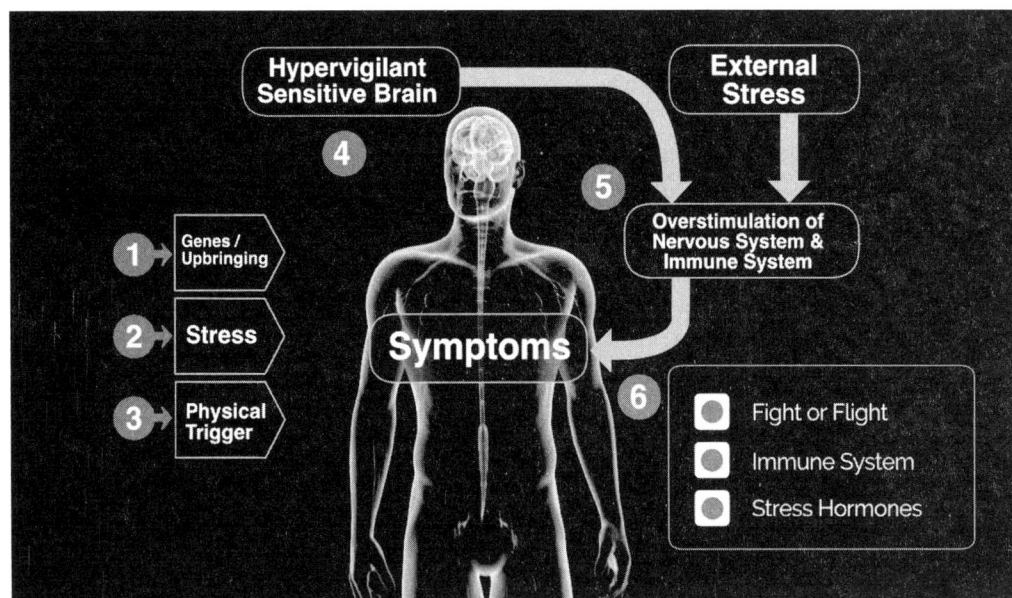

If we have an excess of stress chemicals in the body, the front of the brain can actually shrink, especially the areas around the prefrontal cortex. We also get reduced blood flow to the brain. The prefrontal cortex acts as our rational thinking mind, so we might get brain fog, difficulty thinking, or difficulty remembering things.

The area of the brain called the hippocampus also shrinks. The hippocampus is responsible for memories and can also act as a brake on the fight-or-flight system, but shrunken, the hippocampus cannot fulfill those two roles, causing more stress. Also, we may find it difficult to recall information or events, and thinking in general can become a bit fuzzier, which we refer to as "brain fog."

When these systems become over-triggered, the system eventually becomes so exhausted and depleted that the body can no longer respond effectively to stress or to diverse situations. We may actually have very low levels of stress hormones like cortisol and adrenaline when we are trying to do a task or exercise, because our system has no resources left. We are running on empty.

This hyperstimulation leads to symptoms at step 6, and potentially, secondary conditions at 7 as a result of the ongoing overstimulation of the nervous system and the immune system.

This leads to a vicious cycle of reactivity:

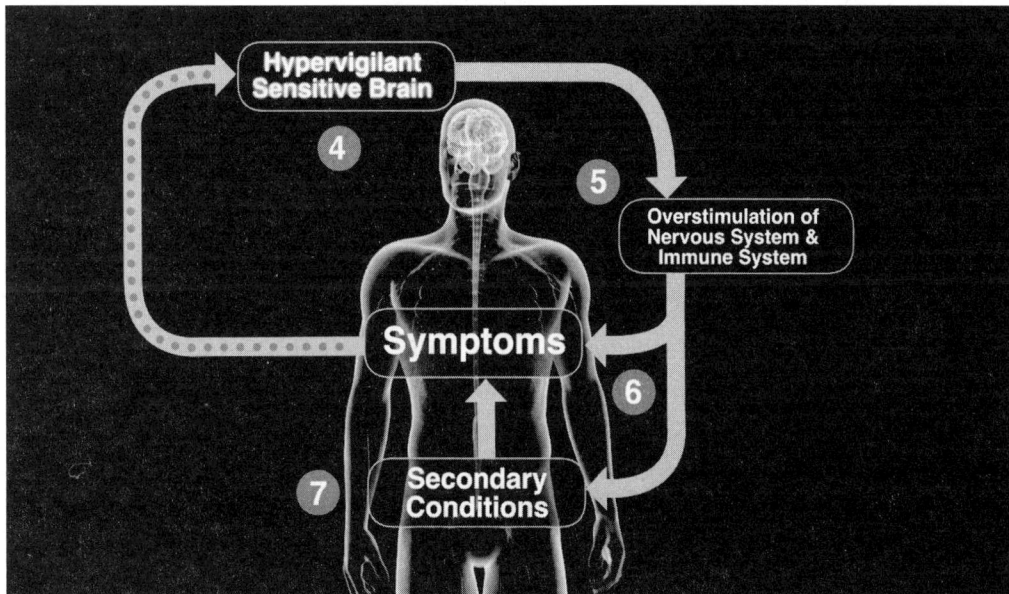

The brain may also learn to become hypersensitive to the symptoms of a sensitivity reaction itself, because when there are symptoms in the body, it indicates to us that we are in imminent danger, unless we tell the brain something different. So, at step 8, those very same symptoms that are being caused by overstimulation loop back to the brain and tell the brain that we are still in danger, thus triggering new defensive responses. The signals from the body become magnified, and are easily detected by what is now a very sensitive brain.

In MCS, mold toxicity, and electrical sensitivities, the signals of immune reaction indicate either that a chemical or stimulus may still be present or we are about to have a strong reaction, and this becomes a snowball of triggers and reactions. In IBS and food sensitivities, those gut reactions indicate that that food is still dangerous or that our gut is about to react.

In this explanation of sensitivity reactions, it is very important to emphasize that it is *not* "all in the mind!" These reactions are not the patient's fault, are not imagined, but are real physical reactions.

In conclusion, sensitivity illnesses are caused by an initial single or multiple exposures to a trigger, which then causes a shift in the wiring in the brain. The brain learns to react to even small traces of the original trigger, leading to ongoing illness.

But Isn't My Condition Caused by the Trigger?

The main question we are asked at our clinic is, "Is it not the trigger that is causing my illness? Do I not need to remove myself from the triggers?" Many well-meaning support groups insist that a person can never recover until all triggers have been removed, but for many patients, until they retrain their brain to realize that the stimuli they are experiencing are far safer than they thought, removing the triggers will be too difficult unless retraining comes first.

We certainly don't advocate ignoring the triggers at the start of retraining. A person can minimize exposures at the beginning of retraining to give themselves space to learn the tools. Of course, it can be impossible to completely remove triggers from our environment, so we can do what is practically possible without disrupting life too much.

Then we can realize that although what we are sensitive to may trigger a reaction, the strength of that reaction is due to the conditioning in our brain, because due to its hypersensitivity, the brain is now reacting to low levels of that trigger in our environment, and is being hypersensitive as part of an over-the-top evolutionary protection mechanism that the situation does not warrant.

Brain Retraining and Neuroplasticity for Recovery

Brain retraining involves repeatedly training the brain to no longer be sensitive to the triggers, and to get out of symptom-perpetuating brain loops. These tools support the brain and body to gradually relax and feel safe in the presence of triggers. For example, one tool uses visualization to envision the future desired state; that is, feeling strong and healthy in the presence of something the sensitive patient previously reacted to.

The sensitive patient can focus the retraining tools on whatever they are most reacting to. For example, they could focus on mold, a specific chemical, particular foods, or electromagnetic fields. Step by step, they can reduce their sensitivity to each environmental factor they are reactive to.

We notice that many of these patients have an underlying feeling of lack of safety in the world, and many carry a previous trauma around this, often dating back to before the initial exposure or trigger occurred. So, restoring a sense of safety in one's body and safety in the world is key. To support this, some patients may require a combined approach of the Gupta Program and some one-to-one support with an experienced coach or therapist on some of the deeper layers. These might include any previous traumas such as the traumas of initially getting sick, not knowing what their options for treatment are, and feeling unsupported by the medical profession or by family and friends.

Another layer the program invites patients to work on is those parts of the personality that can perpetuate stress in the patient's belief system, and were likely a contributing element to the creation of the illness in the first place.

The parts of the personality that we find often need to be addressed to maintain health after recovery are: the Over-achiever part that wants to achieve so much and has such high expectations that as soon as symptoms resolve a bit, the patient gets too busy and active too quickly; the Over-helper part that feels a compulsion to focus on others' needs over one's own; the Approval Seeker part who constantly wants the approval of others to feel okay about oneself; the Victim part who feels that it's all not fair and wants to give up; the Safety Seeker part, which is particularly relevant to many with environmental sensitivities and don't feel safe in the world at a core level; the Inner Critic part who is actually trying to protect you through internally criticizing and judging you, and the Perfectionist part who wants to be perfect and do everything perfectly, which is unrealistic for all of us.

All of these parts of a patient's personality make sense based on the patient's experience as a sensitive child. As a result of their illness, these parts often need addressing to support a full and lasting health recovery. In our program we use fun puppets to represent these parts.

There is also an invitation in our program to find what sparks joy, and to fill as much time as possible reengaging with activities that bring lightness, a happy mood, and joy. This supports neuroplasticity and makes the brain more flexible, as do relaxation techniques. When in an uplifted state of mind, fear-based thoughts and other stress-inducing patterns naturally fall away.

All of this supports the brain to be retrained over time, so the person can ultimately feel calm and healthy in the presence of what was previously a trigger for their system, and neutralize the loop in the brain that is causing symptoms. A patient gradually retrains the brain to feel safe, that there is nothing to fear, and that it doesn't need to work so hard trying to protect itself anymore—for the patient to feel and embody "I am safe" and "the world is safe."

As I write this, I hear in myself the voices that say, "But chemicals are dangerous, mold is dangerous!" Yes, but the reality is that most people manage to stay healthy even in the presence of chemicals and mold. Of course, prolonged exposure to a toxin, or an undiagnosed or untreated infection, can mean that even the strongest individual can succumb to illness, but most of the time, a person may have had that type of experience once, and from then on their immune system continues to react to very small exposures to err on the side of caution. Understanding and embracing this difference is crucial to recovery from sensitivity illnesses.

We have helped many patients to fully recover their health and even learn how to stop a reaction in its tracks. It is incredibly empowering to know that even in the presence of a triggers, they can train their brains to feel safe and calm despite the trigger.

Below are some patients' experiences that we feel help describe the journey to wellness.

In my mid-twenties, I began noticing physical reactions to food additives—mild at first, but over the years, the reactivity became more and more extreme, uncomfortable, and life limiting, and it expanded to include some fragrances as well. Unfortunately, around age fifty, I was chemically poisoned at work, causing the sensitivities to expand to include mold, all chemicals, synthetic fragrances, some natural fragrances, many more food intolerances, IBS, and other symptoms and conditions. I was no longer able to work, have people in my home, eat out, or go into any building without having a reaction. My life became very small.

Over the course of several years, I sought help from several doctors, none of whom were able to help with the sensitivities. Fortunately, my primary doctor had recently learned of the brain retraining program from one of her patients who also had not recovered with the doctors' protocols and treatments. She pointed me to the Gupta Brain Retraining Program, and within just a few hours of retraining, I noticed a huge shift in reactivity to fragrances. Within a few weeks I was able to go into public buildings, shop, eat at restaurants, and even socialize with groups of people. I was so encouraged and hopeful that I continued with enthusiasm and conviction, knowing that the program really works! I have not only reached full health but am so grateful and inspired by the program that I trained to become a certified Junior Gupta Program Coach! It is my passion and purpose to help others in their own recovery journey!

—S. H., USA

Many MCS patients are concerned with letting go of their knowledge that chemicals are "bad" for us when they retrain their emotional response to their hypersensitive reaction to chemicals. When I was personally struggling with these issues, I used to remind myself that I was knowledgeable enough to know that the average amount of chemicals out in the world is generally not harmful. Yes, large amounts of chemical from autos in the shop being lacquered or airplanes spraying pesticides are not reasonable levels of chemicals to choose to be around; however, the average floor cleaner, air freshener in the bathroom, perfume on the person nearby—all are reasonable levels of chemicals to be around. I had to intellectually override my MCS reactions using the techniques but also to satisfy my former learned behavior that *all* chemicals needed to be avoided and I was not betraying my body to abandon my old beliefs as well as to retrain out of my body's reactions.

I retrained around sensitivities to electromagnetic things. I reminded myself, from my training as a Reiki practitioner, that electrical fields move through our bodies in order to ground out into the earth. The reason I was feeling so ill around electrics was due *not* to any inherent danger from computers or electric trains but from my body's own electrical field, which was in a state of disarray from my electrical brain connections being hyperactive and stuck in excess mode. I reminded myself that retraining would bring order to my body's electrics, which would allow for external electrical frequencies to move smoothly through my body and ground out efficiently, and to remember that an unpeaceful brain would cause extremes in emotions, and hypersensitive emotions can represent stuck energy.

I also encouraged myself to *not* make significant changes to my world while retraining. So, I think it is important for an MCS patient to maintain a simplistic environment from which explorations into the outside world can be accomplished; and in the beginning, confidence in the retraining x is easier if you know that you have your clean space to go home to. As the retraining takes hold and wellness comes, more and more outer experiences bring confidence that the clean space can now be modified to include electronics, things with odors, etc. I believe the confidence while retraining grows gradually, and I believe that for the MCS patient, trust in that growth is best accompanied by a steady relinquishment of the clean bubble space. I believe the immediate introduction of the "normal" world is too jarring for the recovery/retraining process. You are cautioned not to change much in the beginning of the retraining process. I think this is very wise, especially for the MCS patient.

I also think that, unlike the ME and CFIDS patient who looks at their body for signs of distress from activity, the MCS patient looks at the world as a potential source for bodily reactions to cause severe harm. I constantly used the Soften and Flow to loosen up my body out in the world, and used my knowledge that my liver enzymes have almost always shown to be normal, so I chose to trust that my detox capabilities were indeed not compromised, despite how my body felt, and that my reactions were due to my brain. I had to rethink how I had learned to perceive the outside world as the danger, and to trust that my body was manifesting faulty wiring, and that was the true source of my reactions.

The key to the MCS patient doing well with retraining is to learn, retrain, and do the Accelerator technique around one's learned perceptions, which have been reinforced by one's bodily symptoms, that the world is indeed a safe place to thrive. The trending mindset supported by the media can at times echo that chemicals are not safe and electronics cause brain tumors, etc. This seems to be the factor that works against the MCS patient in retraining, since so many voices support the perception that the abovementioned stimuli are truly "bad" for your health. The MCS patient has to overcome what the media enforces—that the chemical world is dangerous and unsafe. The platform from which the MCS patient can create wellness in is to rely on their own discernment that extremes of almost anything are not necessarily good. In moderation, however, most things in the world are truly safe and our bodies can handle them, So, the MCS patient finds wellness in trusting their knowledge that staying out of extremes and dwelling in moderation is a trustworthy concept from which to incorporate successful brain retraining.

As I was recovering, I had occasion to have my new understanding reinforced. I was setting up an air conditioner, and the old patterns in my brain were telling me I might have a problem with the plastic off-gassing from the warmed wires in the unit's motor. As I ran the air conditioner, I began to smell something; I "knew" it was the warm plastic and that I would eventually not be able to use the unit. I went into my kitchen to retrieve a phone directory to call the local hardware store for tools with which I would take the thing apart and try to make adjustments to it when I noticed that there was a glass saucepan on the stove that I'd forgotten about and all the water had boiled off. The hot electric burner was creating an overheated smell from the glass pot—not a bit of plastic involved—but my body went into the very same reaction that

I used to experience when I was severely sensitive to any plastic! It was so powerful for me to witness my body having a clear, recognizable reaction to plastic when in fact it was a generic "smell." My focus on the new air conditioner had convinced by body to have a full-blown plastic reaction, and when I realized my perceptual error, my reaction immediately resolved!

What a powerful story I now tell about my focus, my perception, and my body's compliance with what I feared was true, despite its all not being reality!

—BF, Connecticut, USA

In Summary

Whatever sensitivity reaction you are experiencing, we want to give you the certainty that recovery is possible. That there is nothing "wrong" with you. You are simply experiencing an evolutionary mechanism that is overprotecting you and simply needs to be reset. Thousands before you have taken this path to recovery, and so can you!

If you think neuroplasticity and brain retraining could support your healing from a sensitivity illness, you can take a free 28-day trial of the Gupta Program online. You can watch videos about what may be causing your condition, and learn from others' experiences.

You can sign up for the 28-day free trial at www.GuptaProgram.com, or, if you have questions, you can email info@guptaprogram.com.

The Gupta Program contains fifteen interactive video sessions, over thirty audio exercises, a loving support group, and weekly webinars with Ashok.

You can also download the free app by searching "Gupta Program" on the App Store or Play Store.

About the Authors

Ashok Gupta, MA (Cantab), MSc, is the founder and CEO of the Gupta Program. He suffered from ME/CFS when he was studying at university, and through neurological research managed to get himself 100% better and set up a global neuroplasticity clinic to support others with chronic illnesses.

Ashok is trained in many healing modalities, including clinical hypnotherapy, meditation, NLP, breathing techniques, and many others. He published the online Gupta Program to support patients worldwide. He lives in London and continues to deliver weekly webinars for patients.

Ashok's program has benefitted thousands of people with sensitivity illnesses and other chronic illnesses. In addition to clinical work, he has also published and contributed to several medical papers, including randomized controlled trials showing very promising results. He and his team continually initiate further trials to prove the efficacy of this new approach.

FRANCES GOODALL is an official Gupta Program Coach. Frances had ME/CFS herself for five years, and has enjoyed many years of full recovery. She has developed a full-health coaching practice that supports others to recovery, and has undergone Gupta Program Training and intensive training in many coaching and therapeutic modalities.

Papers by Ashok Gupta

"Unconscious amygdalar fear conditioning in a subset of chronic fatigue syndrome patients", Ashok Gupta, Medical Hypotheses, (2002), 59 (6):727-735

"Can amygdala retraining techniques improve the wellbeing of patients with chronic fatigue syndrome?", Ashok Gupta, Journal of holistic health care, Volume 7 Issue 2 September 2010

"Mindfulness-Based Program Plus Amygdala and Insula Retraining (MAIR) for the Treatment of Women with Fibromyalgia: A Pilot Randomized Controlled Trial", Sanabria-Mazo, JP, Monterro-Marin, J, Feliu-Soler, A, et al., Journal of Clinical Medicine, 2020, 9, 3246, doi:10.3390/jcm9103246

Chapter 3: Polyvagal Theory and Sensitivity

Stephen W. Porges, PhD,
and Neil Nathan, MD

When we raise the subject of the vagus nerve, please don't be intimated by what might look like complex medical science. We've done everything we can to make this information as clear and useful as possible. Let's review why it's so important to understand this subject.

One major function of the vagus nerve and its intimate connection to the autonomic nervous system (ANS) is to serve as an element in our perception of our *safety*. How do you know at any given moment that you're actually safe? Whether you're aware of it or not, your nervous system is examining the stimuli it receives and analyzing them for safety. This includes *sound* (What a loud noise!), *light* (It's so bright out here I think I need sunglasses), *touch* (Ouch!), *smell* (What's that perfume she's wearing?), and *taste* (Yum!). This extends into our connections with people and animals: Is it safe for me to spend time with this person? Does this situation feel similar to one that caused me harm in the past?

In previous chapters, we learned the importance of the limbic system in analyzing these stimuli and monitoring them for safety. The limbic system works closely with the vagus nerve (the tenth, or X, cranial nerve) and the other cranial nerves that are connected to it. This wasn't widely realized until 1994, when Dr. Stephen Porges began to write a series of papers that revolutionized our grasp of the process. He called it *polyvagal theory* and taught us how critical it was to our understanding of trauma and safety.

A key component of polyvagal theory was that our earlier learning about the vagus nerve (what I learned in medical school) was that it was a single nerve with a single physiology. The vagus is the longest cranial nerve in the body and regulates an array of vital functions (see illustrations 1 and 2).

It's primarily a sensory nerve, meaning that it receives input about what's happening from a lot of important organs: the heart, lungs, esophagus, stomach, small intestine, most of the large intestine, the ear, throat, spleen, thymus, and the lymphatic tissue around the intestines called the GALT (gut associated lymphoid tissue). To a lesser extent, the vagus sends information *to* those tissues that helps them function properly.

Dr. Porges discovered that the vagus nerve was actually composed of not just one branch but two separate branches with somewhat different functions. The branch that originates in the dorsal portion of the brainstem is the one we studied in medical school. There was, however, a second branch, originating in the ventral portion of the brainstem, that coordinates different neurological activities; hence the term "polyvagal."

Without going deeply into the anatomy, when faced with any kind of threatening situation, we have just three choices. We can flee the threat or attack it directly. To do so, we mobilize what's called the sympathetic nervous system, often described as the "fight or flight" system, which uses the dorsal branch of the vagus nerve. Or, we can freeze in place, "play dead," and hope the threat just goes away. That method uses the ventral branch of the vagus nerve. These strategies for dealing with threat have been hardwired into our nervous systems for millennia, and shared with most of our vertebrate ancestors that evolved hundreds of million years before humans and other social mammals.

Dr. Porges not only recognized these neurological connections but also realized that these threat responses also incorporated our ability to perceive safety by paying attention to the facial and vocal features of whatever was before us, as would any animal in the wild that came in contact with another animal.

How does an animal recognize safety in this situation? By noticing the *muscles of the face* and the acoustic features of vocalizations (e.g., a dog growling or a lion roaring), which reflect accurately how the other animal is responding to its presence. There's a direct connection between the vagus and the muscles involved in facial expression and vocalization. Those muscles are regulated by neural pathways that travel through several cranial nerves, including cranial nerves V (the trigeminal), VII (the facial), IX (the glossopharyngeal), and X (the ventral branch of the vagus nerve). Within the brainstem area in which these cranial nerves originate, there is constant interneuronal communication, which enables coordination among the muscles regulated by these cranial nerves and the ventral vagus. "Ventral vagal complex" is a shorthand label for this area. This coordinated system enables humans to broadcast their autonomic state via facial expressions and voice. When another person approaches us, whether we're aware of it or not, we pay attention to the other's facial expression and detect acoustic features from their voice.

If friendly, their facial expression and vocal intonation reflexively trigger in us a feeling of comfort. If not, we're more wary. There's a phrase I've read in many novels: "His smile never reached his eyes." In that situation we see the person's lips curl upward, but the facial muscles correctly tell us, "Be careful."

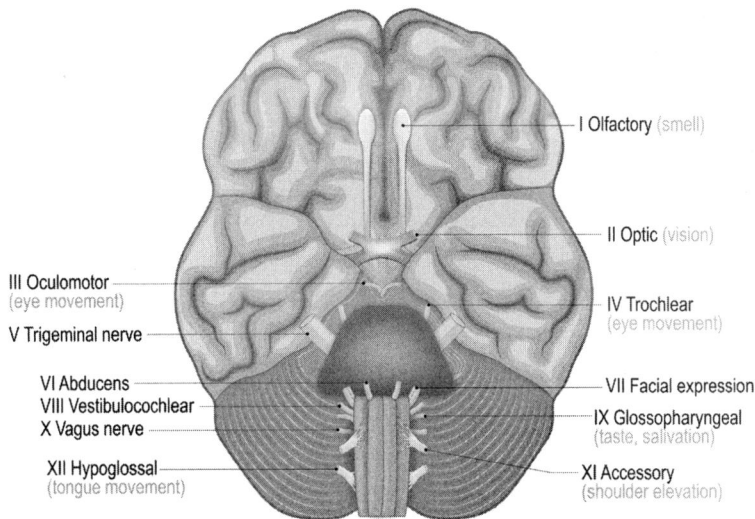

Cranial nerves

In light of that information, you can see how COVID has profoundly affected our feelings of isolation, in that the facemasks we all wore decreased our ability to make these decisions. If the individual wearing a mask also wore sunglasses, we'd be unable to read them at all. The pandemic markedly influenced our connections to family and friends, as did the profound fear the media disseminated.

The essence of human society is, as with most mammals, interconnectedness. In our complex world, where would I be without the efforts of countless people who've contributed to my well-being? This interconnectedness is a precious gift that often goes largely unrecognized, but COVID has actually brought it into our everyday awareness.

The heart of this discussion is our view of how safe we feel. As Dr. Porges points out, this perception of safety has been in the process of evolving from all life experiences we bring to the table. It's a rare person who's had an ideal childhood. To varying degrees, our needs were met or not met depending on our home life, our parenting, and our experiences, some of which may have been traumatic. For example, children who had various kinds of recurrent infections and had to take round after round of antibiotics, or those who needed surgical procedures, or those with asthma or other conditions that required hospitalization, or who experienced abuse of any kind—emotional, or sexual— would have had to constantly assess how safe they were in these situations. As they grew older, each subsequent traumatic event gradually made their limbic systems and vagal systems more and more hypervigilant. Keep in mind that the vagal system and limbic systems are essentially protective. They're not trying to hurt us, but trying to alert us to possible dangers by getting our attention. With each episode of threat, both systems react more and more strongly and grow more and more vigilant—to the point of becoming overreactive. This sets the table for what can happen later in life, when we're exposed to a toxin or an infection and our health is threatened in a different way.

The triggering event may be a leaky water heater that exposes you to mold, or a tick bite, or the newly installed smart meter in your home that creates a large increase in EMF exposure. By themselves, these experiences might not seem like much; they might not have affected you if you hadn't had a lifetime's preparation of a limbic/vagal system that was set on edge by prior events. Now, though, these events can have powerful, even catastrophic, effects on your nervous system such that you don't feel safe at all. Your nervous system has taken on the responsibility of analyzing every stimulus you're exposed to, both internal (all that you feel coming from inside your body) and external (the lights, sounds, touches, smells, and tastes you're constantly exposed to). Your nervous system is no longer certain about how safe those stimuli are, and it warns you with attention-getting symptoms so you'll avoid them.

The longer this process goes on, the more vigilant your nervous system becomes, and for some this becomes extreme to the point that debilitating sensitization occurs. In this state, the constant inflammation triggered by mold toxicity or Lyme disease and other inflammatory conditions becomes intolerable.

As described by Dr. Robert Naviaux in his Cell Danger Response model, on the cellular level (extending to the whole organism), we can't heal until we feel safe, so the first order of business is to restore our perception of safety, or at least improve it. Many patients are unable to tolerate or respond to treatment of the inflammation until they first do that. Only when some semblance of safety has been restored can they respond to appropriate treatments and get well.

As Dr. Porges expanded his ideas, he recognized that nearly all kinds of trauma impact the vagal system. This includes posttraumatic stress disorder (PTSD) and every type of injury, so that in any patient who has been injured in any way, vagal dysfunction should be considered essential in the treatment. Any significant stressor (and some relatively minor ones) can create vagal-system dysfunction, and for any chronic illness, we must consider treating this system for healing to occur. This is particularly true of sensitive patients, in whom vagal dysfunction is the rule rather than the exception.

Here we have a key interaction between the dorsal and ventral branches of the vagus and the sympathetic nervous systems. In this context, the dorsal branch is the more primitive, and the ventral branch has evolved to regulate these other components of the autonomic nervous system. Hence we should emphasize the profound role that the ventral vagus has in "containing" and repurposing the reactions of the sympathetic and dorsal vagus to support *mobilization without fear* and *immobilization without fear*. This means that activities that stimulate the ventral vagus, such as play, or dance, or moments of intimacy and connecting with others, improve our ability to deal with stresses that might otherwise cause us to freeze or flee. The opposite is also important: Suppression of the ventral vagus by fear or danger optimizes access to the fight-or-flight sympathetic nervous system and inflammation. I emphasize that the vagal anti-inflammatory reflex is compromised when the autonomic nervous system is responding to stress and threat. When locked in a state of chronic defense, which characterizes many of our patients, the autonomic nervous system is functionally supporting inflammation. From a medical perspective, we can see the comorbidity of inflammation with atypical and frequent disruptions in the regulation of the visceral organs contributing to all the adverse effects we write about in this book.

As Dr. Porges has shared with me: "I believe that the sensitive patient is 'locked' into a chronic state of defense with a predictable autonomic profile that fosters constant detection of danger on every level of their experience including physiological, psychological, and behavioral, while compromising the homeostatic functions of health, growth, restoration, and even sociability."

With this grasp of the importance of polyvagal theory, let's go deeper so we can understand how to approach treatment. So far, I've simplified this discussion, but like most everything, the more you study it the more complicated it gets.

We've focused on the vagus nerve so far, but the vagus, like the rest of our nervous system, doesn't function in isolation. It's closely connected to other cranial nerves, so we can more accurately think of it as the "vagal nerve system." The vagus comes out of the brain stem very close to the IX cranial nerve (glossopharyngeal nerve), the XI cranial nerve (spinal accessory nerve) which supplies the important muscles of the shoulder (the trapezius and sternocleidomastoid muscles), and the V and VII cranial nerves (refer to cranial nerves illustration earlier in this chapter). To make this a bit more real, let's review some of the symptoms that dysfunction of these nerves can produce (see cranial nerves illustration).

Symptoms of Vagal Nerve System Dysfunction

Chronic Physical Conditions

- Tense, hard muscles (especially neck and shoulders)
- Migraines
- Clenched or grinding teeth
- Cold hands and feet
- Difficulty swallowing
- Lump in the throat
- Dizziness

Emotional Issues

- Anxiety/Fearfulness
- Depression/Hopelessness
- Cognitive Dysfunction
- Emotional Lability
- Fatigue
- Insomnia/Nightmares

Heart and Lung Symptoms

- Chest Pain
- Asthma
- Shortness of breath
- Arrhythmias
- POTS
- High or low blood pressure
- Labile blood pressure

Gastrointestinal Symptoms

- Constipation
- Diarrhea
- Gastric Reflux (GERD)
- Nausea
- Loss of appetite

There are two ways to get a feel for how affected the vagus nerve might be. If we examine the mouth and throat, we can see, hanging down at the back of throat, an anatomical structure called the uvula. If you ask a healthy patient to say "Ah, ah, ah," the uvula will bob up and down actively. In someone with a compromised vagal system, it will often barely move, or move just a little.

Another simple way is to ask the patient to take a deep breath, put a finger into their mouth, and try to gag. Many will say, "Oh, I can't do that; I might throw up." To honor that, I bring out a wastebasket, just in case. Having done this with thousands of patients, I have yet to see anyone actually throw up. Rather, patients—even those with a strong history of chronic nausea—are surprised that they can't elicit a gag reflex. This is another indication of a compromised vagal system.

In addition to these observations, branches of the vagus nerve go to the spleen, thymus, and gut associated lymphoid tissue (GALT), all of which play an important role in inflammation. Just recently recognized, this is referred to as the *vagal inflammatory reflex,* which is now being taken seriously as a major component of inflammation and provides an exciting way to treat it. Some of the treatments below take advantage of this process.

Treatment of Vagal System Dysfunction

Only recently did we realize the need to reboot the vagal nerve system when it has become dysfunctional. Early recognition of this need was explained in an excellent YouTube video by Datis Kharrazian, DC, called "The Gut-Brain Axis." He describes using gagging, gargling, and singing to help restore vagal function. For many years this was our major intervention, but over time we have found an array of treatments to be more helpful. Here are some that I've found most effective:

1. "Cues of Safety *Are* the Treatment" is the vital first step Dr. Porges emphasizes. It means that the *setting* you bring a patient into is crucial to establishing a sense of safety for them. When they come into your office (or you see them via telemedicine), the tone and timbre of your voice begin this process. Are they soothing or strident? Calm or excitable? The office décor—your paintings, photographs, items in view, the color of the walls, the desk, which may be between you or off to the side, and whether you're typing into a computer with your back turned or facing the patient with nothing in the way, are vital to their perception of how safe you and your office are. This extends to your staff, your waiting room décor, how the patient is treated on arrival and departure. All matter, because they set the table for the patient to decide whether this is a safe place to be.

2. To heal a dysfunctional vagus system, Dr. Porges developed a sound-based method called "Safe and Sound," which has helped countless patients heal. It's available at contact@unyte.com.

3. A good starting point for treatment is to get a copy of Stanley Rosenberg's *Accessing the Healing Power of the Vagus Nerve.* The book contains a series of exercises that take only 5 minutes a day to begin the process of treating vagal dysfunction.

4. Rosenberg was a Danish craniosacral therapist, and designed his exercises to complement that form of treatment. I encourage patients to find an osteopathic cranial practitioner to work with. The best approach I've found is the one developed by the late James Jealous, DO. At his website, https://traditionalosteopathyedu.com, you can find practitioners he has trained. Another excellent resource: contact the Osteopathic Cranial Academy for a list of physicians they've trained in this treatment.

5. Frequency Specific Microcurrent (FSM) is a unique medical device that provides miniscule amounts of electrical current in two different frequencies simultaneously, and has a wide range of clinical benefits. For the sensitive patient, specific programs for the vagus nerve, concussion, and mast cell activation are the first step, followed by programs that help with detoxification for those with mold toxicity, and pain relief for those who suffer pain. Find a list of practitioners at https://frequencyspecific.com

6. Brain Tap is a medical tool that looks like a virtual reality device, by which different frequencies of sound and light can be delivered to the eyes and ears simultaneously. This might not work well for patients with sound and light sensitivity, but for those with other sensitivities, using Brain Tap to quiet the autonomic nervous system and get to sleep can be very helpful. Their programs are short (about 20 minutes) and can be bought for home use.

7. Emotional Freedom Technique (EFT) is a method by which tapping on specific points on the face and shoulders can reboot the vagal nerve.

8. The GammaCore is a medical device developed by Peter Staats, MD, at Johns Hopkins. A handheld instrument designed to be placed directly over the vagus nerve area in the neck, it has proven very effective in treating a broad spectrum of vagal-related conditions.

9. The ApolloNeuro, a band worn on the wrist or ankle, stimulates the vagus nerve. Sensitive patients should start using it for just two to three minutes once a day, then slowly increase as their tolerance allows.

Many of our patients who have experience with meditation and other relaxation techniques are unaware that these approaches, though helpful, are not as specific for optimal benefits in either vagal or limbic treatment, and that some combination of vagal and limbic rebooting is essential for all of our sensitive patients.

Bear in mind that the vast majority of our patients have both limbic and vagal dysfunction, which are intertwined at a deep level. Once they've become hypervigilant, treating only the vagal system or only the limbic system is unlikely to be sufficient: *both* need to be treated concurrently for maximal improvement.

It's nonetheless helpful for patients to add any type of relaxation they are drawn to. This could include tai chi, yoga, deep breathing techniques, or chi gong, among many others.

We hope we've made it clear that vagal dysfunction is a key element in patients who've been unusually sensitized, and that treating it is vital to improve their health.

Resources

Stephen Porges and Deb Dana, *Clinical Applications of the Polyvagal Theory*, 2018
    Stanley Rosenberg, *Accessing the Healing Power of the Vagus Nerve*, 2017
    Robert Naviaux, et al., "Metabolic Features and Regulation of the Healing Cycle—A New Model for Chronic Disease, Pathogenesis and Treatment, *Mitochondrion*, 2018, 1-18, https://doi.org/10.1016/j.mito.2018.08.001

STEPHEN W. PORGES, PhD, is Distinguished University Scientist at Indiana University where he is the founding director of the Traumatic Stress Research Consortium in the Kinsey Institute. He is Professor of Psychiatry at the University of North Carolina, and Professor Emeritus at both the University of Illinois at Chicago and the University of Maryland. He served as president of the Society for Psychophysiological Research and the Federation of Associations in Behavioral & Brain Sciences and is a former recipient of a National Institute of Mental Health Research Scientist Development Award. He has published more than 350 peer reviewed scientific papers across several disciplines including anesthesiology, biomedical engineering, critical care medicine, ergonomics, exercise physiology, gerontology, neurology, neuroscience, obstetrics, pediatrics, psychiatry, psychology, psychometrics, space medicine, and substance abuse. His research has been cited in more than 10,000 peer-reviewed publications. He holds several patents involved in monitoring and regulating autonomic state and originated the Polyvagal Theory, which emphasizes the importance of physiological state in the expression of behavioral, mental, and health problems related to traumatic experiences. He is the creator of a music-based intervention, the Safe and Sound Protocol,™ which is used by more than 2,000 therapists to improve spontaneous social engagement, to reduce hearing sensitivities, and to improve language processing, state regulation, and spontaneous social engagement. He is the author of *The Polyvagal Theory: Neurophysiological Foundations of Emotions, Attachment, Communication, and Self-Regulation, The Pocket Guide to the Polyvagal Theory: The Transformative Power of Feeling Safe,* and *Polyvagal Safety: Attachment, Communication, Self-Regulation,* and is co-editor of *Clinical Applications of the Polyvagal Theory: The Emergence of Polyvagal-Informed Therapies.*

Chapter 4: Mast-Cell Activation and the Sensitive Patient

Beth O'Hara, FN

Dr. Nathan's Introduction

This chapter is intentionally a bit longer than many of the others in our book, simply because this topic, mast-cell activation, is crucial to understanding and treating sensitive patients. Here, Beth gives a beautifully detailed description of exactly what mast-cell activation is, what triggers it, and how to treat it effectively, using her own experiences to emphasize the important points of discussion. Beth has done a particularly fine job of integrating this subject with the other chapters in this book: limbic and vagal dysfunction, structural issues, oxalates and salicylates, to help you to segue into the interconnected complexities we are laying out for you here.

✿ ✿ ✿

To begin, I'll share parts of my own experience of becoming an extremely sensitive patient. My health crises helped me understand what was happening for my clients and I believe made me a better practitioner. Clients have often shared with me that hearing my story helped give them hope that they too could heal. May my story bring you a deeper sense of understanding and compassion for what's happening for you (or for your patients), as well as bring you hope that healing is not only possible but highly probable!

"What am I going to do?" This question kept rolling through my head. I was desperate. I had become progressively more sensitive to a point where living outside the controlled confines of my home became increasingly more challenging.

My eyes burned and I got nauseous and lightheaded anytime I smelled fragrances, paint, VOCs, or any number of other chemicals. Certain food smells could make me instantly nauseous and force me to run to the bathroom. One time I accidentally inhaled some gas fumes. My legs stopped working, and I had seizure-like spasms for two hours.

EMF sensitivities kept me from going to concerts or plays or wherever there were a lot of cell-phones. My joint inflammation was out of control, and I could barely hobble around if I used a cane. I had constant burning joint, muscle, and nerve pain. My GI tract was a mess, and no matter what I ate I had bloating, abdominal pain, and reflux. My hands and fingers became hot, red, and swollen within minutes of eating, even with low-histamine foods.

I couldn't sleep. This wasn't your average insomnia, though. I hadn't had deep sleep for four years, and I had to rely on Benadryl just to be able to get drowsy and nod off a little. I was severely fatigued at the same time. It was a living nightmare to be so tired for years yet unable to rest.

The anxiety made me feel like I was coming out of my skin, and no amount of meditation or gentle yoga could settle it down. I had panic attacks trying to drive to the grocery. Several times I got to the parking lot and had to turn around and come straight home again.

My brain often felt like I had fireworks going off inside my head, with intense pain and neurological "flashes" of activity I couldn't control. I developed significant light and sound sensitivity—I had to wear sunglasses inside the house with the lights dimmed. I couldn't listen to music, TV, or movies because it was painful to try to process those stimuli. Even the sound of my husband's breathing or chewing was immensely painful.

The least of my worries were the head-to-toe itching 24/7 and intense flushing, rashes, hives, and eczema. The debilitating three days a month that menstrual cramps left me flattened seemed mild compared to some of my other symptoms, as did the urinary burning and urgency, breathing challenges, constant postnasal drip, and the ringing in my ears.

The most worrisome part, though, was every time I tried to add just a little sprinkle of quercetin or curcumin, anything that might quiet that inflammation, my symptoms cranked up several notches. Numerous practitioners had told me I was the most sensitive person they'd ever seen. Others said no one could be this sensitive, that I must be making it up.

What none of us understood at the time was that my mast cells were completely out of control. Fortunately, it was this knowledge that finally allowed me to start to unlock my health mysteries by learning what triggered my mast cells and drove all these symptoms and sensitivities. Understanding Mast Cell Activation Syndrome allowed me to find my way out of the complicated maze of being highly sensitive and get back to living a full and joyous life.

If you've dealt with numerous sensitivities, and/or have inflammatory symptoms in multiple systems of your body, knowing about mast cells may be a game changer for you as well.

In fact, if you're dealing with any kind of inflammatory chronic illness, you'll want to at least consider the possibility of Mast Cell Activation Syndrome, which is incredibly common and is on the rise. Population studies have shown that between 9% and 17% of the general population have it—that's about 1 in every 10 people, up to possibly more than 1 in every 6. We still need research to validate this observation, but my colleagues and I have noted that up to 80% of those with chronic illness are likely dealing with some level of mast cell dysregulation. This makes Mast Cell Activation Syndrome one of the most common, yet underrecognized, conditions that affect people.

To understand what's happening in Mast Cell Activation Syndrome (MCAS), we need to learn about mast cells.

What are Mast Cells?

Your mast cells are types of white blood cells, and function as some of the major front-line defending and sensing cells of your immune system. You can think of them as involved in protecting and healing your body. They're kind of like the guards at the castle gate and some of your immune first responders all rolled into one.

They are made in your bone marrow and then migrate to nearly every tissue in your body, with the exception of your retinas. Here are some of the places your mast cells are found:

- Mucosal and epithelial tissues such as the lining of the nose and sinuses, eyes, mouth, lining of the digestive tract, lining of the bladder and urethra, and lining of the lungs
- Vascularized tissues (anywhere with blood vessels)
- Connective tissues such as ligaments and tendons of the joints, bones, bone marrow, lining of your blood vessels, lymph vessels, hair follicles, and skin
- Your entire GI tract (mouth, esophagus, stomach, intestines)
- Along your blood vessels
- In and around your muscles, tendons, ligaments
- Your brain, including your limbic system
- Lining every nerve sheath and nerve ending

Your mast cells have more than 200 types of receptors that are found all along the outside of the cell membrane, and they contain hundreds of chemical mediators in tiny granules that they can release, depending on what's occurring in or around your body. In fact, mast cells have over 1,000 mediators! These are stored in granules, which are basically little pouches within the mast cells. Release of these mediators is called degranulation. Mast cells can release these mediators selectively (selective or piecemeal degranulation) or all at once (total degranulation).

The mast cell receptors sense and respond to everything that's happening both inside and outside your body. Then, depending on what triggers the receptors, they can release their mediators. This gives the mast cells an enormous range of responsiveness and communication abilities within your body.

Your mast cells sense every molecule of air you breathe, everything you put in your mouth, and everything you swallow. They respond to thyroid and steroidal hormones, and to what's moving through your bloodstream. You've probably heard that everything in your body is connected; mast cells play significant roles in these connections, particularly in the psychoneuroendocrinoimmunological (mind, nervous system, hormone system, and immune system) axes.

Here are some of the roles that your mast cells are major players in:

- Immune function
- Defending against infections – such as viruses, bacteria, mold, candida, and parasites
- Venom detoxification –Bee sting, mosquito bite, spider bite, snakebite
- Wound healing and tissue repair
- Helping build new blood vessels (angiogenesis)
- Widening or constricting blood vessels, playing a role in blood-pressure regulation
- Creating new brain cells (neurogenesis)
- Menstrual cycle regulation
- Circadian rhythm regulation
- Pregnancy, in fetal growth and development
- Cancer

Here's a small sample of the huge array of the types of receptors mast cells have:

- FcεRI (pronounced Fc epsilon RI) – involved in IgE allergic reactions
- H1, H2, H3, H4 histamine receptors – respond to histamine levels
- TLRs (toll-like receptors) – immune response to pathogens, including bacteria, viruses, molds, candida, parasites, also lectins
- FcγR (pronounced Fc gamma R) – involved in IgG reactions in sensitivities to pathogens, medications, foods, etc.
- KIT receptor – responds to stem cell factor in mast cell division and growth
- Cytokine and T-Cell Receptor – respond to various immune cell communications

- CB1 (cannabinoid receptor) – respond to THC, CBD, CBG, etc.
- Hormone Receptors – respond to hormones like estrogen, progesterone, and testosterone
- Various neurotransmitter and neuropeptide receptors – interact with the nervous system and various neurotransmitter-affecting medications
- Receptors for pressure, injury, heat, cold, sunshine, etc.
- CRF receptors (Corticotropin-releasing factor) – respond to stress, trauma

You've probably heard of one of the most commonly discussed mast cell mediators, which is histamine. You may also be familiar with IgE antibodies, which were at one time thought to be the most significant of the mast cell mediators.

Today, however, we know that mast cells can release over a thousand different mediators.

Here is a small selection of them:

Amines
    Histamine
    Polyamines
    Proteoglycans
    Heparin
    Chondroitin sulfates
    Serglycin
Lysosomal enzymes
    β-Glucuronidase
    β-Hexosaminidase
    Arylsulfatase
Proteases
    Tryptases
    Chymase-1
    Cathepsin G
    Granzyme B
    Carboxypeptidase A3
Serotonin
Leukotrienes
Prostaglandins
VEGF
PDGF
Cytokines
    TNFα
    TGF-β1

IFNγ
βFGF
Interleukins such as IL-4, IL-6, IL-10, Il-13, etc.
Chemokines
SCF
Substance P

These mediators have various roles in your body:

- Histamine – numerous roles including in immune functioning, sleep, digestion, etc.
- Certain prostaglandins, leukotrienes, platelet activating factor – blood vessel constriction or dilation, narrowing of bronchial passages
- Cytokines – inflammation increase, inflammation reduction, cell signaling
- Growth factors – growth of different cell types, new blood cell formation, blood vessel dilation
- Neurotransmitters and neuropeptides – signaling with the nervous system
- Tryptase – allergic responses and immunity
- Platelet-activating factor – inflammation, anaphylaxis, platelet functioning, immune defense

Now that you understand more about mast cells, let's dive into what Mast Cell Activation Syndrome (MCAS) is.

Mast Cell Activation Syndrome is a type of mast-cell disorder defined as a multisystemic inflammatory condition of inappropriate mast-cell activity. This can occur with or without allergic-type symptoms and with or without anaphylaxis. Symptoms must occur in at least two or more systems (i.e., the GI tract and nervous system, or the skin and urogenital system).

Unlike rare mast-cell disorders such as mastocytosis (a type of cancer), MCAS is quite common and the types of presentations quite varied. Remember that there are mast cells in nearly every tissue in the body, combined with over 200 receptors and over 1,000 mediators. Can you imagine the number of possible permutations among mast-cell locations, receptors, and mediators to arrive at the number of symptoms a person can have? This is why symptom presentations in MCAS vary widely from person to person and why this condition has so long been mystifying. Symptom presentations depend on which mast cell locations are being affected, which receptors are being activated by which triggers, and which mediators are being released.

It's usually easiest to explore possible mast-cell symptoms by looking at them system by system. Many people with MCAS don't have involvement of all these systems, but some of the worst cases, like mine was, have symptoms in every category. This is not an exhaustive list, but it includes the most common symptoms linked to MCAS.

Systemic Symptoms

- overall fatigue
- inflammation
- swelling
- weight changes
- sensitivities to foods, medications, environment, chemicals, EMFs, etc.

Musculoskeletal Symptoms

- osteoporosis/osteopenia
- arthritis that moves around
- muscle and/or bone pain
- hyperflexible joints

Skin Symptoms

- itching
- flushing
- hives
- rashes
- hair loss
- rosacea, psoriasis, eczema

Cardiovascular Symptoms

- fainting or feeling faint
- chest pains
- heart palpitations
- dizziness
- low or high blood pressure

Digestive Symptoms

- mouth burning
- diarrhea and/or constipation
- nausea
- reflux or heartburn
- food sensitivities
- IBS
- throat/tongue swelling
- onset of symptoms within 15 minutes of eating

Urinary Tract Symptoms

- inflammation of tissues
- burning sensation

- pain with urination
- infection-like symptoms of the urinary tract

Brain and Nervous System Symptoms

- brain fog
- difficulty paying attention
- headaches, migraines
- depression, anxiety
- tingling and numbness
- tinnitus

Lung and Respiratory Symptoms

- congestion
- coughing
- shortness of breath
- asthma

Reproductive System Symptoms

- endometriosis
- painful periods
- male and female infertility
- hormone imbalances

Eye Symptoms

- eye pain
- redness
- trouble focusing
- inflammation in the eyes
- blurry, itchy, watery eyes
- Irritated eyes

Anaphylaxis or Anaphylactoid Reactions (can be life threatening)

- difficulty breathing
- itchy hives
- flushing or pale skin
- feeling of warmth
- weak and rapid pulse
- nausea
- vomiting
- diarrhea
- dizziness and fainting

Again, most people don't have all those symptoms, but in MCAS, there are symptoms in at least two of the categories listed above. Most people with MCAS have several symptoms. MCAS has classically been thought of as involving, at a minimum, allergy-like symptoms, skin symptoms, and anaphylaxis, but not everyone with MCAS has those.

For example, one client I worked with had symptoms related to her GI tract (diarrhea, reflux, abdominal pains), urinary system (urinary pain and burning with urgency), fatigue, and brain fog. She didn't experience any skin or allergy symptoms and didn't suffer from anaphylaxis.

Because of the major role mast cells have in the neuroendocrinoimmunological axes, MCAS rarely occurs in isolation. Here are some of the most common conditions that are often related to MCAS and may represent a misdiagnosis when MCAS is the true issue:

- Fibromyalgia/ME
- Chronic fatigue
- Interstitial cystitis
- certain cancers
- Crohn's disease
- Diabetes
- Ehrler's Danlos Syndrome (EDS)
- Postural Orthostatic Tachycardia Syndrome (POTS)
- Many forms of autoimmunity, such as rheumatoid arthritis, lupus, Hashimoto's thyroiditis, and multiple sclerosis
- Autism spectrum disorders

How Do These Mast Cells Get So Dysregulated?

In normal mast cell activity, the mast cells are stimulated by a trigger that may or may not cause the mast cells to activate and release certain appropriate mediators. For example, if you twist your ankle, causing injury, your ankle may get red, hot, and swollen. Your mast cells (and other related immune cells) are on the scene to protect your body and create inflammation to evoke a healing response. Likewise, if you cut your finger and it gets infected, it may get hot, red, and itchy. Again, your mast cells and other immune cells are there sensing the injury and for pathogens to protect you while directing the rest of your immune network to attack the infection and initiate healing. If you catch a respiratory virus, your mast cells will be involved in creating inflammation in the mucosal tissues of your sinuses, nose, and throat to protect you. If you get food poisoning, your mast cells will be a big part of the response of vomiting and diarrhea that help you purge the pathogenic bacteria.

Most people have experienced these various types of normal mast cell activation. If you don't have MCAS, then once your ankle or cut heals, once you get over the cold or food poisoning, your mast cells calm down again and usually forget that anything happened.

What's happened, though, is that we now live in a world where we're bombarded by mast cell triggers all the time. We're surrounded by both chemicals and artificial EMFs at levels we've never experienced in history. Our food, air, and water supply is highly contaminated with pesticides, herbicides, microplastics, pharmaceuticals, heavy metals, and a number of other toxins. Due to a variety of factors, environmental mold is at epidemic levels. The incidence of Lyme and other tickborne infections has skyrocketed. We now have super viruses, super bacteria, and super molds. Candida has become more resistant and widespread as well. Technology has forced upon us a constant stream of sensational, stressful news. Pandemics have contributed to a global level of traumas. What's considered a "normal" lifestyle of working 40–55 hours a week, driving kids across town to extracurriculars every night in rush-hour traffic, trying to cram in a healthy meal, and pack lunches while barely able to catch our breath is a highly stressful way to live.

These stressors deplete important nutrients, creating numerous cascading biochemical imbalances. All of these factors contribute to epigenetic expression of a number of genes, including those for mast cells, histamine regulation, detoxification, and so on (see chapter 19 for a discussion of the role of genetics).

Mast cells these days have a constant onslaught of triggers. As the underlying toxin, pathogen, and stress loads pile up, many people's mast cells can no longer keep up. Some people are more genetically predisposed, but even without genetic predispositions, we all have a certain threshold of how much of these triggers our bodies can handle.

When mast cells are continually triggered, they start to lose their fine tuning. Their ability to stabilize themselves decreases. The mast cells' receptors become overly sensitive and overly responsive, releasing inappropriate numbers and types of mediators. Think of it like this: If the guards at the castle gate must be on duty 24/7 for weeks, months, and years on end, you can fully expect they'll get wonky. It's as if your mast cells are on a hair trigger and can no longer tell the difference between the real threats and the butterflies, so they start to fire machine guns at everything.

When you add to the picture how much mycotoxins, tickborne infections, constant stress, B1 deficiency, and trauma dysregulate the nervous system, signaling the mast cells to continue sounding the alarm bells of danger, you can see how mast cells can become so dysregulated, develop hypervigilance for triggers, hypersensitivity to triggers, and over-responsiveness in their mediator release.

To recap, here are the most common root triggers I've seen in the MCAS population I've worked with over the last several years:

- Mold Toxicity
- Tickborne infections – Lyme and *Bartonella*
- COVID
- EMFs
- Food triggers
- Chemical toxicity (such as glyphosate, organophosphates, perchlorates, etc.)
- Heavy metal toxicity
- Nutrient imbalances
- Hormone imbalances
- Epigenetic factors
- Physical stressors (surgeries, illnesses, injuries, airway obstructions)
- Chronic emotional and/or mental stressors
- Toxic relationships
- Traumas

How Is MCAS Diagnosed?

MCAS only received a diagnostic code in 2016, giving it a bit of "official" status. For a few decades before then, there were case presentations, theories, and preliminary research. There is naturally still a lot of debate occurring in terms of what technically constitutes MCAS.

There are two types of diagnostic criteria being debated, what are called consensus-1 and consensus-2 criteria.

The current, and more strict consensus-1 criteria requires all three of these criteria be met:

1. MCAS-associated symptoms in two or more systems, with periodic flares;
2. Increase in serum tryptase during a flare, having already excluded other differential diagnoses that could explain these symptoms; and
3. Improvement in symptoms with H1 or H2 receptor-blocking medications or mast cell-targeting medications.

The current consensus-2 criteria requires:

1. MCAS-associated symptoms in two or more systems, with periodic flares, having already excluded other differential diagnoses that could explain these symptoms;
2. Increase in one of these mast cell mediator markers during a flare:
   - Chromogranin A

- Leukotriene E4
- Total serum tryptase
- 11-β-PGF2α
- Heparin
- Histamine
- Urinary 24-hour N-methyl histamine
- Urinary PGD_2

3. Improvement in symptoms with H1 or H2 receptor-blocking medications or mast cell-targeting medications (minor criterion, not required);
4. Tissue biopsy with CD 117 staining (skin, GI tissue, etc.) (minor criterion, not required);
5. Certain genetic variants in the more rare clonal MCAS disorders (minor criterion, not required),

Just like with any good research, this healthy debate will continue to evolve and expand as more information becomes apparent. There have been some challenges with testing in MCAS and with getting a positive response to medications that are still being explored. These include: Mast-cell blood markers can elevate and then return quickly back to a normal level in the blood *within minutes,* begging the question of whether these mediators are sometimes missed due to the timing of blood draws.

What if the handful of accepted mediators aren't the ones that are problematic for that particular person? What if some of the 990+ other mediators that can't yet be measured are the ones that are actually elevated?

Blood and urine samples have to be kept chilled and processed by cold centrifugation to be reliable, yet most labs still don't have this equipment.

The mast cell and antihistamine medications as formulated have likely mast-cell triggering excipients (dyes, titanium dioxide, corn starch, plastic residues). This means they may not help because the excipients, rather than the substance itself, may be triggering a reaction and masking improvements.

Compared to the diagnosis of more established chronic illnesses such as diabetes or Parkinson's, Mast Cell Activation Syndrome is still in its infancy. Further, it takes years for medical schools to update their curriculum with the significant amount of emerging research. Regardless, huge strides continue to be made in diagnosing and addressing MCAS, and I fully expect that understanding, awareness, and effectiveness will only continue to grow as time goes on.

How Can MCAS Cause Sensitivities?

Those of us with Mast Cell Activation Syndrome are not unique. We've often been called the "canaries in the coal mine," and I find this an apt descriptor. Today, we live in a world with astronomical levels of toxins, full of ever-evolving superbugs, laden with unnatural types of EMFs, and facing a disconcerting levels of stressors, all of which we've never experienced before in history. If you can ever step off this merry-go-round for just a few days by entering into a technology-free, pristine natural setting and slow down, then coming back to the way we live is absolutely shocking. Many people got a glimpse of this during the pandemic when everything shut down, and I've seen the juxtaposition of that slower pace with returning to "life as usual" cause many meltdowns from the stress of this lifestyle.

Our toxic world is actually harming all of us, and it's catching us unprepared. High levels of toxins are found in the cord blood of infants, where they can pass through the placenta. Most forms of chronic illness, along with cancers, have been dramatically on the rise for the last few decades, and the complexity of chronic illness has also risen exponentially. Children are substantially more ill than a few decades ago, and it's not uncommon now for children to have been ill since birth.

All to say, those of us with MCAS aren't experiencing something bizarre and unusual. To the contrary, we're simply the ones who are sounding the alarm about our toxic environment faster and louder than others. We're the ones saying, "danger, danger, something has to change." While we may be more sensitive than most other people, it's important to remember that those of us with MCAS are not the only ones being affected by this toxic world. For others, the effects may smolder for decades only to show up as cardiovascular disease or cancer or neurodegeneration down the road. No matter how our illnesses show up, we're all being affected and we're all in it together.

For those of us who develop MCAS as a result of the imbalanced world we're living in, we can develop all kinds of sensitivities to foods, chemicals, supplements, medications, allergens, mold, even EMFs. With mast cells being part of your body's sensing, protection, and defense systems, it's hardwired into your mast cells to detect things that may potentially be harmful to you and create protection and defenses for you. The bottom line is that no matter what your mast cells are doing, they're not trying to hurt you. If you have MCAS, your mast cells are working very hard to *protect you* from the major categories of triggers: pathogens, toxins, and/or stressors.

One of the roles of mast cells that I find most fascinating is their relationship with the nervous system. In addition to being closely connected to the network of other immune cells, mast cells are also intricately interwoven into your nervous system, occurring along every nerve sheath, at every nerve ending, and even within your brain, particularly in your limbic system. Then, when there is neuroinflammation, even more mast cells will migrate across the blood-brain barrier and into the brain to protect and defend from anything that may affect your brain.

Mast cells function as an interface between your nervous system and the rest of your body. Because of this interrelationship, the immune and nervous systems have to be considered as an axis that always operates in tandem. Your mast cells have receptors for many neurotransmitters and neuropeptides released by your neurons, and their granules also contain many of these chemicals, which they can release to communicate with your nervous system. Your neuronal endings also have receptors for various mast-cell released neurotransmitters and neuropeptides. Thus there is constant cross-communication between your mast cells and your nervous system.

This is how your mast cells can so quickly respond to smells, stress, and even to your thoughts. Let's consider my client "Frannie" who was particularly sensitive to onions. She would start to get acid reflux, abdominal pains, and nausea as soon as she smelled onions; she didn't even have to register the smell. Soon after exposure Frannie would have diarrhea. She could be in a grocery store, and if there was a sample table with freshly cut onions, she'd start to react before she even knew the onions were there. Contrary to what some people in her life thought, Frannie wasn't crazy and wasn't a hypochondriac. It's common for people with Mast Cell Activation Syndrome to have reactions to smells of triggering agents, whether foods, fragrances, paints, gasoline, etc.

How can this happen so quickly and sometimes without Frannie's consciously knowing the onions were there? Consider again that there are mast cells in the limbic system in your brain. Your limbic system plays a major role in monitoring your environment for safety and in protection and defense. Your limbic system and mast cells work together to remember historic events that caused you harm, whether real or perceived, and create changes in your behavior in avoiding toxins, allergens, and too much stress. Guess which nerve runs directly to the limbic system—the olfactory nerve in your nose. This means that the limbic system and mast cells in your brain can respond to smells in seconds and signal through the nervous system to mast cells throughout your body that there is danger. Frannie's mast cell/nervous system axis signaled danger particularly to her GI system. I've seen other people who would break out in hives, have breathing problems, brain fog, get muscle and joint pains, or any other number of symptoms within seconds to a few minutes in response to olfactory triggers.

Sometimes your limbic/mast cell axis can misidentify triggers as well. To illustrate, I'll share a story from my life. I spent some time in India a couple of decades ago, and while I was there I made the mistake of eating a salad with raw vegetables at an Italian restaurant. In India, this is a big no-no for westerners because our GI systems aren't used to the bacteria in raw produce there due to the lack of purified water available for irrigation and washing produce. I had some mild GI distress afterward, but it wasn't until three days later that I developed severe dysentery and dehydration. It was clear I had gotten ill from the salad, but when I was so sick, friends brought me traditional Indian foods that would be gentle on my GI tract. I was so nauseated and dangerously ill that I could barely eat; however, I forced myself to get down something during those days. My limbic system naturally came to associate the nausea, GI pain, and severe diarrhea with Indian food. After the illness, every time I smelled Indian food I got nauseated and developed abdominal cramping, yet I have no problems eating Italian food. This is because my limbic/mast cell axis incorrectly identified the Indian food as the cause of my dysentery. Even though I was fully aware of what the trigger was, the pattern mis-recognition by my limbic system and mast cells happened anyway. This pattern recogni-tion in sensitivities is below the level of conscious thought, but these sensitivities can be reprogrammed (see chapters 1 and 2 on the limbic system).

This cross-talk with the nervous system and mast cells is actually very good news for those of us with Mast Cell Activation Syndrome! It means that even for the most sensitive people who can't tolerate any supplements or medications orally, you can still make a significant impact on your mast cells by supporting your nervous system.

Here's a very simple example of how powerful this can be. I noticed many years ago that when I became stressed about something, my knuckles would start to swell, but if I started resonant breathing and deep relaxation, the swelling would go down within minutes. This alone convinced me of the power of rebooting the nervous system in MCAS!

Next, let's look at some of the other sensitivities that can develop. Beyond sensitiv-ities to individual foods, there are some common larger food categories that can trigger mast cells in some people. Foods high in histamine are common triggers in many people with MCAS (though not all). This is because mast cells have four types of histamine receptors (H1, H2, H3, and H4), which are triggered when there's too much histamine in your body.

High-histamine foods and histamine-liberating foods include aged beef and bison, most fish and seafood, citrus, strawberries, pineapple, vinegar, spinach, tomatoes, egg-plant, cashews, peanuts, walnuts, cloves, cinnamon, and fermented foods such as kom-bucha, kefir, and raw sauerkraut. This is just a small selection, but a full list based on extensive research data is available on my website.

Other, more common, food categories that may trigger some people with MCAS (but again not all) include oxalates, lectins, FODMAPs, and salicylates (read more about salicylates and oxalates in the salicylate and oxalate chapters of this book). If you suspect you have issues with oxalates, please read about this carefully and find someone to guide you through reducing them. You can go off of high-histamine, high-lectin, or high-salicylate foods safely by stopping them right away, but you should carefully wean off oxalate foods to avoid the terrible experience of oxalate dumping. You can learn more about these potential food triggers and find foods lists on my website.

I want to caution you, though: It's a very slippery slope to refrain from every food you think might be offending you and soon whittle down to too few foods. I did this until I was down to just ten foods, not counting seasonings. I've worked with many people who'd cut down to two foods—usually chicken and rice—for years. When this hyper-vigilance develops, we naturally start looking for every possible trigger and try to avoid it, but this can lead us to making incorrect associations to foods that aren't triggers. This is particularly a problem for people whose mast cells start reacting to everything they consume, even water. Whether or not your mast cells react, and to what extent, can vary day to day depending on the total inflammation load and trigger exposure you have that day. One day, you might feel just fine eating broccoli, carrots, and lamb. A few days later, maybe it rained and mold counts are higher, you got a stressful bill in the mail, and you didn't sleep well; then you might react eating the same foods that were no problem a few days earlier. Generally, with this kind of mast-cell reaction to eating, the symptoms will develop within thirty minutes or less, as opposed to reactions to histamines, salic-ylates, oxalates, lectins, or FODMAPs, which can take thirty minutes to a few hours to even a couple days to develop. It's very important to keep as much variety in your diet as possible, and some of the tips in the next section might help you tolerate foods better. Also, I've seen in thousands of cases that MCAS can be dramatically improved, if not reversed, if the underlying root triggers are fully addressed.

What Can You Do About MCAS?

Mast Cell Activation Syndrome can be tricky to manage, and sensitivities can compound these challenges; however, with good guidance, perseverance, persistence, and courage, you have great odds of improving significantly. We practitioners develop approaches that work best for the populations we work with. The practice I run typically serves very sensitive people dealing with MCAS, mold toxicity, tickborne infections, and signifi-cant levels of nervous-system dysregulation.

There are many approaches to MCAS, and what I'm going to present is the method I've been using in my own practice with great success with the population I see. This, however, is certainly not the only way to work with MCAS, and other practitioners have had success with different models. The key is to find a practitioner and an approach that fits who you are and where you are in your journey.

I've found over years with the sensitive population that there is a very important order of operations regarding which layers sensitive bodies are able to address first and which are usually best left for later. I conceptualize this in what I call the MC360™

method, which provides the overall framework we use in our clinic for those with MCAS and sensitivities.

Stabilization
Gentle detox of mycotoxins and chemicals
Cleanup of infectious layers and heavy metals
Rebuilding systems where needed (i.e., GI tract, bone integrity, cell membranes, etc.)
Optimizing for long-term health

For those who are sensitive, it's very important to remember that even within this framework, much has to be customized for individual sensitivities and triggers. There just isn't a one-size-fits-all approach that works with sensitive people with MCAS. Some have such severe sound sensitivity that they're unable to do the vagal listening programs and need other options for the vagal system. Some have salicylate intolerance or severe SIBO and won't tolerate certain supplements. Some have trouble with even the most hypoallergenic excipients. Others are so sensitive they need to start with six to twelve months of nervous-system rebooting work before they move into working with homeopathics or topicals.

In this chapter, I'll focus primarily on the stabilization phase of this method, as the other phases are either covered very well by other authors or are outside the scope of this book. It would still take an entire volume to adequately describe the various options that can be used in this stabilization phase and how they can be customized, so I'll present a selection of options within the context of each phase of this approach.

The stabilization phase provides critical support to prepare your body to be able to address underlying root factors. This phase is especially important for sensitive people, and is often a major missing step for those who have struggled to detoxify, methylate, and repair mitochondria. Most of the clients I work with have several systems of their bodies stuck in Cell Danger Response 1, where their bodies won't allow them to detox until they can feel safe to do so. (For an in-depth discussion of Cell Danger Response, I refer you to Neil Nathan's book *Toxic*.) The top priority for this phase is to create a deeply felt sense of safety, on the emotional, mental, spiritual, and energetic levels, that trickles down to the cellular and biochemical levels. I've seen remarkable results in people who previously couldn't move forward with their health until this phase was adequately supported. The stabilization phase has five steps:

Stabilizing the nervous system;
Calming mast cells;
Supporting digestion and elimination;

Identifying and removing external mast cell triggers; and

Supporting adrenals, hormones, and sleep, where possible.

Let's explore each of these steps, with the most emphasis on specific considerations for sensitive people in working with the nervous system and calming the mast cells.

The Nervous System, MCAS, and Sensitivities

I recommend starting by stabilizing the nervous system. In this step, I focus on the limbic, vagal, and structural aspects of the nervous system, and if needed, trauma. The vagal and limbic systems are directly linked with mast cells in their involvement in sensitivities, and this neuroimmune axis has major roles in regulating fear and monitoring for safety.

I refer you to the chapters on the limbic and polyvagal systems for more detailed descriptions of these systems and techniques. For our purposes in this chapter, recall that mast cells line the nerve sheaths and nerve endings, and there is continual cross-communication between the nervous system and mast cells. For sensitive people, working with the nervous system is a powerful way to begin to calm sensitivities. I strongly recommend combining vagal-support modalities with limbic modalities for those with MCAS. It's often tempting to want to shortcut this step by working solely on the limbic or vagal system; however, it's critical to work on both systems simultaneously. If you reset the limbic system but don't work on the vagal system at the same time, the vagal system will take the lead in sensitivities. It's also very important that you work on nervous-system techniques that specifically target these systems. These days you can access myriad nervous-system techniques, which is great, but if you're dealing with sensitivities, you need to fine-tune of the areas of your nervous system that are governing your reactions. You wouldn't walk into a supplement store, blindly grab anything off the shelf, and assume it will work for you, and the same is true for rebooting your nervous system. Yoga, meditation, and guided relaxation are wonderful tools, but they don't specifically target the limbic and vagal systems. You need to choose what helps the limbic and vagal systems.

Ultimately, your sensitivities developed as a result of your body's working incredibly hard to protect you and keep you safe from the overwhelming levels of pathogens, toxins, and stressors that have accumulated in it. Many people who have become sensitive feel betrayed by their bodies, and come to see their bodies as an enemy, which makes the journey much harder. Also, if you see your body as an enemy, it's very hard to feel safe. As a part of recovering from sensitivities, it can greatly help you to befriend this part of yourself with appreciation and gratitude for how hard your body works to take care of you and protect you. I often recommend that my clients speak to themselves with lovingkindness, gentleness, and a soothing tone as they would to a beloved two- or three-year-old who is scared, sick, and exhausted. I often have them conjure a specific child in their lives, practice seeing themselves as this vulnerable child, and give themselves the love, care, and concern they need. During the worst of my illness, I noticed how much I was whipping myself to try to function and how much extra stress this created. A high-achieving, highly motivated person, I beat myself up mentally when I couldn't get things done. Some days I was so exhausted I couldn't brush my hair.

My self-talk was a clear mast cell trigger in itself, though. I decided to work on changing this and practiced calling myself "sweetheart." When I was in severe pain and exhausted and had to get myself to an appointment, I would gently cheerlead myself every step of the way. "Sweetheart, you're doing great. Let's get your jacket on. That took a lot of effort. You did a really great job. Now, let's get your purse. Very good. You can do this, sweetheart. You're doing great. Let's just see if we can walk to the car. Let's just do that much."

If this kind of practice resonates with you, consider some version of it for yourself. Lovingkindness for yourself can give you a good bit of fuel for the road ahead, and provides a starting point for limbic-system rebooting. Then, be sure to work with a limbic rebooting program to deepen this work.

On the vagal side, there are many modalities that can be used. Some are more effective than others, but the more different vagal supports you use the better. If you don't have sound sensitivities or trouble processing music, then BrainTap and Safe and Sound Protocols are often helpful. There are targeted vagal acupressure points that can be helpful, and the Emotional Freedom Technique is another method that can work effectively with both the vagal and limbic systems. A breathing technique called alternate nostril breathing can also support vagal signaling, and for those who aren't EMF sensitive, Frequency Specific Microcurrent has several programs for the vagal nerve and the nervous system in general.

On the structural side, many sensitive people have cranial, cervical, and jaw dysfunction that puts pressure on cranial nerves involved in regulation, proprioception (knowing where you are in space), and a sense of physiological safety. It's very common for cranial bones and cervical vertebrae to be out of alignment, affecting the craniosacral rhythm and putting pressure on cranial nerves. The nerve endings to the jaw are also critical in feeling comfortable and safe in your body, and even slight misalignments can create feelings of anxiety, irritability, and general unease that again communicate to your neuroimmune system that you're not safe and further perpetuating sensitivities. See the chapters on dental components and structural components for more details.

Finally, trauma is another element to consider in sensitivities, given its significant impact on the nervous system. In the MCAS population, there's a much higher percentage of people who have experienced trauma than in the general population, indicating that trauma is another contributor to MCAS. Traumas can include physical, mental, emotional, sexual, or spiritual abuse (and even witnessing abuse), accidents, surgeries, losses, war, natural disasters, severe illnesses, and medical traumas. The pandemic that started in 2020 created a global sense of trauma that affected nearly all people. Medical traumas have become almost ubiquitous in this population. Trauma isn't as much about the event that happened as it is about the resiliency of the nervous system and perception of the experience.

Two people could experience the same fire or earthquake or abuse and one is traumatized while the other isn't. For those with cumulative traumas, this can lead to complex PTSD (cPTSD), which could need skilled support to unravel. Incredible breakthroughs can happen, though, and I see it daily. Determination and persistence are two of the key personality qualities that predict whether someone can recover from trauma. One of the other key determinants is not being attached to the story of the trauma. Processing the trauma can be helpful to develop a sense of context and understanding of the event, but your limbic system can't tell the difference between telling the story and the trauma reoccurring. The most effective techniques have been somatic-based therapy and mind-body techniques that help you release the trauma at a physiological level. These include somatic focusing and trauma-informed mind-body work. Very low-dose IV ketamine has also helped many with PTSD. During this stabilization phase, it's very important to focus on soothing trauma rather than unearthing and processing it, as you're also working on calming your limbic system. Discernment and carefulness are needed in determining when to work directly on trauma in those with significant chronic illness and sensitivities, and sometimes this isn't needed if a deep sense of safety can be restored through somatic-based and mind-body techniques.

I'd like to address toxic relationships, which are related to trauma. I've seen that a high percentage of people in the MCAS population our practice serves are empaths and are often in personal or professional relationships with personality-disordered or toxic people. These may be family members, friends, acquaintances, colleagues, or bosses. If you come from a childhood background of abuse, then this kind of treatment might feel "normal" or familiar to you, but it perpetuates the sense of a lack of safety, and if you're an empath, it may be impossible to keep yourself grounded. For your body to feel safe enough to stop reacting so much and to be less sensitive, you need true safety in your life. I refer you to Neil Nathan's book, *Energetic Diagnosis,* for more information. Many of my clients in relationships with toxic people have also found Margalis Fjelstad's book, *Stop Caretaking,* helpful.

One last practice that has been life changing for me and many of my most sensitive clients has been connecting with the Earth and with nature on a daily basis or as often as possible. The vast majority of sensitive people have the capacity for a tremendous amount of energetic sensitivity. As a species, we're hardwired to be in touch and in tune with nature, but we've lost this with our rubber-soled shoes, concrete foundations, and the electrical fields that surround us. For those who are energetically sensitive, this loss of attunement with nature is very hard on our systems. Realigning ourselves to our natural state in tune with the Earth's and natural energies can bring a tremendous sense of peace and deep relaxation that's otherwise hard to attain. This can be as simple as finding a quiet space outdoors where you feel safe, and allowing yourself to deeply relax into the Earth while you sense the pulse and energy of the natural world around you. Please see the chapter on emotional, energetic, and spiritual considerations for more details.

If you're a sensitive person, you might need to start slowly with these techniques. Don't feel pressured to start with twenty or thirty minutes. The most sensitive people I've worked with had better results starting with just one or two minutes a day and very gradually layering in other techniques. The more sensitive you are the more locked down your nervous system/mast cell axis is, and you'll want to unlock it gently. It could help you to think about shifting your nervous system with a feather by adding modalities slowly and gently, rather than try to shift your nervous system with a sledgehammer by adding in numerous things all at once. As you build up your time and your techniques, however, you might need anywhere from twenty to sixty minutes, once or twice a day, of various modalities, depending on how stuck your nervous system has been.

Calming Mast Cells Directly

While the nervous system modalities will help calm mast cells indirectly, there are many ways to work on them more directly. The most sensitive person might need to work on the nervous system for two to six months before moving to this step, while those who are tolerating some gentle mast-cell supports can work on both stabilizing the nervous system and calming mast cells simultaneously.

There are many ways to work with supplements and medications for those with MCAS, including oral, topical, and olfactory. Traditionally, oral supplements, medications, and homeopathics are used, but some people have such dysregulation of the GI tract that they can't tolerate anything orally and may need to work with topical, IV, or olfactory delivery. I've had other extremely sensitive people who started in an energetic way. I'll describe more about each of these delivery mechanisms next.

Beginning with oral delivery, many sensitive people continue to start with too large a dose, but in sensitive people less is usually more. Somewhat paradoxically, lower doses often have a better effect in sensitive people than higher doses. In significant limbic and vagal dysregulation, the neuroimmune axis can register any new substance as a threat. I often describe the limbic/vagal/mast cell axes as super-beefed-up guards at the castle gate that have become so hypervigilant, concerned, and overprotective that they defend you from everything and anything. Even the butterflies are suspects. If you come charging up to the castle guards on an elephant, there is no way they'll step aside and let you in without a fight. This is the equivalent of starting with a whole or half a capsule of a supplement or medication. It's much more effective to sneak a little mouse under the door undetected, like starting with an eighth or a sixteenth of a capsule or perhaps even a sprinkle of a supplement or medication, an amount equal to a few grains of sand. The more sensitive you are the smaller a dose you start with. I've even had very sensitive people get success starting with what I call "sips of sprinkles," where you put a sprinkle in water, stir it, and just take a sip. Some people find adding the supplement or medication to food works better than water. Sometimes people can start with teas or glycerin tinctures or add fresh herbs to soups.

Another delivery method is topical. I often recommend the most sensitive clients start with a topical homeopathic ointment called Inflamyar (made by Pekana) applied behind the ears and at the top of the back of the neck to support the cranial nerves in that area. Then, if this is effective, we layer other homeopathics or supplements in powder or tincture form into the cream. Some who can't tolerate anything orally have been able to work with medications this way as well. Adding fresh herbs to baths with filtered water sometimes works; adding fresh rosemary or lavender, for example, can be gently supportive. About 80% of the extremely sensitive clients I work with do very well with this, but the rest seem to react even to topicals. This is most often a sign that the nervous system hasn't been adequately rebooted and that there are environmental triggers that haven't yet been fully resolved.

IV delivery has worked well for some people with severe GI issues. I've been pleasantly surprised at how well some do with IV medications and nutrients, though this isn't right for everyone. Even with IV, sensitive people usually do best starting with low dosing.

Another less commonly considered administration route is olfactory. This works for those who aren't sensitive to the aromas of essential oils or teas. Many studies have shown that essential oils can support the limbic system via the olfactory nerve. Brewing a cup of tea and inhaling the steam, or diffusion of mast cell-supporting essential oils is another route that may be effective for some people. There's an art to onboarding supplements when you're sensitive. Befriending yourself, listening in, using good judgment, and being willing to experiment will take you a long way.

For those with MCAS, in choosing supplements, it's important to avoid triggering excipients and high-histamine ingredients. Not everyone reacts to the same things, but these are the most common excipients that can be troublesome for those who are sensitive with MCAS:

- Carrageenan
- Citric Acid
- Citrus Oils
- Lactose
- Potassium Sorbate
- Potassium Triphosphate
- Sodium Benzoate
- Sodium Triphosphate
- Talc
- Titanium Dioxide
- Xanthan Gum

In very rare circumstances, I've worked with people who were quite sensitive to any form of cellulose, including microcrystalline cellulose, particularly those with severe pine or other tree allergies. This has occurred in fewer than ten clients, but it can make sourcing supplements a challenge. I've also had one client who was clearly sensitive to silicon dioxide. As you can imagine, it can take a good bit of detective work to determine whether sensitivities are due to the active or inactive ingredients in a supplement. This is why I recommend sensitive people start with single-ingredient supplements and keep what I call a changes journal, tracking every new supplement, food, or lifestyle change along with symptom changes. This journal has a particular focus on changes, not on writing down every symptom or every substance consumed, which could lead to an undesirable hyperfocus on symptoms. The journal should be easy and quick to keep up, taking only a minute or less per day, but it is invaluable in tracking down triggers.

In addition to checking excipients, some active ingredients can be triggers, particularly for those who are also histamine intolerant. Here are some of the most common ones:

- High-dose Niacin – increases PGD2 from mast cells and decreases methyl cofactors needed for histamine degradation
- Ascorbic Acid (Vitamin C) from fermentation – high histamine
- Ascorbyl Palmitate (Vitamin C) from fermentation – high histamine
- High dose methyl folate (unless needed for a specific purpose) – increases mast-cell activity; often not tolerated in CDR1
- Supplements or powders with dried spinach, strawberry, or pineapple – high histamine

- Collagen – high histamine
- Citrates – high histamine due to fermentation
- Supplements with citrus oils, clove, cinnamon – histamine liberators
- Probiotics *L. bulgaricus* and *L. casei* – well known histamine-raising strains

Now that we've explored what potentially may be problematic, let's look at which supplements and medications are often best tolerated. I must preface this by saying that anyone with MCAS can react to anything, even the most benign agents. What's listed below is merely a starting point for exploration, but in my practice with extremely sensitive people, there is nothing that everyone has tolerated. I've worked with people who couldn't tolerate the cleanest unrefined sea salt, who couldn't handle a tiny sprinkle of baking soda, and even patients who were triggered by every form of filtered water. The key is to keep a journal, look for patterns when there are reactions, and if you're quite sensitive, take your time and start onboarding things very slowly. I spend a lot of time reminding people to go slower than they think they need to.

Homeopathics, as appropriate to the case, are often well tolerated by sensitive people if there aren't triggering excipients. Alcohol in homeopathics can be flashed off by preparing a mug of boiling water, then adding the remedy to the hot water, and allowing the alcohol to evaporate for ten minutes. This preparation can be consumed all at once or slowly throughout the day.

For those with low blood pressure, unrefined sea salt in water works not just for improving blood flow but also as a natural antihistamine. Further to this point, water is also a natural antihistamine, and I'm frequently surprised with how well educated and motivated our client population is, that many aren't drinking enough water. We aim for at least ½ body weight in ounces if not more. Dehydration is a mast cell trigger.

Bicarbonates are often a gentle way of supporting mast cells. Bicarbonates reduce the release of pro-inflammatory cytokine IL-1β that can recruit more mast cells, along with reducing IL-18, which also triggers increased inflammation. Sodium or potassium bicarbonates can be used, considering both blood-pressure status and electrolyte balance. A higher sodium ratio is often helpful in low blood pressure, while a higher potassium ratio often helps in high blood pressure. Some people with very low stomach acid might not tolerate bicarbonates until stomach acid levels can be improved. I recommend working with your healthcare provider to find bicarbonate amounts and ratios appropriate to your situation, as overdoing these can cause problems in some people.

Perilla seed extract is a favorite of mine. It's derived from an Asian herb perilla, also called shiso. Perilla is high in apigenin, luteolin, and rosmarinic acids, which can support mast cells. Studies have demonstrated that perilla can reduce histamine, the cytokine TNF-α, and arachidonic acid, decreasing inflammation and mast-cell activation. This is usually the first herb I try with sensitive people, as long as they don't have salicylate intolerance, as perilla does have salicylates. If this is well tolerated, the next herbal I try is quercetin, considered one of the most important flavonoids in MCAS. Quercetin has been shown to reduce the inflammatory cytokines IL-1 β, IL-6, and IL-8, as well as reducing chemokines and tryptase. Quercetin can reduce the conversion of the amino acid histidine to histamine by blocking the enzyme histidine d-carboxylase (HDC), and can also block the FcεRI receptor on mast cells. I often start with the isoquercetin form, which is more bioavailable and can be used to good effect in much lower dosages in sensitive people. I've found that this form is often better tolerated in the sensitive population than forms like quercetin dihydrate; however, I've had a handful of cases in which the opposite was true, and I always stay open to individual biological uniqueness. Both of these supplements can be helpful systemically and, when taken about thirty minutes before meals, can be supportive with GI symptoms and food intolerances.

When there are any GI issues or food intolerances, I often recommend the DAO (diamine oxidase) enzyme as well, also called histaminase. DAO is naturally made in the brush border cells of the small intestine and ascending colon, but GI inflammation reduces the ability of these tissues to produce it. The more histamine can be reduced in the intestines the less histamine there is to trigger the mast cells lining the GI tract or spill across the intestinal lining into the bloodstream, which can increase systemic mast-cell activation and worsen nighttime waking. Further, just the act of digesting, even of the most low-histamine foods, will still trigger histamine release in the gut. For all these reasons, if DAO is well tolerated, I recommend taking it regularly, not just before eating high-histamine foods. The optimal time to take it is about ten to fifteen minutes before eating, but it can still be helpful even if taken with the meal or after. While it's import-ant for sensitive people to start everything slowly, once DAO is tolerated, most people do best with between two and four capsules before meals. It can be increased to four to eight capsules if eating a higher histamine meal is necessary, such as when traveling or at a family event, but DAO supplementation can't fully offset high-histamine foods, and shouldn't be used as an excuse to regularly eat those foods if they're triggers. DAO supplements are generally derived from pork kidney, but for those with pork allergies, DAO is also found in beef kidney to a lesser degree, as well as in pea shoots.

Baicalin is another favorite herbal supplement of mine. This is an extract of Chinese skullcap root (*Scutellaria baicalensis*), also called Baikal skullcap, This is a different spe-cies than American skullcap (*Scutellaria lateriflora*). While full-spectrum Chinese skull-cap root can be hard on the liver in higher doses in the longer term, Baicalin extract has been shown to have significant hepatoprotective effects. It's available as alcohol or glycerin tincture, powder, or in capsules. It's very important to get a clean, high-quality source. Baicalin has neuroprotective properties, can help regulate HPA axis functioning, and has been shown to inhibit mast-cell degranulation, reduce IgE food response, and decrease a number of inflammatory mast-cell mediators. It can also be taken thirty minutes before meals to further support the GI tract.

Quail egg extract functions as an important tryptase inhibitor for those who can tolerate eggs; however, the most effective version of this product does also contain some quercetin in the form of isoquercitrin, so there has to be tolerance to both for a sensitive person to take it. In addition to helping systemically, quail egg extract can be taken thirty minutes before meals for GI support.

Cortisol is stabilizing to mast cells, and low cortisol is a common trigger. Adrenal cortex (not the full glandular) has often been well tolerated when indicated, taken first thing upon waking and again at noon if needed. Rhodiola is a great adaptogen that can support improved HPA axis signaling, and simultaneously has likely mast cell-stabilizing effects by reducing pro-inflammatory cytokine production.

Omega-3 fatty acids have many helpful actions, including reducing inflammation and IgE activation of mast cells. Omega 3s also help improve barrier tissue function, which can decrease the triggering of mast-cell activation by allergens. Fish oils are rather high in histamine, but many sensitive people can better tolerate the SPM (specialized pro-resolving mediators) form of Omega 3s. This form seems to be lower in histamine, but it's unclear why. EPA and DHA omega 3s are converted naturally in your body to SPMs, which are then responsible for reduction of inflammation, but EPA and DHA aren't completely converted, so they require high doses. SPMs often have improved benefits with lower dosing than EPA and DHA, which can be helpful for sensitive people.

Mast cells are dependent on a number of nutrients as well. Some of the better tolerated ones are vitamin D3, magnesium, zinc, vitamin E, and vitamin A. Vitamin C can also be helpful, but needs to be unfermented. Ascorbates and camu are usually well tolerated. B1 is essential to proper function of the neuroimmune axis, and I refer you to the chapter on thiamine deficiency for more information.

Here's a list of the supports covered above, with those that are low salicylate marked with the letters LS:

- Homeopathics – LS
- Unrefined Sea Salt – LS
- Ample water consumption – LS
- Bicarbonates – LS
- Perilla seed extract
- Quercetin as Isoquercitrin
- DAO – LS
- Pork sensitivities
- Pea derived DAO
- Baicalin
- Quail Egg extract
- Adrenal cortex – LS
- Rhodiola
- SPMs – LS

- Vitamin D3 – LS
- Magnesium – LS
- Zinc – LS
- Vitamin E – LS
- Vitamin A – LS
- Vitamin C as ascorbates – LS
- Vitamin C as camu
- B1

There are of course hundreds of other mast cell-supporting supplements, but these tend to be better tolerated as a starting point for those with sensitivities. You can learn more about these supplements and more through the resources on our website.

Mast cells have over 200 receptors and 1,000+ mediators, so mast-cell activation can require a multifaceted approach to manage until the root causes are addressed and the mast cells can re-regulate. This is why most people dealing with complex MCAS do better with a synergistic protocol of targeted supplements and medications. There are many medications that can be helpful for MCAS. I've observed that sensitive people tend to do better with lower dosing and compounded materials, as well as starting with the gentler medications before moving into the heavy hitters.

As a consulting practitioner, I don't prescribe, but I have significant experience working alongside prescribers, and the medications listed below have been better tolerated in our sensitive MCAS population. It can, however, still be hit or miss, requiring a few trials to find what works. For those with excipient sensitivities, medications may need to be compounded. Many sensitive people have been able to successfully onboard medications with the same slow and steady approach discussed earlier—starting with sprinkles or a drop and building gradually.

H1 blockers like cetirizine, fexofenadine, levocetirizine, or loratadine work systemically by blocking H1 histamine receptors and can be taken once or twice per day. These are found over the counter or may be compounded. H2 blockers like famotidine block H2 histamine receptors, which are found in high concentrations in the GI tract but also in the bladder and other tissues. Many with GI symptoms have found better relief with taking H2 blockers thirty minutes before meals. These too are available over the counter or may be compounded.

Ketotifen has selective H1 blocking activities and is also anti-eosinophilic (reducing histamine release from these cells), with anti-leukotriene properties. It is most commonly prescribed at 1mg, which is usually too strong for most sensitive people. It can also be compounded at 0.25 or 0.1 mg for those who are more sensitive to medications. Many with food intolerances and other GI symptoms have found it helpful to take thirty minutes before meals. It can also be taken at bedtime to support deeper sleep. In the United States, ketotifen is available orally only if compounded. Outside the US, it is widely available as a prescription formulation, but may need to be compounded if the excipients are a trigger. Watch out for potassium sorbate or sodium benzoate in liquid preparations.

Cromolyn sodium is a mast cell-stabilizing medication that can be delivered as an oral solution, nasal spray, eye drop, or inhalation solution. The prescription oral solution is most commonly used in this population, followed by the over-the-counter nasal spray. There can be an adjustment period for the autonomic nervous system with the oral solution, which can be avoided by onboarding it very slowly. There are no excipients other than purified water in the oral solution, and most sensitive people tolerate the solution as formulated, but a select few may have trouble with the plastic lining for the ampules and need to have it compounded in capsule form. For those with GI symptoms, the oral solution can be taken thirty minutes before each meal.

Low-Dose Naltrexone (LDN) can help modulate immune functioning and reduce pain perception. It is often prescribed to be taken at night, but those with sleep disturbances sometimes find taking it in the morning more helpful. As with Ketotifen, avoid potassium sorbate or sodium benzoate in liquid preparations. Compounded capsules are usually better tolerated. *The LDN Book,* Volumes 1 and 2, are a great resource on the uses of LDN.

Hydrocortisone is well known as an over-the-counter topical cream, but it's also available orally as a prescription. When taken orally, hydrocortisone is a bioidentical replacement for cortisol and can be useful in HPA axis dysfunction (often called adrenal fatigue). Hydrocortisone, when used for someone with low cortisol, has a mast cell-stabilizing effect. *Safe Uses of Cortisol* by endocrinologist William Jefferies, MD, is an excellent resource.

There are certainly many more mast-cell medications available, such as aspirin, diphenhydramine, hydroxyzine, doxepin hydrochloride, montelukast sodium, imatinib, and omalizumab to name just a few. Some sensitive people tolerate these well, but they've been more challenging than the medications mentioned above. The key is to work with your licensed medical provider on what may be the best agents for your unique case and to listen to your body when onboarding anything.

Removing Triggers

Last but certainly not least in the stabilization phase is identifying and removing triggers. We discussed triggers in depth earlier. In the stabilization phase, we work on the external triggers. Testing and remediation for toxic mold and toxic chemicals in the environment are very important. We focus on improving air quality, addressing mold, pollen, dust, VOCs, pollution, toxic cleaning supplies, fragrances, etc. We check water quality and make sure drinking water is adequately filtered; it's quite surprising how often even expensive water filters fail to filter out toxic chemicals and pharmaceuticals. We also check for food triggers. This includes removing pesticides and processed foods as well as looking at whether histamines, oxalates, lectins, salicylates, FODMAPs, sulfur, or other food intolerances may be a concern. Triggers to the nervous system need to be considered as well, and can include overly stressful lifestyles or jobs, EMFs, toxic relationships, and stressful forms of entertainment such as violent movies. Once the stabilization phase is in place and symptoms have calmed down a few notches, then it's time to move on to the underlying internal root triggers. The stabilization phase generally takes three to six months for most sensitive people, depending on how long mold remediation takes. I've had some people take less time, and for others it has taken one to two years before they could move forward to detoxification. The overall process generally takes sensitive people two years at a minimum, and can take up to six years or more, contingent upon the levels of sensitivities, the complexity of the case, and how long triggers go unidentified (like environmental mold exposure, often the most problematic). This can seem like a long time, but the vast majority of sensitive people get gradual improvements over this timeframe, while a very small percentage of sensitive people may not feel significantly better until they've fully addressed their major root triggers.

Ending with Hope

Healing from MCAS takes time. Mast cells are among the longest-lived cells in the body, with a lifespan of over a year. It takes a few years for dysregulated mast cells to turn over and for the dysregulated programming to be changed. The journey from being a chronically ill person with MCAS and sensitivities isn't for the faint of heart. It takes patience, perseverance, courage, dedication, and keeping hope alive. That said, this is very doable with a trusted guide who can help you navigate when the seas get rough. I opened with the struggles of my own health story, and I'll now share my successes. I not only got my health back but got my life back, and I've been able to pursue my dreams and mission in life. I can travel, eat in restaurants, go hiking, ride a bike, go dancing, and run a full-time practice. I was able to return to graduate school for two graduate degrees, and now work on very complex cases that require a lot of brainpower.

I'm not eating pizza and candy bars; I'm not partying and drinking. I eat very cleanly, I take supportive supplements, and I get quality sleep. I exercise, meditate, and support my nervous system. I drink good-quality purified water and use great air purification. I try to avoid EMFs and furnishings that off-gas VOCs. If I could go back and choose whether I'd be as sick as I was, I don't think I'd choose that nightmarish road, but I'm grateful for the lessons I wouldn't otherwise have learned about self-care, self-love, compassion, and the importance of work-life balance.

That mindset will carry you a long way, and it can help to think of your MCAS and sensitivities not as your enemy but as your body working extremely hard to take care of you and protect you from the pathogens, toxins, and stressors that have overwhelmed your system. In fact, without your mast cells you wouldn't be able to survive outside a bubble; they're that essential to your survival. It's easy for many of us who've dealt with these issues to feel sorry for ourselves, and it's okay to have those days. I had many meltdowns and many days of wanting to just throw in the towel, but ultimately I'd remember that giving up wouldn't get me anywhere. One of my mantras every time I thought I couldn't keep going was to say, "Well, Beth, what else are you going to do?"

Keep putting one foot in front of the other and, no matter what, find a way to continue moving forward. You might very well be the most sensitive and ill person you know, yet there are hundreds of thousands of people in the same boat. Here is a selection of case stories to inspire you:

A young woman had multiple seizures daily; she was unable to walk or communicate, struggled to tolerate the supplements and medications she needed, but recovered and has been able to return to college. A mother who was so chemically sensitive, fatigued, and brain fogged that she couldn't leave her home was traveling with her daughter and eating in restaurants a couple of years later. A young child covered head to toe with hives, unable to sleep, and struggling with foods, chemicals, and mold allergies, was completely hive free and off medications in one year. A man with severe GI symptoms who was down to two foods was eating normally again within three years. The mindset they all had in common was that they were determined to keep going, and had the patience to see the process through.

One of the ways I've kept myself going through my health battles was to remember that I'm not a victim, and that what I'm experiencing was not happening only to *me* (or to you) but happening to all of us in one form or another. The ways our toxic world have affected my health are much bigger than what I could control, but I focused on how I could make the world a better place and be an advocate to support others to live healthier lives. The more of us who refuse to buy toxic products, refuse to eat toxic foods, refuse to participate in crazymaking stress levels, and understand mold and EMFs, the more we will naturally influence those around us, which will continue to trickle out and change the world not only for ourselves but for our children, our grandchildren, and many future generations to come.

If you keep putting one foot in front of the other, no matter if it takes one year or ten years, you'll get there. Remember: We're all in this together. Believe in yourself. Believe in the others who've already gone through this and gotten better. Believe that we as a human race can make this world better. I'll be right here, believing along with you.

BETH O'HARA is a Functional Naturopathic Consultant, specializing in complex, chronic cases of Mast Cell Activation Syndrome, histamine intolerance, and mold toxicity. She is the founder and clinical director of Mast Cell 360, which she designed to be the kind of practice she wished had existed when she was severely ill with MCAS, histamine intolerance, mold toxicity, neural inflammation, Lyme Disease, fibromyalgia, and chronic fatigue. Beth's mission today is to be a guiding light for others with Mast Cell Activation Syndrome, histamine intolerance, and related conditions in their healing journeys. She holds a doctorate in Functional Naturopathy, a master's degree in Marriage and Family Therapy, and a bachelor's degree in Physiological Psychology. You can find a number of resources at mastcell360.com, including blogposts, courses, and information about the Mast Cell 360 practice. You can also join her community and get access to a number of free educational videos by liking the Mast Cell 360 page on Facebook.

Chapter 5: Spiky-Leaky Syndrome As a Trigger for Sensitization

Andrew J. Maxwell, MD, Deborah Wardly, MD, and Neil Nathan, MD

Drs. Andrew Maxwell and Deborah Wardly have made some seemingly disparate but very important observations in a unique description that pulls together an array of medical conditions into one unified theory that they call the Spiky-Leaky Syndrome (SLS). They have allowed me the opportunity to try to make this fascinating discovery accessible to patients so it can be understood as another component of what creates sensitization, and from this understanding, how to approach treatment from yet another perspective. Please note the continuing interwoven concepts and processes that underlie all of these chapters: here we will unite physiology with mast-cell activation, inflammation, and body structure.

We'll first provide an overview of this concept, and then go into a bit more detail. If at first the overview seems to contain some medical information you're not familiar with, bear with us as we bring it all together. This chapter is bit more technical than most of the others in this book. Given the complexity of body systems that comes into play here, we'll do our best to make these concepts clear. Some of this information might not apply to all of our sensitive patients, but to those whom it does apply to, it will help them and their physicians to understand their symptoms and learn about a novel approach to treatment.

Overview of the Spiky-Leaky Syndrome

The starting point of this idea springs from mast-cell activation and inflammation, both major components of everything we write about in this book. In a genetically susceptible patient who has a chronic inflammation created by mold or other environmental toxicity, or has an infection such as Lyme disease and has developed mast-cell activation, this combination (so common in our sensitive patients) will lead to the development of a hypermobile state (loose ligaments), often seen in patients with the diagnosis of Ehlers-Danlos syndrome. This in turn leads to a structural instability at the base of the skull (where it connects to the first cervical vertebra) and facial bones. This creates a phenomenon of musculoskeletal, vascular, lymphatic, and nerve injury in the upper neck; analogous to carpal tunnel syndrome of the wrist, it might therefore be considered "carpal tunnel syndrome of the neck." This creates a cascade of events that causes dysautonomia (dysfunction of the autonomic nervous system) and daytime/nighttime cycles of hyperventilation (breathing too fast) and hypopnea (shallow breathing due to increased airway resistance).

The result is a significant difference in carbon dioxide levels in the blood during the day and at night. To understand the significance of these shifts, it's important to understand that the carbon dioxide level in the body is what drives respiration. Our bodies give great weight to this because when CO_2 levels are high, we breathe faster and more deeply to lower them, and when CO_2 levels are low, our breathing becomes more shallow; hence, faster breathing lowers the carbon dioxide levels and raises oxygen levels. You might be unaware of these shifts as you sleep and go about your daytime activities, but your body must respond to this differential. Excessively fast breathing while awake occurs as a natural response to the dysautonomia. This is called sympathetic overdrive. It causes low carbon dioxide levels all day while you're awake and while you consciously or subconsciously protect your airway. Doing this chronically likely leads to the body being more sensitive to these changes in blood CO_2 levels. Shallow breathing with hypopnea in sleep will increase those levels and increase blood flow to the brain, which can raise intracranial pressure unless cerebrospinal fluid (CSF) can rapidly drain out of the skull via several different pathways.

The unstable anatomy at the base of the skull and facial areas in these patients may then also cause compression of the veins and lymphatic vessels in the neck, thereby interfering with the normal flow of spinal fluid and lymph out of the cranium and thus create an increase in intracranial pressure (the Spiky phase). Think of this as a rise, or spike, in that pressure. The body must find a way to release it. The normal pathway is via something called arachnoid granulations, which filter the cerebral spinal fluid and drain it onto the veins that help it leave the cranium. When this pathway is obstructed, there is an alternate pathway through the lymphatics, the potential cerebral-spinal fluid space along the cranial nerve sheaths. In SLS patients with compromised connective tissue, however, it can do this by leaking fluid through ruptures in the tight junctions of the cranial nerve sheaths, notably through the olfactory nerve into sinus and facial tissues where it leaks out through the nose and ears, into facial tissue, or down the throat (the Leaky phase). In a patient, this would appear in the morning as swelling of the face and sinus tissues in the nose, or fluid leaking from the ears or nose, and sometimes a metallic-tasting fluid leaking down the back of the throat.

Accordingly, Drs. Maxwell and Wardly have termed this Spiky-Leaky Syndrome, and have found that this explanation has helped them understand a wide variety of medical conditions that had not previously been understood. For many years I've had patients complain of fluid leaking from the ears and eyes; it made no sense to me, and I wrote it off as water that remained in their ears after a shower, but now we have a better explanation. I've also had patients with swelling of the face, sometimes quite severe, for which none of my treatments made much difference.

Given this information as a starting point, let's explore these concepts more deeply. To make this information accessible, I will at times oversimplify a much more complicated process. For greater depth, I encourage medical practitioners to contact Drs. Maxwell and Wardly directly.

Spiky-Leaky in More Depth

The observations Dr. Maxwell made on his patients are similar to mine and my colleagues'. We're dealing with a state of chronic inflammation, largely triggered by toxins and infectious agents, and usually accompanied by Mast Cell Activation Syndrome. Most have dysfunction of their autonomic nervous system (think limbic and vagal), which often shows up as POTS and blood pressure fluctuations, Chronic Fatigue Syndrome, and gastrointestinal dysfunction, plus many have hypermobility. In addition, Dr. Maxwell has noted that a great many of his patients have some form of sleep-disordered breathing. Obstructive sleep apnea is also known to cause chronic inflammation, and hypoxia has been noted to trigger mast-cell degranulation. Obstructive sleep apnea is a significant cause of intracranial hypertension, which produces headaches, tinnitus, visual changes, fatigue, and dizziness, symptoms common to the chronically ill.

In this setting (see chapters 15 and 16 on jaw dysfunction and structural issues), many of our patients have been seen to have cranio-cervical instability (CCI) and TMJ. From this information, Drs. Maxwell and Wardly have realized that there are important interconnections among all of these phenomena that not only allow us to understand what's happening at a deeper level but also lead to an expansion of our treatment options.

Signs and Symptoms of Spiky-Leaky Syndrome (SLS)

Hypermobility, often meeting criteria for Ehlers-Danlos Syndrome which often results in:

- Temporomandibular joint instability (TMJ)
- Cranio-cervical instability (CCI)
- Vertebrobasilar insufficiency (poor blood flow from the vertebral and basilar arteries to the brain)
- Myofascial Pain Syndrome
- Compression of veins, lymphatics and important nerves traversing in the space between the neck bones or cervical vertebrae from the back of the neck against the ligaments in the front of the neck. We call this space the "Eagle Space."
- Dysautonomia (with swings in blood pressure)
- Chronic inflammation
- Mast Cell Activation Syndrome
- Leaky gut
- Neuroinflammation secondary to leaky blood-brain barrier, which in turn may lead to:
- Anxiety
- Depression
- OCD (Obsessive Compulsive Disorder)
- Autism spectrum disorders
- Extreme unresponsiveness to therapies that would ordinarily work when directed at the causes or triggers for these conditions (e.g., mold or other environmental toxicities or Lyme disease). The frequent occurrence of these symptoms in other family members (no surprise, given that environmental exposure is a major trigger for this pathophysiology, plus the craniofacial structure that predisposes to sleep-disordered breathing is at least in part inherited from our parents.)
- PANDAS or PANS

PANDAS (Pediatric Autoimmune Neuropsychiatric Disorders Associated with Streptococcal Infections) and PANS (Pediatric Acute-Onset Neuropsychiatric Syndrome) usually occur after a strep infection. Brain inflammation occurs when the body's immune system mistakenly attacks healthy brain cells, leading to autoimmune effects on the central nervous system. An affected child generally has a sudden change in personality, displayed as obsessive-compulsive disorder (OCD), anxiety, tics or other abnormal movements, decline in math and handwriting abilities, acute-onset food restriction (associated with fear of contamination, poisoning, or choking,) sensory sensitivities, and more. Research suggests that in the U.S. alone, 1 in 200 children have PANDAS—a stunning number, especially considering that many doctors, medical professionals, and clinicians don't recognize PANDAS as an autoimmune disease. Sadly, many children go untreated, and sometimes experience debilitating symptoms for years until they're taken to see a PANDAS specialist.

Symptoms that Reflect Both Intracranial Hypertension and CSF Leak

- Severe headaches upon awakening
- Pulsatile tinnitus – rhythmic thumping, whooshing, or throbbing in one or both ears
- Fullness and pressure in the head
- Restless sleep with anxiety when attempting to lie flat
- Preference to sleep with the head elevated at 10 degrees or more
- Bruxism (clenching of the jaw while sleeping)
- Obstructive sleep apnea (OSA)
- Upper airway resistance syndrome (UARS)
- Restrictive movement of the tongue
- Non-migraine headache described as "bobblehead" or "my head feels like a bowling ball"

Pain In the Throat

- Aching pain at the back of the throat or base of the tongue with the feeling of a mass at the back of the throat on swallowing (globus)
- Sharp, stabbing pain at the front of the throat made worse when turning the neck
- Fullness, tightness near the lymph nodes in the neck
- Pain and sensitivity of the scalp, which might appear to be occipital neuralgia
- Extreme pain and tightness of the trapezius muscle (the thick muscle at the top of the shoulder

Ear symptoms

- Sensitivity to sound (hyperacusis)
- Tinnitus and/or vertigo
- Pain in the ear canals or middle ear

Symptoms of Vertebrobasilar Insufficiency

- Brain fog
- Headache
- Fatigue
- Decreased vision in the sitting position relieved by upward cranial traction
- History of sudden "drop attacks"
- History of narcolepsy or cataplexy

Symptoms Similar to Chiari Malformation

- Pressure headache aggravated by Valsalva maneuver (a forceful attempt to exhale against a closed airway, done by closing the mouth and pinching the nose shut)

- Numbness, tingling and weakness in the arms and legs
- Loss of hand grip strength
- Swallowing difficulties
- Speaking difficulties or hoarseness
- Fine hand motor skills
- Nystagmus (repetitive, uncontrolled eye movements)
- Signs of sacral nerve dysfunction (occult tethered cord, fixation of the terminal end of the spinal cord)
- Irritable bladder and bowel
- Constipation
- Ataxia
- Low end-tidal carbon dioxide measurement in daytime
- History of chronic sinusitis
- Worsening of symptoms after sinus surgery or orthodontic procedures

While some patients may exhibit a variety of these symptoms, the point in laying this out is to consider the possibility that symptoms that have previously been unexplained, or baffling, might now come into clear focus with the delineation of this model.

Physiological Interactions of the Spiky-Leaky Syndrome

While the comprehensive model proposed by Drs. Maxwell and Wardly is beyond the scope of this chapter, I'll briefly explain some of these interactions to introduce the reader to the process described here.

For most patients, the onset of their difficulties begins with single or multiple triggers in genetically predisposed individuals. That illness creates a chronic inflammatory response, which in turn triggers significant mast-cell activation. In addition to setting off a leaky gut and compromise of the blood-brain barrier, these inflammatory processes weaken, or "tenderize," the ligaments, resulting in craniocervical instability (CCI), which leads to three major phenomena:

1. Upper airway resistance syndrome (UARS)
2. Sympathetic overdrive (stress response promoted by the sympathetic nervous system)
3. Jugular venous and lymphatic compression

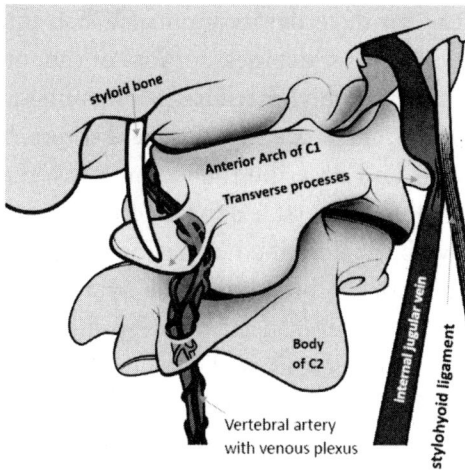

Craniocervical Instability with Vascular Compressions: *Anterolateral view of the C0-C1-C2 joints showing anterior slippage of C1 (atlas) relative to C2 (axis) causing the transverse process(es) of C1 to compress the internal jugular vein (uni- or bilaterally) into the styloid bone or stylohyoid ligament thereby obstructing venous return causing back-pressure on CSF drainage. Vertebral venous plexus drainage is also likely compromised. The vertebral arteries and venous plexus are also stretched and compressed (uni- or bilaterally) leading to vertebrobasilar insufficiency. The anterior slippage is thought to occur from various weakened ligaments responsible for stabilization in this region. This has been called 'jugular vein bone nutcracker' or Eagle Jugular Syndrome or Styloidogenic Jugular Venous Compression Syndrome*

In this figure, note especially the compression of the internal jugular vein (on the right of the image) compressed by the stylohyoid ligament. This will give you a better picture of the type of compressional forces involved in this model.

The sympathetic overdrive is a natural reflex to parasympathetic dysautonomia resulting from vagal nerve injury or dysfunction, and results in chronic hyperventilation driving down carbon dioxide as well as setting off anxiety, racing heart, and insomnia.

The large difference between daytime and nighttime CO_2 levels causes a dramatic increase in nighttime cerebral blood flow and blood volume. The displaced cerebral spinal fluid (CSF) cannot filter by normal means due to jugular and epidural venous backpressure. Hence CSF pressure rises and displaces into cranial nerve sheaths (the Spiky phase).

CSF pressure rises, causing intracranial hypertension until it is released at the end of the cranial nerve-sheath cuffs, notably the end of the olfactory nerve (the Leaky phase).

Part of the mechanism for how SLS creates a sensitive patient is in this idea of cranial nerve edema resulting from the spike and leak process. This has been termed the Wardly Phenomenon, the presence of symptomatology referable to the dysfunction of multiple cranial nerves, and which our authors propose is then suggestive of a process involving an elevation of intracranial pressure. For example, one might have odor hypersensitivity and auditory hypersensitivity, referable to swelling of both the olfactory and the auditory nerves. Involvement of the vestibular nerve might produce vertigo or balance issues, and involvement of the vagus nerve can produce dysautonomia. When intracranial pressure is very high, it can even cause blindness, deafness, or loss of the sense of smell, but in SLS patients the pressure never gets so high because it "pops-off" and drains out before that can happen. The sensory problems are therefore less severe, but unfortunately, as patients express their concerns and describe their symptoms, these may be invalidated by health professionals who don't understand these concepts.

Patients with intracranial hypertension have been described as having these types of sensory problems, as have patients with disordered breathing. The symptoms of insomnia and anxiety seen in sensitive patients can be caused by sleep-disordered breathing. In one study, 90% of nocturnal awakenings were caused by sleep-disordered breathing. If, therefore, a sensitive patient has such symptoms, a good sleep study would be an important part of their evaluation. SLS is a narrow subset of a type of sensitive patient, but it encompasses various pathophysiologies that by themselves can produce such sensitivity.

Some of this might be a bit much to take in all at once, but the point of this discussion is to help the reader understand that, thanks to Drs. Maxwell and Wardly, we now have a clear and plausible explanation for exactly how these physiological shifts occur, so we can understand some of the underpinnings of sensitization and now move on to some possible therapeutic interventions to help our patients.

Diagnostic Clues for the Spiky-Leaky Syndrome

The tests currently available to make this diagnosis are just generally suggestive, so this is now primarily a clinical diagnosis. That doesn't change the importance of making this diagnosis or empirically treating it. The kinds of tests that will, we believe, ultimately be developed to be able to make this diagnosis are:

1. Identifying the presence of CCI with accuracy will require appropriate imaging. Much of the imaging that leads to satisfactory diagnosis is still a work in progress. MRI images in various positions with and without traction might be revealing but are often not. Digital Motion X-Ray (DMX) might add further to the diagnosis. Some of the most reliable imaging has been from Cone Beam CT Scans (CBCT), which allow simultaneous assessment of the cervical bones for signs of instability as well as the soft tissues of the mouth and neck, including the airway. CT Scans of the cervical spine with contrast can show arterial and venous compression; however, the risk of exposure to CT contrast must be weighed against the value of obtaining such results. An MRI or other forms of imaging would include performing that test with and without traction, and supine compared to upright. Ultrasound imaging of the spinal cord of the C1 and C2 nerve roots would be helpful.

2. Studies to accurately identify increased intracranial pressure or CSF leak are not often helpful as these patients tend to have high CSF pressure only while deeply asleep at night while retaining carbon dioxide. Furthermore, evaluation by lumbar puncture risks causing a chronic CFS leak in EDS patients. Doctors often look for signs of increased CSF by looking at the retinas of their eyes. This is to look for papilledema. This too can be tricky because the pressure is only high when the patient is deeply asleep.

3. Studies of carbon dioxide levels while asleep and awake (continuous TcO2 and TcCO2 monitoring), to complement a full polysomnogram, which includes evaluation for UARS. There are various ways to measure daytime CO_2 with monitors as well. Dr Maxwell uses a full metabolic exercise test so he can look at the hyperventilation under resting and exercise settings. Resting values can be easily altered by the patient's current state of anxiety, but it is difficult to alter the CO_2 state during exercise no matter one's state of anxiety or any other state that might alter daytime CO_2 levels.

4. Continuous intracranial pressure measurements

5. Continuous intrathecal lumbar pressure measurements

Potential Treatments for Spiky-Leaky Syndrome

Dr. Maxwell has already successfully used some of the following strategies to treat this syndrome, which adds a great deal of weight to these hypotheses. A description of possible treatments includes:

1. Noticing that patients who are being treated with BiPAP do much better than those who use CPAP (because CPAP can elevate intracranial pressure in susceptible patients due to an increase in Valsalva compared to BiPAP).
2. Surgical maxillomandibular advancement may correct the anatomical problem that predisposes to both airway resistance and impaired jugular venous drainage.
3. Tongue retaining devices may help.
4. Surgical corrections in restrictions of tongue mobility, via release of tongue-ties, might help.
5. Orofacial myofunctional therapy might help.
6. Correction and strengthening of the TMJ is important.
7. Enhancement of head and neck lymphatic drainage is important.
8. Stylohyoid ligament release may relieve internal jugular and lymphatic drainage. Some have found that side-to-side or lateral expansion of the oral palate can achieve this same effect.
9. Methods of reducing CSF production and circulation are important.
   a. Carbonic hydrase inhibitors may be helpful, at least in the short term.
   b. Methods for reducing carbon dioxide levels at night and increasing them by day would be helpful.

10. Methods of early intervention would be ideal:
    k. Avoidance or removal of environmental triggers;
    l. Treatment of Mast Cell Activation Syndrome with the appropriate medications and supplements; and
    m. Early treatment of craniofacial issues in children with such modalities as tonsillectomy/adenoidectomy, expansive orthodonture, and myofunctional therapy as described above.

You can see how well this model dovetails with much of the information presented throughout this book. The discussion of triggers, including mold toxicity, environmental toxins, and infections, is clearly relevant here. The discussions of jaw physiology and osteopathic treatments, as well as the information on mast-cell activation, again help us integrate this information with this model.

ANDREW J. MAXWELL, MD, FACC, is a pediatrician and pediatric cardiologist practicing in Northern California (Heart of the Valley Pediatric Cardiology). He received his training at Johns Hopkins Medical School and The University of California at San Francisco, with fellowships in Pediatric Cardiology and Cardiovascular Research at Stanford University and Children's Hospital of Philadelphia.

His research interests include study of endothelial control of vasomotor tone, nitric oxide, sports cardiology, dysautonomia, POTS, Mast Cell Activation Syndrome, and hypermobile Ehlers Danlos Syndrome, and their relationship to environmental exposure.

DEBORAH WARDLY, MD, is a board-certified pediatrician and Fellow of the American Academy of Pediatrics. She practiced general pediatrics from 1991 to 2009. She has been involved in research and hypothesis work, and has published papers on the topics of sleep-disordered breathing and intracranial hypertension.

Chapter 6: The Biochemistry of Sensitivity

Kurt N. Woeller, DO

Dr. Nathan's Introduction

The underlying cause of dysfunction in the limbic system, the vagal system, and in mast-cell activation is inflammation. Virtually every chapter of this book includes references to the pivotal role inflammation plays in the initiation and persistence of sensitivity. For some of you, just understanding that is sufficient. For those who wish to dig deeper into the process, Dr. Woeller helps us grasp the newest information available to put the entire subject of inflammation into fuller perspective. This includes dissecting the immune system into its innate and adaptive components and learning about PAMPS, DAMPS, HAMPS, and APCs, with the idea that once we comprehend these elements, we can have a better understanding of how inflammation leads directly to sensitization. Using a patient's case study, he amplifies this discussion and then provides a blueprint for leading a healthy lifestyle.

✪ ✪ ✪

For many individuals with chronic health problems, particularly those exposed to environmental toxins and/or biotoxins, the prevalence of physiological sensitivity is a reality in their daily lives. It can manifest in various ways, intensifying or diminishing for unknown reasons, and might change in its nature over time. I first recognized this early in my career when I was trying to help a woman with debilitating fatigue and environmental sensitivities following mold exposure in her condominium. Her list of complaints:

- Food sensitivity described as a burning sensation in her mouth, throat, and stomach
- Light sensitivity that would lead to headaches and mental fatigue
- Intense mental fogginess and lethargy after exposures to perfumes, colognes, laundry detergent, air fresheners and other synthetic chemicalized scents, e.g., scented candles
- Immediate skin itching on eating foods such as fruits and high-oxalate vegetables, e.g., kale
- Fluctuating muscle and joint pain that worsened with consuming raw vegetables or vegetable juice
- Histamine reactions when stressed

Of course, an extensive list of physical sensitivities can manifest in different individuals for various reasons. With no two people exactly alike, the symptom picture of sensitivity can be complex and confusing; however, it's not uncommon for a physically sensitive person to exhibit a few or more of the following complaints:

- Allergic reactions such as hives, inflammation, itching, and swelling
- Acid sensation in the mouth, throat, esophagus, and/or stomach, often described as a burning sensation
- Muscle burning
- Urinary discomfort and/or a feeling of pressure or achiness in the kidneys
- Electrical, buzzing, or vibrating sensations along the spine, neck, and head, which can reverberate into the extremities
- Crawling sensations on the skin
- Shooting pains in muscles and/or joints
- Muscle twitching or spasms
- "Strange" taste in the mouth
- Light sensitivity leading to headaches and mental or physical fatigue
- Phantom smells

Definition of Sensitivity

The definition of sensitivity changes depending on how it's applied and in which context it's used. In general, sensitivity means "the capacity to respond to changes in the environment." With regard to a living organism, this translates into the ability of an organism or sense organ, e.g., olfactory system, to respond to stimulation. The stimulation that triggers a response can be chemical, electrical, pressure, temperature, etc. Here our emphasis is on physical sensitivities, not emotional or mental ones. It needs to be emphasized, however, that all of us are complex beings who exist moment to moment within the intertwined physical, mental, and emotional realms. These cannot be separated, but there can be pure physical manifestations, i.e., cramping pain, or twitching in a muscle, which can occur outside the realm of the psyche. By sheer confluence of cellular reactivity and chemical signaling, along with disruption in cellular homeostatic control mechanisms, certain "physical" imbalances causing a muscle spasm or pain can manifest on their own.

From a biological or physiological standpoint, the term "sensitivity" takes on a different meaning for an organism as it relates to its environment. For example, many of our cells are sensitive to changes in pH (the chemical nature of acidity and alkalinity), sugar levels, and electrolyte balance (sodium and potassium concentrations), and through this recognition a variety of cellular mechanisms are initiated. A good example is the process of eating food. The physiological act of eating involves many sensory organs and cellular chemicals, along with the motor control over chewing, swallowing, and digesting of foodstuffs. Here's how it works:

At the smell of some delicious food (either alone or in combination with visual recognition), chemicals from the food interact with cellular receptors (aka chemical receivers) within our nose. These receptors transmit a chemical signal through the olfactory nerve to the brain.

Upon receiving this chemical signal, the olfactory nerve has its cell membrane change in its chemical equilibrium (aka depolarization), causing an influx of extracellular (outside the cell) sodium and an outflux of internal potassium. This chemical switch triggers electrical movement through the olfactory nerve to centers in the brain. Different areas of the brain, including cells in and around the hypothalamus, receive the signals from the olfactory nerve. Messages for appetite, salivation, and gastric contraction are then sent to many of the digestive organs, including the stomach, in preparation for the incoming food.

As food is placed in the mouth, salivary digestive enzymes have already been triggered. At the same time, additional nerve signals are sent throughout the digestive system in preparation for this food moving into the stomach and small intestine for eventual digestion and assimilation of nutrients. *Which of us hasn't felt the gurgling and growling of the stomach from just the sight and smell of food?*

The physical act of chewing requires both motor control of the mouth muscles and proprioceptive nerve feedback to the brain for continued smooth and coordinated movement of the jaws. Once the food in the mouth is sufficiently broken down, it moves to the back of the throat, which triggers the swallowing mechanism to move the bolus of food into the stomach.

There, already prepped by the early signaling from the brain, parietal cells release hydrochloric acid (HCl) and chief cells release pepsinogen. These two chemicals are linked with the goal to enhance protein breakdown. The pepsinogen, under the influence of the acid nature of HCl, is converted into pepsin, which chemically acts on food protein to split it up into smaller components.

In the stomach, this bolus of food, now called chyme, is moved toward the distal end of the stomach, aka pylorus region. As it passes through the pyloric valve into the first part of the small intestine, it's met by additional enzymes and acid buffers produced by the pancreas.

From there, the chyme continues to move through the small intestine for nutrient absorption, and eventually moves into the large intestine where the remaining substances coalesce into fecal matter.

Except for the process of physical chewing and swallowing, this entire process acts automatically as a coordinated dance between the complex nature of the sensory, motor, and autonomic (aka automatic) nervous system relationships. In general, the biochemistry of sensitivity is not always something under our conscious control.

When Sensitivities Go Wrong

The sensing aspect of biology is established within the fundamentals of cellular and molecular biology. This science has emerged over the past several decades through advanced technology and greater understanding of biochemistry, receptor sensitivity, intracellular communication systems, and much more. I'll focus only on a few important aspects of these complex interactions as they relate to the biochemistry (aka chemistry of biology) of sensitivity. Even a basic understanding of these following systems can provide an individual suffering from chronic illness with a deeper understanding of how the body is supposed to function, recognition of overlapping systems, and certain strategies for helping reestablish normal (or improved) function.

The section title "When Sensitivities Go Wrong" is not meant to insinuate that our biology is doing something inherently wrong. Rather, it's acting in a way that's appropriate to its inherent nature, but the ramifications for us as individuals might not always feel good or be desired. For example, when we encounter an environmental allergen such as pollen from a spring bloom, certain body cells, called mast cells, become sensitized and release histamine, which triggers a series of appropriate biochemical reactions intrinsic to its nature, but the symptoms that ensue—nasal congestion, cough, itching, and sometimes hives—are unpleasant. Taken to an extreme, overactivity of mast cells and the associated chemistry can trigger acute anaphylaxis, or even an insidious chronic condition of heightened cell sensitivity called Mast Cell Activation Syndrome (see chapter 4 for a detailed discussion).

It's important to understand that a symptom is a manifestation of a biochemical reaction causing a cellular change as a reflection of that cell's response to a changing environment. The environment where the cell lives and functions includes not only other cells in its immediate environment but the fluid dynamics outside and inside the cell. A confluence of symptoms might therefore be difficult for us as individuals (including doctors) to figure out, but a symptom (or multiple symptoms) is a message sent by the body that certain cellular and biological systems are reacting and responding to various changes.

Cellular Mechanisms as They Relate to Biochemical Sensitivity

For this discussion, there are three fundamental components that can increase physical sensitivity in the chronically ill, particularly with regard to environmental sensitivity, which can manifest in various ways such as fatigue, brain fog, and food reactions. The three components are abbreviated PAMP, DAMP, and HAMP; which I'll describe, and the key to this discussion is that *these are all aspects of inflammation.* To understand inflammation we need to examine the workings of the immune system.

Before I detail the relationship between PAMP-DAMP-HAMP, we need a basic understanding of immune function as it relates to cell-to-cell communication, as well as systems within the cell that register imbalances in homeostasis (defined as state of equilibrium maintained by self-regulating processes).

The immune system is highly complex and involves multiple cell types that coordinate to recognize, and initiate acute and long-term defenses against, a variety of pathogens that exist in our world. As a brief overview, I'll describe the basic function of the main categories of the immune system, which are called *innate* and *adaptive*. Then we'll dig a bit deeper into the ways in which the immune system recognizes pathogens, toxins, etc., and coordinates this information for a broader integration of homeostatic control. *At the core of this process, we're looking at an inflammatory process that is essentially out of our control.*

Overview of Immune Function for Pathogen Detection and Inflammation Activation

The human immune system is well adapted to recognize and respond to the various pathogens it encounters. There are three main categories of immune function: *physical barriers, innate, and adaptive.*

The physical barriers of our body are made up of the skin and mucosal surfaces (those cells that line our bladder, digestive system, nose, sinuses, upper and lower respiratory tract, urethra, and vagina). Our skin provides a barrier defense against opportunistic pathogens, but when the skin is breached by a pathogen, either from inflammation or injury, anti-pathogenic chemicals are produced at the barrier level. If these don't work to stop the infection, our innate immunity steps in.

The innate immune system includes white blood cells such as neutrophils, monocytes, and macrophages (aka "big eaters") that are not intrinsically affected by prior pathogen or toxin exposure (these are often referred to as antigens). An antigen is a substance—usually foreign, such as bacteria, foreign blood cells, toxins, or viruses—that, when introduced into the body, stimulates an immune reaction. Innate immunity responds similarly with each encounter, and does not need to be trained by prior exposure. A good example is the mast-cell reaction mentioned earlier when we're exposed to a pollen.

The adaptive immune system, also referred to as acquired immunity, is highly specialized to react to various pathogens. This includes the B-cells (derived from *b*one marrow) and T-cells (derived from bone marrow but matured in the *t*hymus gland). Adaptive immunity has a primary immune memory capacity for pathogens of previous exposure.

When considering both systems, innate and adaptive, it's the adaptive that has millions of options for immune-system diversity through its multitude of chemical configurations. The innate system is more limited in its scope of diversity of immune activity. Interestingly, the adaptive component is a more recently evolved immunological system (in relative biology terms, which can mean thousands of years); whereas the innate system is ancient, primitive, and has likely been at work in various life forms, e.g., microorganisms, for millions of years.

These systems complement one another, and both are essential for a healthy and robust immune system, but they play different roles within the body, and imbalances in either can create problems. For example, with regard to our previous discussion of mast cells and pollen exposure, these innate immune cells respond pretty much the same way each time we encounter a pollen: with a release of histamine and the corresponding symptoms of allergy.

Problems that occur within the innate system can cause increased reactivity of mast cells and aggressive production of histamine; or the problem could lie within the adaptive immune system through an antibody protein called IgE. IgE is a type of immune protein (aka immunoglobulin or antibody) that is produced because of prior exposure to a pollen.

IgE can activate mast cells in response to a pollen as part of the coordinated communication between the innate and adaptive immune systems. Like everything else in the body, nothing exists in isolation, and through complex and multi-diverse biochemistry there are a multitude of communication mechanisms for whole-body integration.

A key to this whole-body integration are the receptors found on the outer surface of each cell or buried inside the cell either as free-floating receptors or those attached to various organelles (cell organs). Certain receptors can float freely in body fluids too, which includes antibodies like IgE. You can think of antibodies (IgA, IgD, IgG, IgE, and IgM) as specialized receptors involved in immune function. It's critical to understand that a receptor is a cellular component that recognizes and responds to other cellular signals (chemicals) to initiate some type of cell activity.

A receptor is a door to the cell; the door is opened by chemical stimulation and allows entry of a substance into the cell or triggers downstream chemical reactions that influence a specific cell response. For example, each mast cell has receptors for IgE. When IgE binds to the mast cell, this interaction causes a downstream effect within the mast cell to release histamine.

Before we move on, I'll briefly describe an important aspect of cell biology, immunology, and tissue reactivity called inflammation. We've all experienced inflammation, whether it was itchy, red eyes from allergies, nasal congestion from a cold, or a swollen ankle after accidently twisting it. Inflammation is normal and a necessary component of immune function; however, too much inflammation can be problematic and lead to tissue damage, scarring, or in extreme cases autoimmunity, in which the immune system attacks the body's own tissue.

Within the category of the innate immune system are polymorphonuclear (PMNs) cells such as basophils, eosinophils, and neutrophils. Macrophages, either as tissue-resident cells or derived from circulating monocytes (another cell within the innate immune system), play an important role in engulfing (aka phagocytizing) antigens (e.g., pathogens) that have first been processed by tissue-infiltrating neutrophils. For the sake of this discussion, the focus here will be on the relationship between neutrophils and macrophages in a process called apoptotic (programmed cell death) PMN activation for macrophage engulfment.

When a bacteria or fungus pathogen invades a tissue such as the skin or lining of the digestive tract, certain immune chemicals are released that call into action blood-circulating neutrophils to infiltrate the tissue area and destroy the pathogen. Once the neutrophil has "neutralized" the pathogen, it transforms into an apoptotic PMN (e.g., apoptotic neutrophil).

Apoptosis is a process in which a cell dies naturally through intrinsic cell mechanisms that trigger this event. Apoptosis is a normal, natural, and highly desirable process. For example, there are mechanisms in the immune system that can trigger apoptotic mechanisms in abnormal cells before they become cancerous. The apoptotic neutrophil has a limited amount of time to be destroyed and cleared from the tissue area before it begins to degrade, releasing its internal enzyme granules. An important role of a macrophage is to engulf the apoptotic PMN before it degrades, and clear it from the tissue area via the locally available lymph system. If the apoptotic PMNs are not cleared efficiently, they will break down, release their granules, and cause more tissue inflammation.

There is a key element to this discussion that must be understood: A cell that is undergoing apoptosis will not trigger inflammation (or at least significant inflammation), but a cell that has been damaged by infection, injury, or surrounding tissue inflammation can go through necrosis (death of cells through injury or disease, especially in a localized area of a tissue or organ). Tissue necrosis can engage the immune system in nefarious ways and lead to the potential for autoimmunity.

In many situations it's desirable to have the innate immune system take care of the infectious problem. It can act quickly and efficiently without too much cellular chemical complexity. There is, however, a time and place to activate the adaptive immune system too, to help form long-term immune memory against a pathogen, or if the innate system is overrun and further help is needed. Remember also that the innate immune system may be limited in its capacity to recognize and deal with the multitude of pathogens or other non-pathogenic antigens; therefore, there needs to be a way to connect the innate and adaptive immune systems so they can work together seamlessly to integrate the receptors and chemical signaling mechanisms. For this next part of our discussion, I'll focus on specialized receptors called PRRs (Pattern Recognition Receptors) and their recognition of Pathogen Associated Molecular Patterns (PAMPs).

Pattern Recognition Receptors and Pathogen Associated Molecular Patterns

Our immune system is linked to various tissue receptors, such as those in the gastrointestinal (GI) tract, that contain what are called PRRs (pattern recognition receptors). There are receptors throughout the body, not just the digestive system; however, I'll use the GI tract as an example of a PRR and pathogen associated molecule pattern (PAMP). Each PRR is unique for a specific PAMP. For example, the *candida* species, which can be normal inhabitants within our digestive system, contains various layers to its cell membrane.

An important inner layer called β-glucan (beta-glucan) is a type of PAMP that our GI cell PRRs can recognize. The *candida* organism tries to shield the β-glucan PAMP from our host immune surveillance system (innate and adaptive immunity).

When a fungal organism such as *candida* contacts the epithelial surface of a GI cell, various PAMPs are recognized by host cell PRRs, which elicits an innate immune response. Unfortunately (and this is just one aspect of the invasive diversity of *candida*), the initiating act of this organism interacting with an epithelial cell also triggers a series of chemical reactions within the *candida* organism to become invasive. The PRR-PAMP interaction is critical with regard to immune recognition and action against a pathogen.

Within the innate immune system are additional cells called antigen presenting cells (APCs) which relay information about a specific PAMP to a naïve (aka virgin) T-cell, which is part of the adaptive immune system. A naïve T-cell is an adaptive immune cell that has not been previously presented with an antigen. Macrophages (innate immune cells) can act as an APC, but it is the dendritic cell (DC) that plays the primary role as an APC.

The naïve T-cell links to various other T-cell types such as cytotoxic T-cells (CD8) and T-helper cells (CD4) like Th1 and Th2. There are also other T-cells that are important, including T-regulatory (Treg) and Th17 cells. The implications of these different cells can be important for immune system reactivity to various types of pathogens and toxins. The coordination between these varied T-cell types is beyond the scope of this discussion, but for the sake of completion, here's a brief description as it relates to immune surveillance of intracellular and extracellular pathogens and immune tolerance:

- Th1 cells are directed toward intracellular pathogens such as viruses. For many years Th1 cells in excess were felt to play a major role in autoimmune reactions.
- Th2 cells are directed toward extracellular parasites and can be involved in allergy and asthma.
- Th17 cells are directed toward extracellular bacteria and fungus. They are now recognized to play a significant role in autoimmunity. Th17 cells are important for mucosal reactivity against fungus, e.g., *Candida albicans, Aspergillus,* or *Penicillium.*
- Treg (T-regulatory) cells are regulators of overall immune responses, immune tolerance (to aide against immune attack against self-tissue), and homeostasis.

The relationship between these T-cells is a complicated dance coordinated by immune chemicals, cell membrane receptors, and second messenger reactions (additional chemical chain reactions within the cell), including various transcription factors that induce protein production through DNA and RNA genetic influences.

Bringing this discussion back to our primary objective with regards to the biochemistry of sensitivity, I want to introduce a few other components as they relate to cellular and molecular biology. I have briefly described PAMPs (pathogen associated molecular patterns), which are unique molecular patterns of various pathogens that our innate immune system recognizes through our cells' PRRs (pattern recognition receptors).

Damage to a cell from disease or injury can lead to necrosis. This unfortunate event can also trigger innate immunity to try to clean up the area, but instead of a potentially advantageous PRR-PAMP interaction, what ensues is a PRR-DAMP interaction. DAMP stands for Danger Associated Molecular Patterns. The DAMPs are associated with self-components of cells normally sequestered away from the immune system. It is the PRR-DAMP reaction that may trigger more tissue inflammation mechanisms and/or autoimmune reactions. In brief, autoimmunity is a condition in which one's immune system attacks self-tissues. Some examples of autoimmune disease are rheumatoid arthritis, lupus, and Hashimoto's thyroiditis. The problem with autoimmune reactions is they lead to autoinflammation, which is defined as inflammation caused or exacerbated by an autoimmune reaction.

Both the PRR-PAMP and PRR-DAMP scenarios may cause or worsen a sensitive individual's condition. Dysfunctions in the immune system can lead to conditions in which communication between the innate and adaptive immune systems is not normal, and triggers disadvantageous chemical reactions within cells that drive the biochemistry of sensitivity.

There is one other mechanism I want to introduce that likely plays a fundamental role in sensitivity issues and cellular imbalances. It is called HAMP (Homeostasis Associated Molecular Patterns).

The concept behind HAMPs comprises the cellular components, e.g., organelles, chemical messenger systems, receptors, and various molecules, all being involved in the communication network that maintains harmony within the cell. When there's harmony, there are usually pro-harmony chemicals released by the cell; these then signal other cells to act in a unifying harmonic way. When components of the cell are altered by imbalances, however, e.g., nutritional, environmental, or genetic, then homeostatic control can be altered. When homeostasis is out of balance, the cell gives off chemical signals that the immune system can recognize as abnormal. It is possible that HAMPs may drive cellular imbalances outside the usual PAMP and DAMP mechanisms. Still, there are consequences for the individual in feeling the symptom effects of imbalanced homeostasis mechanisms at the cellular level.

A multitude of pathogenic environmental toxins and exposures can trigger HAMPs within the body, including:

- Biotoxins, e.g., animal or insect poisons
- Electromagnetic fields (EMFs), 5G, etc.
- Environmental chemical toxins, e.g., glyphosate
- Heavy metals
- Hormone disruptors
- Mold and mycotoxins
- Nutritional deficiencies

It's possible that cellular components themselves can trigger HAMP reactions such as adenosine triphosphate (ATP) release from the breakdown of mitochondria or changes in pH, fluid dynamics, and electrical potentials. Mental and emotional stressors may also signal cellular imbalances through receptor engagement from stress hormones and altered chemistry.

It's quite possible that the newly appreciated area of cellular biology linked to HAMPs and the complex interaction between our environment (both internal and external), along with unique genetic variants and intracellular self-preservation defense mechanisms, all linked through the PAMP-DAMP-HAMP relationship, is central to an individual's biochemical sensitivity.

My Patient With Mold Exposure

Earlier, I described a woman who developed significant environment illness from a chronic mold exposure. Many of her complaints can be linked to a PAMP-DAMP-HAMP interaction. For example, her issue of food sensitivity causing mouth, throat, and stomach burning is sometimes seen with mold exposure leading to infection. The mold organism (in her case the common opportunistic mold *Aspergillus* encountered in water-damaged building material) can colonize the digestive system, triggering a PAMP-PRR reaction. This interaction increases immune activity that tries to control the mold by attacking it with proinflammatory chemicals; however, the chronicity of the infection and subsequent prolonged inflammation can lead to DAMP expression, which further exacerbates the situation.

Because fungal organisms have various ways of infiltrating tissues, including the lining of the digestive system, chronic inflammation leads to increased intestinal permeability. This increase, called leaky gut, is another complicating factor seen in chronic fungal infections. With a leaky gut there is enhanced absorption of chemical compounds normally retained in the digestive system. These compounds, which can include various proteins or fragments of cellular debris, interact with the immune system, causing a shift away from normal activity toward autoimmune and autoinflammatory patterns. Her histamine issues, e.g., itching, can also, in part, be linked to imbalances in the digestive system, which allow for increased histamine release following loss of cellular regulatory control.

Oxalate, aka oxalic acid, is a compound found in many types of foods such as almonds, kale, spinach, and soy. Accumulation of oxalate leads to tissue inflammation, joint and muscle pain, and urinary tract discomfort. Kidney stones can occur from high levels of circulating oxalate (see chapter 12).

Aspergillus and *candida* are known producers of oxalic acid. In this woman's case, much of her body pain was linked to elevated oxalate occurring not only from consuming high oxalate foods but from fungal production within the digestive system. To make matters worse, oxalate absorption from the digestive system is enhanced in the presence of a leaky gut.

Oxalate is a chelator (a binder of certain metals) of various minerals such as calcium, copper, magnesium, and zinc. As these nutrient levels are sequestered by oxalate, they become less available for cellular metabolism, including the mitochondrial activity necessary for energy production. This correlates with many of my patient's issues related to fatigue, mental fogginess, and body discomfort.

The HAMP component of her illness, at first glance, can be more challenging to recognize until we appreciate that the cellular mechanisms that control normal cell function are often damaged or hijacked by environmental exposures (in her case mold and mycotoxins), and increase subsequent susceptibility to other entities such as viruses and bacterial infections. As a defense against these, our cells have intrinsic mechanisms that work to protect important biochemical systems. For example, the mitochondria can trigger a necessary and advantageous cell-death response after a toxin exposure that could lead to cancer development. These mechanisms simply shut down vulnerable metabolic pathways for self-preservation.

This cellular self-preservation response, which turns off aspects of normal cell function, has a strong correlation to HAMP and can lead to a host of seemingly unrelated symptoms such as chemical, light, and pressure sensitivity, brain fog, buzzing and vibrating sensations, chronic fatigue, etc., depending on which organ system in the body is being affected.

What complicated this woman's situation was the ongoing mental and emotional stress she dealt with from being the sole provider of her livelihood, and that the condominium mold contamination scenario involved ongoing litigation.

The process of healing in this case took time and involved sacrifice and hard work from the person involved. A synopsis of some of the things done to help in her healing follows. (Some of these steps are discussed in more detail later in this chapter.)

- Removal from place of exposure. This is key for anyone with ongoing mold exposure. If you continue to live in the place that has active mold, the chances of recovery are nearly impossible.
- Treatment of underlying mold colonization through antifungal therapy. This involved prescription medications such as oral nystatin, oral amphotericin B, fluconazole (Diflucan), and itraconazole (Sporanox).
- The combined use of botanical remedies supportive against opportunistic pathogens, e.g., *aspergillus* and *candida,* such as allicin, berberine, caprylic acid, and oregano, along with intestinal binders including activated charcoal, zeolite, and bentonite clay for mycotoxins.
- Nutrient support from a whole-food diet and supportive supplements for mitochondria health, e.g., CoQ10 (ubiquinol), nicotinamide adenine dinucleotide (NAD), riboflavin (vitamin B2), and for liver detoxification and digestion, enzymes and probiotics were essential.

- Calcium and magnesium citrate supplementation, along with a low-oxalate diet, helped reduce oxalate absorption and subsequent inflammation and body pain.
- Multiminerals, including magnesium (glycinate), zinc, and copper, helped replenish sequestered minerals from oxalate binding.
- Natural sunlight exposure for vitamin D activation.
- Consistent hydration through purified water, along with daily dietary fiber to maintain normal daily bowel movements. The two most common causes of constipation are lack of fiber and dehydration. Constipation leads to bowel toxin accumulation and often exacerbates an individual's condition.
- Consistent exercise.
- Consistent sleep and rest.
- Emotional work and counseling therapy to deal with the mental/emotional stress of her situation.

The Nature to Heal and the Inherent Wisdom Behind Biology

Biological systems and the chemistry involved are an interesting point of study and fascinating to evaluate and learn about as they relate to us and the natural world around us. There is no doubt that understanding more about how our cells function and the different biochemical systems involved is crucial to our understanding of health and medicine. The information I have presented here is just the tip of the iceberg when it comes to the complex nature of cellular and molecular biology and how they apply to health and healing. You don't need to be a scientist or doctor to appreciate the intricacies of the systems discussed.

We as individuals, in our unique complexity and diversity, are an integral component of the natural world. Our biology is linked to a boundless spectrum of other life-forms that inhabit our planet. There is a universal wisdom behind what we call science and the physical manifestations we recognize as cellular biology, chemistry, tissue structures, and integrated bodily systems. It appears that we, as individuals and collectively, as living beings with all other living creatures, are a physical manifestation of this creative force. This doesn't mean that biology and chemistry are less real or important in our day-to-day existence. They clearly are, and they can be the central components in physical health and illness. The wisdom I am referring to, however, is beyond the physical; it is a motive force behind the intricacies of cellular function and is bound to the rules and laws of integrated physical systems.

Disease can happen, and is a natural process linked to the physical manifestation in deranged biological systems. Death for us all is an eventual reality linked to the limitations of natural life cycles; however, the universal forces that work through these integrated systems that formed the biological structures of our cells in the first place do not disappear in the presence of disease or ill health. It appears to always be there in the background, trying to return the system to balance. Again, life and death are natural states on opposite sides of a biological coin. If we can remember that we too are manifestations of the universal force behind our biology, we can hope to move ourselves to a higher frequency that is more in line with health. At least this can be a goal in our lives to increase the odds for improved health and well-being, and even recovery from illness.

Strategies for Healing

To end this discussion, here are some basic things to consider for improving health and the potential for healing. Many of these are not new concepts, and you have likely heard them before; however, in many situations with chronic ill health it is the small things done over time that can have a tremendous influence on recovery. The road to recovery is a process that requires diligence, motivation, and consistency. Not everything we do with regard to our diet, lifestyle, and personal pursuits works to the same degree, but often these strategies work in synergy with each other over time.

Suggested Steps to Improve Healing

Eat a whole-food, plant-based (or largely plant-based) diet that's organic and GMO-free. An abundance of nutritious organic plant-based foods provides tremendous nutrition and a variety of phytochemicals. The phytochemicals alone can positively influence mechanisms at the cellular level that move a cellular system to improved function.

Avoid environmental pollutants such as pesticides, herbicides, and other industrial chemicals. For the sensitive person, many of these chemicals can alter signaling mechanisms within cells that alter homeostatic mechanisms and increase the potential for HAMP reactivity.

Prioritize a nighttime sleep routine and periods of rest and recovery during the day. Culturally, here in the United States (and other places throughout the world), the aspect of a midday "siesta" is not appreciated; however, the natural rhythm of cells linked to the natural biological clock is important to pay attention to, and not incorporating restful routines is another contributor to homeostatic cell disturbance.

Avoid stressful and/or disturbing programs, movies, shows, etc., that you know cause mental and emotional distress and turmoil. The chemical response in the brain and nervous system to mental and emotional stress is just as powerful as physical stressors. Every cell in our body has a biological link to this stress response. You particularly want to avoid these stressors at nighttime before bed.

Exercise is critical. This may seem counterintuitive to someone with a chronic illness, but the body, from a fundamental cellular level, is based in movement. It's important to be as active as possible while observing how you feel from the activity. As tolerated, different types of exercise can be implemented to aid in strength, flexibility, and vitality.

Maintain good fluid hydration throughout the day. The human body is mostly fluid, and cellular function is dependent on fluid dynamics in the vasculature and across all cell membranes. Dehydration can lead to poor cellular function and can be another trigger for HAMP reactivity.

Get outside and breathe fresh air, which, with its oxygen, is crucial to our lives. Lack of fresh air is another stressor to our body and can lead to imbalances of oxygen and carbon dioxide, both of which are contributors to homeostasis dysfunction.

Get daily exposure to natural sunlight. It provides photons, which can activate components at the cellular level for increased energy production.

Turn off, reduce, or limit exposure to electromagnetic frequencies (EMF) from wireless devices, 5G, Wi-Fi, etc. For the sensitive person, EMFs are drivers of cellular imbalance, inflammation, and loss of cellular homeostatic balance.

Increase your exposure to natural frequencies (NFs), those that come from the natural world. Spend more time in nature and less time indoors exposed to EMFs. Tend a garden, go for walks in a city park, in the woods, or along a shoreline, or sit quietly beneath a beautiful tree. The frequencies that resonate in nature are the same frequencies that resonate within our cells, as we too are part of the natural world.

Have a purpose to your life, or many purposes. For those with chronic illnesses who struggle to feel well, this can seem like a daunting and unimportant task; however, developing a purpose beyond just dealing with your illness can be satisfying, motivating, and energetically healing.

Incorporate a hobby or hobbies into your life. To pursue something in your life other than just working and dealing with your illness can be extremely rewarding, relaxing, and energetically positive. Dedicate more time to reading, learn to play a musical instrument, or pursue some other artistic endeavor. A hobby should not be viewed as an added stressor but as a critical component of maintaining and engaging in positive life experiences.

Establish positive relationships with likeminded people. You need a support group or an individual who brings positive energy and perspective to your life. Positive people are uplifting and necessary. To make more room for such people, it might also mean avoiding negative influences in your life.

Other things could be added to this list. The point is, the more positive things we can do on a consistent day-to-day, week-to-week, basis the more positive energy gets produced, and, when we think about the biochemistry of sensitivity, what better way to improve cellular homeostasis than through positive and harmonic energy.

All my best to you on your journey of health and healing.

Kurt N. Woeller, DO, is a Doctor of Osteopathic Medicine, and since the late '90s has been in clinical practice as an integrative and functional medicine physician and biomedical Autism Treatment Specialist. He is the author of several integrative medicine books, an international lecturer and educator, and creator and health-education director of Integrative Medicine Academy (https://integrativemedicineacademy.com), an online training academy specializing in functional and integrative medicine courses for health professionals. He is also the co-director—with his partner, Tracy Tranchitella, ND—of Functional Medicine Clinical Rounds (https://functionalmedicineclinicalrounds.com) and Autism Recovery System (https://autismrecoverysystem.com), two additional online educational resources for health professionals and caregivers of individuals with an autism-spectrum disorder. In addition to being the primary education creator for many courses offered through his Integrative Medicine Academy, Dr. Woeller is the Organic Acids Test seminar creator and presenter for the GPL Academy, which is associated with Great Plains Laboratory. He also does educational consulting for BioBotanical Research and other entities in the arena of functional and integrative medicine. He has served as a clinical consultant for various laboratory companies such as Great Plains Laboratory and BioHealth Laboratory. and participates as a scientific advisor for various organizations such as Integrative Medicine for Mental Health. Dr. Woeller is also a member of the American Osteopathic Association. His private practice, Sunrise Functional Medicine (https://mysunrisecenter.com), focuses on specialized diagnostic testing and interventions for individuals with complex medical conditions such as autism, autoimmune and neurological disorders, environmental chemical, mold, and mycotoxin-related illnesses, and other chronic health conditions.

Part II

The Most Common Triggers
For the Development of Sensitivity

Chapter 7: Mold Toxicity

Neil Nathan, MD

How We Learned About Sensitive Patients and How to Treat Them

As I worked with more and more patients with chemical sensitivities, I realized that a common thread was emerging. Almost every patient who presented to me with MCS (multiple chemical sensitivity) turned out to have a significant amount of mold toxicity and/or a *Bartonella* infection. When these patients were successfully treated for their mold toxicity, their chemical sensitivities (and other sensitivities) almost always disappeared within a year of completing treatment. Most began to improve as treatment progressed, and there seemed to be a clear relationship between removing mold toxins from their bodies and a marked decrease in all sensitivities.

At first, I didn't put two and two together, and neither had I realized that the sensitivity being triggered was coming from a dysfunctional limbic system. As I tried to understand these connections, it slowly dawned on me that mold toxins were directly affecting the limbic system, so that every type of sensitivity (sound, light, touch, chemicals, food, and EMF) could be associated with mold toxicity directly. Once I'd made that connection, I found that by adding limbic retraining techniques (see chapters 1 and 2), patients could reduce their sensitivities much more quickly. More important, by introducing limbic retraining early in the course of treatment, my patients could tolerate their treatments much, much better.

With this information and treatment approach already helping hundreds of my patients, I stumbled upon Dr. Porges' polyvagal theory (see chapter 3). It soon became apparent that vagal nerve dysfunction was also a major element in the development of sensitivity, and that the vagus nerve worked very closely with the limbic system in monitoring the body for safety. When either or both systems were dysfunctional, *both* needed to be addressed early on and concurrently for improvement to occur. It had become clear that mold toxicity was directly impacting both systems, and when patients had become unusually sensitive (which was common in my practice), rebooting the limbic system with the vagal system was essential in enabling those patients to tolerate the treatments required for mold toxicity. Ultimately, when the mold toxins were removed, both systems were able to return to normal functioning.

Yet another piece in the sensitivity puzzle emerged when I read Dr. Lawrence Afrin's 2016 book, *Never Bet Against Occam,* a groundbreaking revelation about Mast Cell Activation Syndrome (MCAS). It turned out that most of my sensitive patients (I estimate 70%) with mold toxicity had developed MCAS (see chapter 4) later in their clinical course, which added another level of inflammation and sensitivity to an already inflamed and sensitive system. Again, addressing mast cell activation early on in the treatment program proved to be another key ingredient in quieting that sensitivity and allowing those patients to tolerate the treatments for mold toxicity, which would ultimately cure them. For the vast majority of patients, once the mold toxins were gone, so was the mast cell activation.

For those patients who also had *Bartonella* and/or Lyme disease (see chapter 8), additional treatments for that infection and Lyme disease were also necessary before complete healing could be achieved.

This approach to treating the sensitive patient—finding mold toxicity (and/or Lyme and *Bartonella*) while recognizing limbic dysfunction and vagal-nerve dysfunction and mast-cell activation—essentially revolutionized the effectiveness of treatment for my sensitive patients. We were off to a great start! As with all revelations, given the complexity of the human body, there was still more to be learned. The increase in sensitization produced by COVID, both from the acute infection, Long-Haul COVID, and the vaccines (see chapter 24) taught us a great deal about the inflammatory nature of sensitization and could ultimately lead to other treatments that might augment what we present here.

I was fortunate to become a part of multiple medical networks of pioneering clinicians who were all looking for these answers. Sometimes I stumbled upon an important piece of the puzzle early on; other times my colleagues found those pieces before me. The beauty was that we shared this adventure, each bringing forward important pieces of information. Some pieces, as you might expect, proved more useful than others, as we applied them clinically to patients in our practices.

We learned about the importance of oxalates (see chapter 12), sulfation (see chapter 13), salicylates (see chapter 14), and other environmental toxins (see chapter 11). We learned about thiamine deficiency (see chapter 18) and EMFs (see chapters 12 and 13) as additional triggers for sensitization. We learned that dental issues (see chapter 15) could provoke this sensitization, as can other structural imbalances (see chapter 16). Many of our patients had been placed on antidepressants (especially SSRIs) and benzodiazepines (like Xanax or Ativan), and inadvertent or poorly orchestrated weaning from those medications added another piece of intense sensitization so that withdrawal became another issue that had to be handled as delicately as possible (see chapter 17). Carbon monoxide poisoning (see chapter 22) and secondary porphyrias (see chapter 23) were rare, but occasionally became additional players in this increasingly complex scenario.

We found that EMF sensitivity began to trigger a marked increase in overall sensitivity, especially after the arrival of 5G. Dr. Martin Pall elucidated the biochemistry of EMF sensitivity (see chapter 10), and other pioneers collected evidence of how EMF exposures were having a more profound effect on our health than we had appreciated (see chapter 9). Dr. Ty Vincent developed a method for treating the immune system's role in this sensitivity with low-dose immunotherapy—LDI (see chapter 25). We learned that intravenous ketamine (see chapter 26) was markedly capable of quieting the limbic/vagal systems in many patients.

Looking at the predisposition to this sensitivity, we learned a great deal about genetics (see chapter 19), and Dr. Robert Naviaux provided us a detailed model of how this sensitivity develops, in an orchestrated biochemical cascade called the Cell Danger Response, which I reviewed in my previous book, *Toxic: Heal Your Body from Mold Toxicity, Lyme Disease, Multiple Chemical Sensitivity and Chronic Environmental Illness*.

Both mold toxicity and *Bartonella* (and Lyme disease) are well known to affect the ability of the pituitary gland to regulate our hormones. We noted especially that adrenal, thyroid, and sex-hormone imbalances were present in most of our patients and needed to be treated to facilitate healing (see chapter 20).

In a remarkably short time, we went from a state of confusion as to what this sensitivity was all about, what caused it, and how to treat it, to what we have now: a medical model that allows us to understand many of the triggers of sensitivity and, equally important, how to treat it successfully.

This is great news for those who have suffered for many years, misunderstood and dismissed, but please understand that many, if not most, medical practitioners have not yet encountered this information and are not yet ready to embrace it. You might need to do a little legwork to find a practitioner who has learned how to treat sensitivity. In this book, we have laid out for you the blueprint of how to approach this from every perspective currently available. Considering how much we've already learned, it's almost certain that we'll learn even more in the next few years. We might need to update this information regularly to keep it current, and I hope to do so, but please remember, we already know a lot—enough to help the majority of our patients get well.

Given that much of the epidemic increase in sensitivity we see is caused by our environment, this information comes just in time. It will help not only those who are afflicted with this condition, and those who are on the verge of coming down with it, but will, we hope, also help awaken the entire world to the dangers we face with the ongoing increases in chemical and electromagnetic pollution that play such an important role, so that we can make major strides in doing something about it.

Mold Toxicity: The Basics of Evaluation and Treatment

Having emphasized my own experience of how often I saw mold toxicity as the major trigger for sensitive patients, let's review the key components of exactly how to deal with it. As I assembled this comprehensive book, it became clear to me that every contributing author could write a book on their subject (most have), and we've all striven to distill what we've learned into readable, easily digested chapters. For those who want a more complete discussion of mold toxicity, I would encourage you to read my book, *Toxic*, as well as Dr. Jill Crista's *Break the Mold: 5 Tools to Conquer Mold and Take Back Your Health*. That said, let's dig into this important subject.

For many years, medicine essentially looked at mold issues as primarily involving allergic reactions to mold. Allergists developed a number of tools to help patients become desensitized, which often helped.

We were also aware that a very small number of patients developed a systemic infection from mold species, which required intravenous antifungal medications and months of hospitalization to cure.

The concept of mold *toxicity* is a relatively new one, despite the fact that it is described in the Old Testament (Leviticus). A few medical papers were published in the Scandinavian literature in the 1990s, but it was not until 2003 that Dr. Michael Gray and his colleagues published two papers describing the symptoms unique to mold toxicity and a method for treating them. In 2005, Dr. Ritchie Shoemaker published his groundbreaking book, *Mold Warriors*, which began to bring this important illness to our attention. Shortly after its publication, a patient brought this to my attention and I immediately went to see Dr. Shoemaker at his clinic in Pocomoke, Maryland. That began my involvement in learning about how under-recognized mold toxicity was as a cause of many of my patients' illnesses.

It soon became clear that mold toxicity was a major contributing factor to many common conditions: chronic fatigue syndrome; fibromyalgia; autism; neurodegenerative conditions; and of course, to the process of sensitization. It's now estimated that up to 10 million Americans have some degree of mold toxicity, and the majority have no idea that it's happening to them. Experts now estimate that as many as 30% of all the buildings in this country have a degree of mold toxicity, so once this idea begins to take hold in our consciousness, the extent of the illness should come as no surprise. It is literally an epidemic, and unfortunately, not yet recognized as such.

Let's start with the basics: What is mold toxicity? It is simply the effect that mold toxins have on susceptible individuals. Who is susceptible? It's currently believed that about 25% of the population is genetically unable to process mold toxin; hence, when exposed to enough of it, usually in the form of water-damaged buildings, they may get sick and have difficulty healing from their exposure.

Why can't impacted individuals get well? There are several reasons, but the main ones are that they're genetically unable to make antibodies to mold toxins, hence the toxins stay in their bodies and the body recirculates them. The recirculation involves the fact that the body processes mold toxins, like all toxins, by bringing them to the liver for detoxification, which then brings the toxins to the bile, to which they are bound, for elimination through the stool. The toxins, bound to bile, start their journey through the gastrointestinal tract, but when they reach the small intestine, the natural process of bile recirculation (technically called the enterohepatic circulation) brings the bile, still attached to the toxins, back to the gall bladder where the bile is stored. Thus the toxins persist in the body unless we treat them by the methods described below.

Symptoms of Mold Toxicity

If someone is exposed to mold, how might mold toxicity present itself? The key to understanding the myriad symptoms is that mold toxins trigger a persistent inflammatory reaction in the body, which the body is unable to quiet. For all of the symptoms listed here, inflammation is the common underlying issue. I'll list the symptoms by organ system to make them a little more cohesive.

General Symptoms

- Fatigue, often overwhelming. A common component of fatigue is medically called post-exertional malaise (or post-exertional myalgia); if a patient exercises, they are unusually exhausted or sore afterward, sometimes for days.
- Cognitive impairment. Reduction of memory, focus, and concentration, sometimes referred to as "brain fog," is almost universal. A particular symptom is difficulty with "word finding," in which a person knows what they want to say but can't find the correct word. Difficulties with executive function, organizing tasks (those who were excellent at multitasking find they no longer are), and working with numbers are common.

- Pain: Headaches of every type, sinus headaches especially, are common. Pain in joints, muscles, and tendons are also common, and can affect any or many parts of the body.
- Muscle weakness
- Intense thirst
- Appetite swings and weight gain (or loss)
- Night sweats
- Temperature dysregulation
- Onset of an autoimmune condition
- Increased Sensitivity to:
  - Chemicals/Smells (MCS or multiple chemical sensitivity)
  - Light
  - Sound
  - Touch
  - Food
  - EMFs

Respiratory Symptoms

- Shortness of breath
- Wheezing (looks like asthma, but isn't or, will exacerbate bronchospasm).
- Air "hunger," a feeling that one cannot take in enough air to satisfy their breathing needs.
- Cough

Sinus Symptoms

- Congested sinuses
- Recurrent sinus infections
- Runny nose

Neurological Symptoms

- Paresthesias (numbness and tingling in different parts of the body, sometimes in areas that don't have a neurological dermatome, a pattern of discomfort that doesn't fit known nerve pathways).
- Peripheral neuropathy
- Tinnitus (ringing in the ears)
- Disequilibrium and/or dizziness
- Psychological symptoms
- Anxiety, often with panic attacks
- Depression, often severe
- OCD behaviors (obsessive-compulsive disorders)
- Mood swings
- Irritability, anger, difficulties handling stressors

Gastrointestinal Symptoms

- Bloating, gas, distention
- Diarrhea and/or constipation, often presenting as IBS (irritable bowel syndrome)
- Abdominal pain or cramping
- Heartburn or reflux
- Belching

Pelvic/Urinary Symptoms

- Recurrent urinary infections
- Pelvic pain
- Interstitial cystitis
- Frequent urination
- Irregular periods
- Impotence
- Worsening of PMS symptoms

Many patients have quite a few of these symptoms, based on their own unique biochemistry and genetics. It would be a rare patient who had only one or two. While almost no one has all of them, it's common to see a lot of these symptoms described by patients at their first office visit. As you might imagine, a physician who was not aware of this information would be tempted to think that no one could have all of those symptoms, so this must be psychogenic, or "in their head." It will come as no surprise that the majority of patients I've worked with have been told by one or more physicians that they needed an antidepressant or antianxiety medication or therapy for what they were describing, It will also come as no surprise that those suggestions do not work well, or can even make the patient worse, because their underlying condition has not been recognized and treated.

Diagnosis of Mold Toxicity

The most important component of diagnosis is to understand the symptoms patients experience when they have mold toxicity, so it's paramount to consider the diagnosis based on symptoms and history. This means that once you've begun to learn how common mold toxicity is, you'll begin to ask the important historical questions:

1. Have you ever lived in a moldy environment?
2. Do you currently see or smell mold in your home or work environment or in your car or in a relative's house where you spend a lot of time?
3. Have you ever had water damage to a home you lived in? This could include a leaking washing machine or water heater, basement flooding, poor drainage of the soil around your house when it rains, or a leaky roof or windows.

In my experience, it's common for patients to not recall much of this at our first visit (or even deny it), but once they get a chance to think about it, they often bring it up at their next visit. Then, I hear comments such as "Come to think of it, we did have some black mold growing in our basement in a house we lived in five years ago," or "We had a leak from the water heater, and it took the landlord several weeks to get around to cleaning it up."

Until people begin to understand how important these questions are, and how relevant they may be to their health, many will simply blow off what they thought were minor water-damage incidents, or just paint over areas of mold with Kilz, thinking that will take care of the problem. It won't.

Once you have a history with mold exposure and you realize that your patient's symptoms would be well explained by that diagnosis, then you need to confirm the diagnosis and get going on treatment.

The most accurate method for making this diagnosis is with a simple urine mycotoxin test. You just collect a morning, first-voided urine sample after provocation (described below) and send it to any of several laboratories for analysis. Having done this assay with thousands of patients, using all of the labs currently doing it, I've found that the most accurate lab is RealTime Laboratories, and just behind it was the Great Plains Laboratory (recently renamed Mosaic Diagnostics). Testing can also be done through Vibrant Health, which uses the same technology as Mosaic Diagnostics, or MyMyco laboratory, which uses blood specimens to do antibody testing to mycotoxins. Since these labs use completely different methods for analysis, giving different results, these results cannot be compared, but a positive almost always means that the patient does indeed have mold toxicity.

When these tests first became available, it took us a while to recognize that the very process of mold toxicity interferes with the body's ability to detoxify. This means that having mold toxicity limits the body's ability to mobilize the toxins into the urine, so our first test often yields a lower reading than what actually exists. To improve those initial results, we began to ask our patients to take a sauna or hot bath the night prior to collecting the urine and to take glutathione for several days prior to collecting, which produced much more accurate readings on our first test. (Glutathione is a powerful antioxidant that can help protect the body from disease, slow the progression of cancer, improve insulin sensitivity, reduce cell damage in liver disease, reduce symptoms of Parkinson's disease, reduce damage from ulcerative colitis, and help treat autism-spectrum disorders).

What we get when we run these tests is a clear readout of which mycotoxins the labs are finding and a measurement of how much toxin is present. This makes the diagnosis clear and tells us which toxins are present, which will help guide our treatment.

Currently, the RealTime test measures ochratoxins, aflatoxins, trichothecenes, gliotoxin, and zearalenone. The other laboratories have different panels of mycotoxins that they're able to measure.

There are other tests that can be helpful for diagnosis, and for subsequent treatment, but in my opinion they're nowhere near as specific as looking for the toxins that come directly out of the patient's urine.

An OAT (organic acid test) from Mosaic Diagnostics lab gives us information about possible colonization, the presence of *Candida* as measured by arabinose, and the presence of oxalates, which are usually made by mold species, as well as quite a bit of other information that can tell us a lot about the metabolic issues the patient is facing.

There are several biochemical markers that can provide additional information. These include specialty tests such as TGF beta-1, C4a, MMP9, MSH, and VEGF, which essentially reflect the effects of inflammation and are helpful to suggest mold toxicity, but results could also be elevated by any number of infections or other inflammatory conditions.

Mold toxicity often interferes with the ability of the pituitary gland to regulate hormones, so the measurement of adrenal, thyroid, sex hormones, and ADH can be helpful in understanding what the toxins have done to the patient and how we can move the patient into a greater state of healing by treating them.

Weight gain in the patient is often explained by an elevated leptin level. Other tests may be helpful, depending on the exact issues the patient presents.

Dr. Jill Crista has developed a new questionnaire that can help you and your physician be clear as to whether or not mold toxicity is a likely diagnosis. We've received funding for extensive research as to the accuracy of this questionnaire, and we welcome you to take part, going to an online site where it will be available. If you're interested, please go to my website, www.neilnathanmd.com or Jill's at www.drcrista.com.

Mold Illness Questionnaire

Category 1

General

- Fatigue that doesn't otherwise make sense
- Trouble sleeping
- Worse after eating
- Worse after exercise
- Increased thirst
- Stubborn weight gain
- Anemia

Sensitivity

- Bothered by tags and seams on clothing
- Chemical sensitivities
- Sensitive to light, sound, or touch

Head/Mind

- Slowed thinking or brain fog
- Unsettled feeling, unquieted mind, overwhelm
- Headaches
- Dizziness, vertigo, or drunken feeling
- Unexplained mood changes, anxiety, or depression

EENT

- Allergies/hay fever year-round
- Eye irritation
- Dark circles under eyes
- Floaters in your vision
- Vision blurry, frequently changes, or difficulty reading
- Sneezing or persistent runny nose
- Acute sense of smell for mold
- Recent sinusitis
- Ears feel plugged or clogged
- Itchy or sore ear canals
- Sores in the mouth
- Post-nasal drip or frequent throat clearing
- Chronically sore throat
- Coated tongue

Respiratory

- Easily irritated lungs
- Episodic cough
- Shortness of breath, air hunger, or yawn/sigh often

Cardiovascular

- Easy bruising
- Heart palpitations
- Lower extremity edema
- Protruding veins on limbs

Digestive

- Nausea
- Bloated abdomen or flatulence
- Unexplained change in digestion/bowels
- Recent change in appetite
- Crave carbs, sweets, or alcohol

Genitourinary

- Overactive bladder
- Bladder infections

Skin

- Skin rash, redness or flushing

Immune

- Frequent infections or delayed recovery from colds

Musculoskeletal

- Increased body pain

Category 2

General

- Voice sounds nasally
- Frequent or strong static shocks
- Histamine intolerance
- Non-obstructive sleep apnea
- React poorly to musty spaces

Sensitivity

- Sensitivity to EMFs

Head/Mind

- Migraines
- Difficulty thinking clearly or memory loss
- Confusion or disorientation

EENT

- Allergies are not well-controlled by medication
- Chronic sinusitis

- Nose bleeds
- Ear ringing or ear pain that's new or worsening

Respiratory

- Asthma or wheezing
- Chronic cough
- Burning lungs
- Episodes of fast heart beat
- Chest pain
- Low platelets

Digestive

- Increased food sensitivities
- Frequent vomiting
- Irritable bowel or alternating constipation/diarrhea
- Digestive ulcer or blood in the stool
- Celiac or non-celiac intestinal disease
- Fatty liver
- Liver pain or swelling

Genitourinary

- Unexplained menstrual changes
- Bacterial vaginosis
- Kidney pain or swelling

Skin

- Itchy or burning skin
- Peeling or sloughing skin
- Raynaud's syndrome
- Eczema or psoriasis

Immune

- Epstein-Barr virus activation

Musculoskeletal

- Slow reflexes
- Balance issues or incoordination
- Joints easily injured
- New or worsening nerve pain, numbness or tingling
- Muscle weakness or spasm

Category 3

General

- Current exposure to mold
- Previous exposure to damp, musty or water-damaged building any time in your life
- Mold allergy
- Abnormal reaction to medications or supplements
- Autism or sensory processing disorder
- Chronic fatigue syndrome
- Chronic inflammatory response syndrome (CIRS) or positive Shoemaker tests

Sensitivity

- Feeling of an internal vibration

Head/Mind

- Dysautonomia or Postural Tachycardia Syndrome (POTS)
- Dementia

EENT

- Daily use of sinus spray, sinus prescription, or Neti pot
- Nasal polyps
- Sinus surgery at any time in your life
- Hearing loss
- MARCoNS
- Oral thrush

Respiratory

- Asthma that's difficult to control with medication
- Lung scarring or nodules
- Pulmonary Edema
- Idiopathic Pulmonary Fibrosis
- Respiratory distress or Idiopathic pneumonitis
- Lung cancer

Cardiovascular

- Arrhythmia
- Coagulation abnormalities
- Arteriovenous abnormality
- Churg Strauss Syndrome

Digestive

- Peanut allergy
- Cyclical vomiting syndrome
- Eosinophilic esophagitis
- Non-alcoholic steatohepatitis (NASH)
- Hepatocellular carcinoma or other liver cancer

Genitourinary

- Infertility
- Chronic pelvic pain
- Interstitial cystitis
- History of kidney stones
- Reduced GFR (glomerular filtration rate)
- IgA nephropathy, nephrotic syndrome, nephritis, or other kidney disease
- Kidney cancer

Skin

- Recurrent yeast infections or fungal skin infections, including athlete's foot, jock itch, or yeast vaginitis
- Erythema nodosum
- Toenail fungus

Immune

- Autoimmunity
- Mast Cell Activation Syndrome (MCAS)
- Aspergillosis, current or history of
- Previous or current cancer diagnosis, not otherwise specified
- Aplastic anemia
- Sarcoidosis

Musculoskeletal

- Hypermobility or Ehlers-Danlos syndrome
- Tremors or tics
- Difficulty walking

The MoldIQ Research Initiative is sponsored by Change the Air Foundation.

Now that we have a clear diagnosis based on history of exposure, symptoms, a positive questionnaire, and a positive urine mycotoxin test, along with some other supportive information, we can move on to treatment.

Treatment of Mold Toxicity in the Sensitive Patient

Preparing for Mold Treatment

Most of the patients who are referred to me have already heard about and tried some of these treatments. In sensitive patients, most have already had setbacks because their bodies did not readily tolerate taking these treatments immediately. Discussing with my patients, in detail, exactly what kinds of reactions they had when trying these treatments helps me understand just how sensitive my patient is, and how slowly and carefully we'll need to proceed in order to make progress. In a sense, it helps to define how sensitive my patient is, and that information gives me a pretty good idea of what steps to take next, and in what order. I've found this very important, because if you try to institute a treatment before a patient is ready to receive it, it will usually make them worse, sometimes for weeks afterward.

When we've agreed that we're dealing with a sensitive individual, the next order of business is to identify whether limbic dysfunction, vagal dysregulation, and/or mast-cell activation is present.

If my patient describes any symptoms of anxiety and/or depression, increasing OCD behaviors, mood swings, and irritability coupled with any type of increased sensitivity at all to light, sound, smells, touch, chemicals, foods, or EMFs, then I know their limbic system is involved and needs to be addressed first. If they describe gastrointestinal issues, especially constipation, POTS, labile hypertension, insomnia, or heart palpitations or irregularities, then we're dealing with a vagus nerve component, which will also need to be addressed, preferably concurrent with the limbic issues. I have found that if both the limbic system and the vagal systems are affected (which is almost universal in the sensitive patient) if you treat one of these and neglect the other, then their nervous systems will remain hypervigilant and progress will be difficult, so strategies to treat both are begun at the start of treatment.

At the end of this book I'll outline this approach in an overview of diagnosis and treatment for the sensitive patient (see chapter 27). Each component is discussed in detail throughout this book.

Regarding my own approach, I usually start with one of two limbic treatments. The two that I have the most extensive experience with are the Annie Hopper DNRS program (dynamic neural retraining system) and the Ashok Gupta amygdala retraining program. (The amygdala is another name for the limbic system). By reading the appropriate chapters, you can gain an appreciation for both approaches, and if one or the other resonates with you, I encourage you to trust that feeling.

Both are excellent, and each has helped more than a thousand of my patients. With unusually sensitive patients, however, I encourage them not to jump full-bore into either program, but rather to start slowly and gently. For the DNRS program, that means doing just one or two "rounds" daily, which would take twenty to thirty minutes, or doing twenty minutes of amygdala retraining each day. Daily is important, but if a sensitive patient tries to do more, it will often overwhelm them and set them back. Going slowly and with caution is more effective in both the short and long term.

Once limbic training has begun, I add vagal nerve- retraining programs, depending on my patient's capacities. For almost everyone, I start with the exercises in Stanley Rosenberg's book, *Accessing the Healing Power of the Vagus Nerve*. Rosenberg was a craniosacral therapist who developed his exercises to accompany good-quality cranial therapy.

I encourage my patients to find an osteopathic physician who practices cranial osteopathy—biodynamic osteopathy is ideal. Lists of these physicians can be found on the websites of Biodynamic Osteopathy and The Cranial Academy. These treatments, discussed in detail in chapter 16, are very gentle and effective, and usually should be done no more often than every three weeks.

Other vagal treatments include Frequency Specific Microcurrent, which provides treatment for several aspects of mold toxicity, Brain Tap, Emotional Freedom Technique, and Safe & Sound (described by Dr. Porges in chapter 3).

More recently, I've learned that the vagus nerve is essential in helping the body deal with inflammation. The vagal inflammatory reflex is a name given to the connection that the vagus nerve has with the thymus, spleen, and GALT (gut-associated lymphoid tissue). Those organs are key players in the immune system, and they profoundly influence the inflammatory process, which means that by using direct stimulation of the vagus nerve, we have the opportunity to decrease inflammation. A number of new devices have become available to accomplish this. Two of the ones with which I'm most familiar are GammaCore and ApolloNeuro, both of which have added to our ability to bring inflammation under control. Again, with sensitive patients, these devices need to be used initially at the lowest settings for very short periods of time.

The more of these treatments a patient can work with the faster and more thoroughly they will "quiet" their nervous systems. They'll not only feel better within six to eight weeks but will prepare their body to accept the mold treatments that are essential in their healing.

The third major condition triggered by mold toxicity is mast-cell activation, discussed in detail in chapter 4. A tipoff to the presence of this condition is when a patient describes reacting within a few minutes of eating or drinking anything. This reaction often involves the release of histamine, which presents as heart palpitations, sweating, abdominal pain or cramps, diarrhea, gas, bloating, itching or hives. Patients are often confused by this, because their assumption is that if they react this way they are allergic to the food they just ate.

They often find, however, that a food that seemed like it triggered a reaction one day can be eaten the next day with no reaction. The issue here is that this is not food allergy (though that can also exist and is common in mold toxicity) but has more to do with how reactive the mast cells are at the moment that anything comes down the gastrointestinal tract. This activation, which fluctuates (I suspect with varying levels of mold toxin in the body) is such that if activated at the moment of eating, the patient will react, but if not, they won't.

There are several tests available to make the diagnosis of Mast Cell Activation Syndrome, but they're not very accurate and are hard to obtain. It is easier and more accurate, in my opinion, to treat the condition and see how the patient responds. Details of treatment can be found in chapter 4 and in chapter 24.

Unusually sensitive patients might need to work with limbic and vagal retraining for several months before their bodies will allow them to take the supplements or medications we use to treat mast-cell activation. Others may be able to start those supplements concurrent with vagal/limbic retraining, and if they can, great. The bottom line for sensitive patients is that all three systems must be considered as likely contributors to sensitivity, and unless they're treated first, the patient won't be able to make progress.

Recently, I've found more and more patients who have also been sensitized to EMFs (see chapters 9 and 10). It's helpful for them to get a meter to measure the EMFS they're exposed to in their homes and on the devices they use routinely, so they can properly shield themselves. I find this increasingly important in enabling our sensitive patients to progress.

Treatment of Mold Toxicity

There are three guiding principles in treatment:

1. Evaluate the living/work environment for the presence of mold, and remediate or leave that environment. If the patient cannot, for any reason, get out of their moldy environment, they cannot get well.

2. Use the binders that are specific for the mycotoxins that show up on their urine mycotoxin test to help remove those toxins from their bodies.

3. Colonization refers to the presence of a microorganism on/in a host, with growth and multiplication of the organism, If the patient has colonized (and most patients have), they will need treatment with antifungal medications or biologics and

biofilm-dissolving agents to remove the mold and *Candida* from the areas of colonization, usually the sinus and gut areas. Colonization is an important and sometimes under-recognized issue. With the pioneering work of Dr. Joseph Brewer (see references at the end of this chapter), we've learned that many patients will colonize their sinus and gastrointestinal areas with mold and *Candida* after exposure. Depending on the health of their immune system, they may not manifest symptoms immediately upon exposure to mold, but sometimes will years later. If the colonized areas are not treated, the mold and *Candida* in those areas will continuously produce toxins that will either cause or add to the patient's toxic burden, and they won't be able to heal until this is addressed. This helps explain why many patients do not experience improvement in their symptoms when they leave their moldy home for several weeks—they're literally carrying their toxin source with them.

Evaluating a Home or Office for Mold

A complete discussion of this subject is beyond the scope of this book, and referral to a qualified environmental engineer is the most comprehensive approach for this evaluation; but to begin the process, there are a few relatively inexpensive methods for evaluating a building for safety that consumers can do on their own.

The most inexpensive is to purchase mold plates, which are simply Petri dishes with a medium that enables the growth of molds. One simply places the plate on the floor of a room to be checked, removes the top of the plate, and leaves it off for two hours. Then, marking the plate as to which room has been plated, put the top back on and observe for growth of mold over the next four to five days. If any appreciable mold is growing on the plates (this will be obvious), the plates need to be sent for evaluation to be sure that the growth reflects toxic mold species. More than half of what grows on these plates are nontoxic species, hence of no concern. I have used ImmunoLytics to provide the plates and analysis for many years. In this way, you can check each room in the house, along with the crawl space, basement, attic, or garage, to get an idea of what you're dealing with.

A more accurate but more expensive way is to get an ERMI kit and use a Swiffer or vacuum to collect dust from a room and send it for analysis. Any appreciable mold growth detected by either of these tests needs to be evaluated by an expert. I caution, however, that many who are certified might not have much experience, and most will use air sampling as their major method for analyzing a structure. This is not very helpful, since air sampling takes the sample from the air in the center of a room, but the mold spores are heavier than air, and have mostly already fallen to the floor.

Once you can be assured that you're not being exposed to mold in any ongoing way, you can move into treatment knowing that progress is likely. If you don't leave the moldy environment, you might get a bit better with treatment, but you can't get well.

Avoidance

I hope I've emphasized the importance of being certain that a patient with mold toxicity has no continuing exposure, but this concept has led to a good deal of anxiety in many patients, so I'll discuss it in more detail. Some websites insist that patients can't get well unless they get rid of all of the possessions that may have ever been exposed to mold, and move to the desert.

This is an extreme position; very few patients have needed to do this to get well, and they are vastly outnumbered by the thousands of patients I've successfully treated who did not have to go to such lengths. Given the ubiquitous exposure we humans have to mold, it's close to impossible to avoid all exposure, and most of my patients haven't needed to.

There are three components to mold sensitivity (in addition to allergy) that complicate this issue. First, direct exposure to a moldy building can worsen mold toxicity in patients within five minutes of entering the building.

Some of this is the direct effect of mold toxin on the body, but a secondary component is the sensitization of the limbic system to the smell of mold. As we've learned, the limbic system is directly connected to our olfactory nerves (our sense of smell), so the smell of mold, which unfortunately is enhanced in our limbically affected patients, triggers an immediate reaction that is not toxicity itself. Additionally, we've learned that the smell of mold can affect activated mast cells to produce another immediate reaction.

So, our patients, who are unusually able to detect the smell of mold (not always perceived by their family or friends, which can lead to misunderstandings), could be reacting to the mold directly, or their limbic and mast-cell systems might be reacting to the smell. I believe this has led some to believe that complete avoidance is necessary, but if you've been following our treatment plans, working first on the limbic and mast-cell systems will quiet those extreme reactions, and patients who were unable to tolerate even the slightest whiff of mold can usually (and fairly quickly) reduce that olfactory sensitivity and not only improve from a limbic/mast-cell perspective but progress past danger of exposure from minute amounts of mold in their environment. This means that while most patients do need to be out of a minimally moldy environment to get well, other than the simple precautions that can be outlined by environmental engineers, extreme avoidance is unnecessary. I hope this discussion will help patients who are trying to cope with mold toxicity adopt a calmer approach to improving their environment.

Detoxification

Remember that we must also be mindful of our patients' ability to detoxify and to support it throughout treatment. For specific help in detoxification from the common mold toxins, using both nutritional and botanical supplements, see tables 1 and 2, below. Also, please note the many detoxification strategies described in chapters throughout this book.

Table 1: Detoxification of Mycotoxins
Detoxification by Pathway

Mycotoxin	Detox Pathway	Dietary Supplement	Food
Ochratoxin Sterigmatocystin T-2 toxin (trichothecene) Zearalenone Alternariol DON (deoxynivalenol)	Glucuronidation	Quercetin Curcumin Resveratrol CBD Ellagic acid Astaxanthin	Cruciferous vegetables Turmeric root Curry powder Citrus fruits Grapes, berries Pomegranates, walnuts, black currants, algae, salmon, trout, krill, shrimp, crayfish
Trichothecene	Acetylation	Quercetin	Processed meats, garlic, grilled meats
DON T-2 Toxin	Sulfation	Retinoic acid Caffeine	Fish, arugula, Artichokes, green and black tea
Ochratoxin A DON	Glutathione conjugation	GSH Assist Genistein	Berries, grapes Pomegranates, walnuts, fermented soy, black currants
Aflatoxin B-1	CYP 3A4	Curcumin Resveratrol (−)	Turmeric root Curry powder
Aflatoxin B-1	CYP 1A2	Resveratrol (+) Quercetin (−) Curcumin (−)	Cruciferous vegetables Green tea Chicory root
Aflatoxin B-1 Aflatoxin G-1 Sterigmatocystin	CYP 1B1	Resveratrol (−) Curcumin Indole-3-carbinol	Cruciferous vegetables Turmeric root Curry powder Nuts, maize, rice, figs Wheat, corn, peanuts

Mycotoxin	Detox Pathway	Dietary Supplement	Food
Ochratoxin A	Amino acid conjugation	Glycine Taurine Glutamine Ornithine Arginine	Turkey, pork Chicken Pumpkin seeds Animal protein Meat, dairy, eggs
Ochratoxin A	Microbial hydrolysis (gut)		Coffee, cocoa, beer
Alternariol	Methylation conjugation		Oranges, tomatoes

Table 2
Detoxification by Organ System

Mycotoxin	Organ System for Detox	Supplemental Support
Ochratoxin A Zearalenone Citrinin AFB-1 Patulin	Renal (Urinary)	Renelix Increased fluid intake
Ochratoxin A Zearalenone T-2 Toxin (trichothecene) AFB-1 DON	Gastrointestinal (fecal)	ToxEase GL or caps
Ochratoxin A Zearalenone	Enterohepatic Circulation	Bitters Ox bile Globe artichoke Phosphatidyl choline

Our patients might also be allergic to mold, which is especially problematic if it has colonized and is growing inside their bodies. Immunotherapy for mold allergy can be helpful for many patients. Mold toxins often produce hormonal dysregulation, and treatment of adrenal, thyroid, and sex hormones will facilitate both immediate improvement and long-term benefit. Over the past fifteen years, we've learned much more about which specific binders can work for which specific mycotoxins. Here's a quick summary of that information.

The Use of Binders in Treatment

The use of urine mycotoxin testing has revolutionized our ability to use this specificity in treatment. I recommend that, for each toxin known to be present, you use as many binders as possible, to maximize the body's ability to pull that toxin out.

- For ochratoxin, the best binders are the medications cholestyramine or Welchol (colesevalam). A weaker binder is activated charcoal.
- For aflatoxins and trichothecenes, the best binders are bentonite clay, activated charcoal, and chlorella.
- For gliotoxins, the best binders are bentonite clay, *Saccharomyces boulardii,* and NAC (N-acetyl cysteine).
- For zearalenone, the best binders are bentonite clay, *Saccharomyces boulardii,* and cholestyramine or Welchol.
- For enniatin B, the best binders are bentonite clay and *Saccharomyces boulardii.*

BINDER	DOSAGE	TIMING	NOTES
Cholestyramine	$1/16$ teaspoon of powder once every other day to 4 scoops daily	Taken half an hour before a meal; the patient must wait another 90 minutes before taking anything else (such as a medication or supplement to which it might bind, decreasing its availability to the body)	
Welchol	$1/4$ tablet once daily to 2 tablets (625 milligrams each) 3 times a day	Taken half an hour before a meal; the patient must wait another 90 minutes before taking anything else (such as a medication or supplement to which it might bind, decreasing its availability to the body)	
Activated charcoal	A portion of a capsule (500 milligrams) once daily to 3 capsules a day	Best taken on an empty stomach, 2 hours before or after eating	
Bentonite clay	$1/16$ teaspoon of liquid to 3 capsules once daily	Best taken on an empty stomach, 2 hours before or after eating	

BINDER	DOSAGE	TIMING	NOTES
Chlorella	Vs tablet every other day to 3 tablets (200 milligrams each) once daily	Best taken on an empty stomach, 2 hours before or after eating	Use "glass-grown" chlorella; "natural" chlorella is often grown outdoors in ponds and, as a binder of toxin, may contain excessive amounts of arsenic and aluminum.
Saccharomyces boulardii	¼ capsule (3 to 10 billion units each) with one meal a day to 1 capsule with each meal	Best taken with food	
OptiFiber Lean	¼ scoop mixed in water once daily to 1 scoop 3 times a day	Best taken on an empty stomach, 2 hours before or after eating	This binder, which appears to be useful as a generally applicable binder for all of the named mycotoxins, has been well tolerated by my more sensitive patients. I am grateful to Jill Carnahan, MD, for this valuable suggestion.

While we don't have specific research for other mycotoxins, such as chaetoglobosin, citrinin, mycophenolic acid, and the fungal toxins made by Wallemia, we've learned that the use of generic binders such as bentonite clay, activated charcoal, chlorella, and Saccharomyces has been effective for all of them.

The treatment with binders is straightforward, but not as simple as one might hope. Part of the problem is with the word "binder," which, though technically correct, conveys the idea that the binding is strong and complete. Unfortunately, it's not. For example, activated charcoal "binds" by loosely adhering the toxin to the surface of the charcoal, such that the toxin can easily be dislodged from that surface as it transits the intestines. When the toxin does get dislodged, it can then be readily absorbed through the intestinal lining and back into the circulation. This means that if someone takes too strong a binder, or too much of it, it will essentially mobilize the toxin faster than the body's ability to detoxify that toxin, and the person will become more toxic. This is not rare, which means that it's imperative to approach treatment with binders with great care, especially for sensitive patients. It's essential to start with tiny doses of binders, and slowly increase the dose, carefully monitoring the patient to be sure we're not overdoing it.

We've observed that sensitive patients respond surprisingly well to small doses of binders, so this cautious approach can be very effective if done properly. One of the common problems I've seen is that physicians who don't appreciate how sensitive a patient is jump right in with full doses of binders and thereby set their patients back for weeks, and sometimes even longer. I strongly advise all patients to find a physician with experience in this area to help them work through this. The old TV warning "Don't try this at home!" applies here.

Use of Antifungal Medications in Treatment

If a patient has only recently been exposed to a moldy environment, it's possible that they are reacting only to the toxin that is present, and that they haven't had time to colonize. "Colonization" refers to the ability of mold and *Candida* to begin to grow on body surfaces once they've been introduced into the system. The most obvious places where this occurs is in the sinuses and gastrointestinal tract.

Since it takes some time for sensitization to occur, the great majority of my sensitive patients have indeed colonized by the time they get to my office. For most of them, it's unlikely that the use of binders alone will suffice. Once colonized, the mold will grow and continue to make mycotoxins that will keep our patients ill until we've treated the mold.

For most of our patients, treatment therefore needs to include antifungal medications in the sinus and gut areas. We've also learned that molds produce a great deal of biofilm, a thick, organized coating that protects the mold from attack by either antifungal medications or the body's immune system, so we need to include the use of biofilm-disrupting agents in the sinus and gut regions.

Once established in either region, molds are reluctant to leave the body, so treatment must often continue for a considerable time to be effective. This usually means a year or more, which comes as a surprise to most of my patients. It is important that they understand from the beginning that in order to work, treatment may require more time than anyone hoped for.

A full discussion of treatment options is beyond the scope of this book, but an overview for sensitive patients includes an understanding that we must proceed slowly and cautiously, just as we did with binders.

The strongest treatment for the sinus areas is amphotericin B nasal spray, but it's rarely tolerated by sensitive patients. Depending on the degree of sensitivity, we would use 2% ketoconazole or 1% itraconazole nasal spray in less sensitive patients, and nystatin nasal spray in our most sensitive ones. As a biofilm-dissolving agent, we usually use some form of EDTA, often as BE or BEG spray, which can be gotten from compounding pharmacies. I find hydrosol silver (often called colloidal silver), especially argentyn 23, very helpful for sinus treatments as well.

The strongest treatment for the gastrointestinal area is itraconazole (Sporanox); again, it's sometimes not tolerated by our sensitive patients. Scaling down, we could use compounded amphotericin B in various dosages, even having it made as a 0.06% solution so it can be given in tiny amounts. A biofilm-dissolving agent such as Interfase Plus or MC BFM-1 is also needed here, and other botanical agents have been helpful as well.

Summary and Conclusion

Our understanding of mold toxicity is in its infancy. There is much we need to learn, and a great deal of research must be done to improve our ability to treat this condition more effectively. Still, we've made great strides in the past decade, and I have successfully treated several thousand patients, most of whom presented with great sensitivities. The most important takeaways that I hope I've brought to light here are:

1. Mold toxicity is perhaps the single most common cause for the development of sensitivity, and thus should be a focal point for treatment for most patients.
2. Mold toxicity triggers three other conditions that are critical components in the development of sensitivity: limbic dysfunction; vagal nerve dysfunction; and mast-cell activation. All three need to be treated first (if present) before a sensitive patient can tolerate the treatment for mold toxicity.
3. The use of a urine mycotoxin test is essential in making the diagnosis and clarifying treatment.
4. Treatment involves first being sure that the home and work environment of our patient is safe and free from mold; second, the use of appropriate binders in the correct dosages; And third, the use of antifungal medications and biofilm-dissolving agents.
5. Given how often mold toxicity is a major component of sensitization, a focus on mold treatment should be an important consideration in the evaluation and treatment of every sensitive patient.
6. My final message is that mold toxicity is treatable and there is hope for everyone who has become sensitive that they can get well again.

References

Toxic: Heal Your Body from Mold Toxicity, Lyme Disease, Multiple Chemical Sensitivities and Chronic Environmental Illness by Neil Nathan, Victory Belt Press, 2018. An excellent overview and comprehensive discussion of chronic illnesses and how to evaluate and treat them. An audio version is available for those who cannot focus well enough to read.

Mold and Mycotoxins: Current Evaluation and Treatment, 2022. An e-book of about forty pages, this is a more succinct and focused discussion of mold toxicity and how to treat it. Helpful for families and patients who can't read for extended periods.

Break The Mold, by Jill Crista, Wellness Ink Publishing, 2018. An excellent discussion of how to evaluate and treat mold toxicity from the naturopathic perspective.

Brewer, JH, Thrasher, JD, Straus, DC, Madison, RA, Hooper, D, "Detection of mycotoxins in patients with chronic fatigue syndrome," *Toxins,* 2013, 5: 605-617

Brewer, JH, Thrasher, JD, Hooper, D, "Chronic illness associated with mold and mycotoxins: Is naso-sinus fungal biofilm the culprit?," *Toxins,* 2014, 6:66-80

Brewer, JH, Hooper, D, Muralidhar, S, "Intranasal antifungal therapy in patients with chronic illness associated with mycotoxins: an observational analysis," *GJMR,* 2015, Vol 15, Issue 2: 29-33.

Brewer, JH, Hooper, D, Muralidhar, S, "Intranasal nystatin therapy in patients with chronic illness associated with mold and mycotoxins" *Global Journal of Medical Research,* Interdisciplinary vol 15, Issue 5, 2015.

John C. Banta, CIH, coauthor of *Prescriptions for a Healthy House: A practical Guide for Architects, Builders, and Homeowners.*

Chapter 8: Lyme Disease and Coinfections

Richard Horowitz, MD, and Neil Nathan, MD

In my work with sensitized patients, I've discovered that for most, their sensitivity has been triggered by mold toxicity and/or Lyme disease and *Bartonella,* a common coinfection of Lyme disease.

Many patients are under the impression that Lyme disease is rare, but that's not so. In 2013, the CDC acknowledged that there were 300,000 new cases each year, and in 2022 they acknowledged that this was an underestimate; the number was closer to 476,000 new cases annually. Rare? Lyme disease is much closer to an epidemic, affecting far more patients than AIDS (HIV) ever did. The bottom line: millions of Americans currently suffer from Lyme disease, and many, if not most, are unaware of it.

How is this possible? Why do so many struggle with an illness we can treat? Why do their medical practitioners miss this diagnosis? The answers are important and complicated, so I'll explain how this has come about.

Symptoms of Lyme Disease and *Bartonella*

Let's first clarify the kinds of symptoms someone with Lyme disease may experience. You might be surprised to discover that these symptoms are remarkably similar to those we reviewed when we discussed mold toxicity.

Why would a toxin have the same symptoms as an infection? Because toxins and infectious microbes can trigger the release of similar inflammatory cytokines as the body's way of dealing with those threats. Cytokines, as many have learned from our COVID pandemic, are immune messengers that we produce when exposed to infectious agents and some toxins. They are intended to be a short-term stimulus to get our immune system to deal with those threats effectively, but if, for whatever reason, our immune system is unable to quickly dispose of the offending agent, there's a prolonged release of cytokines that trigger a persistent inflammatory response. That response (see chapter 6 for more details) creates the spectrum of symptoms I'll describe here.

Depending on a patient's unique biochemistry and genetics, the specific symptoms triggered by inflammation will vary. Most patients will exhibit a wide range of symptoms that will appear confusing unless viewed through the lens of persistent inflammation.

Lyme disease may present as some, or all, of the following:

- Fever, chills, day sweats, night sweats (these symptoms may indicate coinfection with Babesia, a malarial-type parasite)
- Joint pain (oftentimes, migratory, i.e., moving around the body with no specific trigger)
- Muscle pain (often migratory)
- Muscle cramping
- Muscle fasciculations or twitching
- Fatigue
- Cognitive: impairment/memory-concentration problems, word-finding problems, disorientation
- Headache
- Swollen glands/sore throat that comes and goes
- Chest pain, palpitations
- Unexplained cough, shortness of breath (this may indicate a coinfection with Babesia if other causes have been ruled out)
- Tendonitis
- Neuropathy (migratory neuropathy, i.e., tingling, numbness, burning and/or stabbing sensations of the extremities and/or cranial nerves that move around the body is a hallmark of chronic Lyme disease)
- Cranial nerve palsies (especially Bell's Palsy)
- Meningitis
- Dysautonomia/dizziness/lightheadedness/poor balance
- Visual disorders (blurred vison, floaters)
- Tinnitus/ringing in the ears/ear pain
- Tremor
- Depression
- Anxiety
- Mood swings
- Insomnia: difficulty falling asleep, frequent waking, or hypersomnolence (sleeping more than twelve hours per day but not feeling refreshed)
- Nausea
- Abdominal pain

- Testicular pain/pelvic pain
- Rashes (especially erythema migrans, the "bull's eye" rash)
- Urinary pain
- Prostatitis

You can readily see the overlap with mold-toxicity symptoms and how it might be difficult to distinguish these diagnoses from symptoms alone.

How Do We Diagnose Lyme Disease?

Here's where medical politics makes this a far more complicated question than it should be. To understand this, we have to go back in history to the way we first began to appreciate what Lyme disease was. An outbreak of juvenile rheumatoid arthritis in Lyme, Connecticut, got some local physicians to suspect that something more than an autoimmune condition was causing this unusual presentation of patients. It was finally described in the medical literature as Lyme disease in 1977. Willy Burgdorfer identified the causative organism as a bacterial spirochete in the family of *Borrelia*, and it was given the formal name *Borrelia burgdorferi* in 1982.

To make the antibody testing as specific as possible for research purposes, strict criteria were eventually placed on the interpretation of these tests—a standard procedure in medicine.

What evolved from this was a two-tiered process for diagnosis. First, a patient was tested for Lyme antibodies, and only if that was positive were they tested with a more complicated Western Blot test. The Western Blot measures what we call "bands," which are pieces of protein from the Lyme bacteria that our immune systems are capable of making an antibody to. There are nonspecific bands (carried on a variety of bacteria), which are bands 41, 58, and 66, and there are more specific bands, unique to the Lyme bacteria, bands 18, 23, 25, 31, 34, 39, and 83–93. To be diagnosed as having Lyme disease, a patient had to have at least five of these bands be positive. Anything less, according to researchers, meant that the patient had not been exposed to Lyme disease.

This was a reasonable place to begin, but unfortunately, as time passed, these criteria were never changed as new information became available. The antibody test for Lyme disease turned out to be quite inaccurate, as the bacteria has many different forms that can't be picked up on one antibody test, apart from its innate ability to avoid immune recognition. Therefore, many physicians who refused to do further testing on patients who had a negative ELISA test missed diagnosing them and countless others with Lyme disease because they didn't understand how inaccurate the test was. Further, based on the rigidity of these criteria, the large number of patients with one or more Borrelia-specific bands were told they could not have Lyme disease.

The Western Blot test was based solely on the *burgdorferi* species of *Borrelia,* and over the past thirty-five years we have learned that there are many other species that cause Lyme disease, none of which were accurately measured by this test. The very nature of *Borrelia* infection is that it weakens the immune system to the point that it becomes unable to make effective antibodies against *Borrelia.* Some patients even become immune deficient due to *Borrelia* affecting their B cells, the body cells tasked with making antibodies. This means that the antibody testing could be negative because of Lyme disease, hence rendering standard testing inaccurate. This led to large numbers of patients complaining of a chronic fatiguing, musculoskeletal illness with neuropsychiatric manifestations and being told it was chronic fatigue syndrome/ME (myalgic encephalomyelitis), fibromyalgia, a nonspecific autoimmune illness, or worse, that it was "in their heads." Inaccurate negative testing led physicians to refuse to treat these patients for Lyme disease, and instead of getting to the source(s) of their illness, just treated their symptoms.

While this is a travesty, it gets worse. Over time, there evolved two factions of physicians who were in complete disagreement over the diagnosis and treatment of Lyme disease.

The IDSA (Infectious Disease Society of America) has long held that Lyme disease is an acute infection easily treated with ten days to three weeks of antibiotics. While they admit that the acute infection can lead to a prolonged illness called Post-Lyme Syndrome, or PTLDS (Post-Treatment Lyme Disease Syndrome), certain leading members of their society do not believe (or admit) that this can be treated by antibiotics or other methods, and patients with this diagnosis are left to fend for themselves. The attorney general of the state of Connecticut (where the city of Lyme is located) has called the IDSA to task for not following the science of Lyme disease or changing their criteria so that more patients could be properly diagnosed and treated. To date, the IDSA has no "official" answers for those suffering from chronic Lyme disease/PTLDS.

In response to this, ILADS (International Lyme and Associated Diseases Society) physicians working with Lyme patients have a completely different viewpoint and experience. Dr. Horowitz was a founding member and past president-elect of ILADS, and we as a group have found that there is indeed a condition of chronic Lyme disease, i.e., a chronic spirochetal infection with associated coinfections that can be effectively treated with antibiotics, herbal supplements, and other methodologies that address multiple sources of inflammation and their downstream components. Dr. Horowitz calls that system of treatment MSIDS (Multiple Systemic Infectious Disease Syndrome). It comprises sixteen different factors that, when properly addressed, often lead to a profound improvement in symptoms and underlying illness. His last book, *How Can I Get Better, An Action Plan for Treating Resistant Lyme and Chronic Illness* (St. Martin's Press, 2017), explains this diagnostic and treatment plan in detail.

All of this historical information has had a profound effect on how Lyme disease may be diagnosed. For patients suffering with chronic Lyme disease, it's of huge importance.

Though our testing is still imperfect, it has greatly improved over the past thirty-five years. Some of the routine Western Blot testing hasn't changed; for a more accurate picture than can be provided by Labcorp or Quest, which check only for one strain of *Borrelia,* most of us in the Lyme community have relied on the IGeneX laboratory, which now offers an upgraded Western Blot called an Immunoblot, which measures many (though not all) of the most common Lyme species and is therefore far more accurate than what was previously available. In the right clinical setting, having ruled out overlapping illnesses, even one *Borrelia*-specific band on an Immunoblot (Osp C, 23 kda; Osp A, 31 kda; Osp B, 34kda; 39 kda, and 83/93 kda) can help establish exposure to Lyme disease.

For the diagnosis of *Bartonella,* some of these same issues apply. There are well over thirty species of *Bartonella*, of which at least eighteen can cause illness, and until recently most labs were able to measure only two species. IGeneX has recently developed an Immunoblot for *Bartonella,* along with a FISH test (Florescent In-Situ Hybridization, i.e., an RNA test) that's far more accurate and sensitive than what we had before.

Other labs are working to develop more accurate testing, but from my experience and that of my colleagues, IGeneX is still among the best. Galaxy Laboratory in North Carolina also has a good *Bartonella* panel that uses antibodies and DNA (ddPCR), and Infectolabs in Minnesota provides another method of determining the presence of *Bartonella* using T-cell reactivity, which can show exposure to Lyme, *Bartonella,* and many other coinfections.

You can see making the diagnosis of Lyme or *Bartonella* is not as simple as we would like. These tests are far more accurate now than before, but they'll still miss many patients who are ill with these conditions. It's important for physicians and patients to realize that the CDC is aware of these issues and has made it clear that *the diagnosis of Lyme disease is a clinical diagnosis,* meaning that if a patient has symptoms of Lyme disease, and perhaps a history of a tick bite (very few patients actually recall the tick bite), *even with a negative test they should be treated if the physician has a high suspicion of clinical Lyme disease.*

Unfortunately, despite these recommendations, many patients with Lyme or *Bartonella* have been denied treatment and continue to suffer a serious and debilitating illness.

To help establish the diagnosis of Lyme disease, Dr. Richard Horowitz has developed a questionnaire, the Horowitz Lyme-MSIDS Questionnaire, which you can take online for free. Just go to his website—https://www.tiredoflyme.com/horowitz-lyme-msids-questionnaire.html—and work with his scoring system to determine your risk for having Lyme disease. This questionnaire has been validated with research in over 1,500 patients, and the results published in a peer-reviewed journal

What are the symptoms of *Bartonella*? Why is it frequently associated with Lyme? For patients who've been sensitized, it's been my experience and that of most of my colleagues that it's *Bartonella,* even more than Lyme disease, that's responsible for their sensitization. Here's a list of *Bartonella* symptoms, which are somewhat similar to those of Lyme disease, with an emphasis on the differences. *Bartonella* can cause:

- Severe fatigue and cognitive/memory-concentration problems
- Increased sensitization to light, sound, food, chemicals, and EMFs
- Intense emotional instability and mood swings
- Intense depression with occasional feelings of hopelessness or despair
- Intense anxiety with "out of the blue" panic attacks
- Depersonalization: a sense that one does not feel like they are present in their own body
- Psychosis and schizophrenia, as well as OCD and other neuropsychiatric symptoms
- An uncomfortable sensation of vibration or trembling, not visible to the naked eye
- Paresthesias (numbness or tingling) especially in parts of the body not normally associated with peripheral nerves
- Pseudoseizures (body movements that look like seizures but do not show up on an EEG)
- Dyskinesias (sporadic unusual twisting movements of the arms and legs)
- Headaches (often localized to the back of the head)
- Joint or muscle pain
- Abdominal pain
- Heartburn or reflux
- Pelvic or bladder pain with interstitial cystitis (inflammation in the bladder leading to frequency and burning, without a clear infection)
- Rashes that look like stretch marks, called *striae,* which can be perpendicular to the skin planes, or horizontal (not associated with weight loss)
- Rashes that resemble granulomas (hard, inflamed nodules), a maculopapular rash (a rash with both flat and raised parts), and/or inflamed blood vessels (vasculitis)
- Rashes that resemble inflammatory breast cancer, lymphoma; with *Bartonella* recently having been found to be associated with melanomas in certain patients

Note that we often lump Lyme disease with what are called *coinfections* of Lyme disease. These infections are *vector-borne,* meaning that a vector, usually a biting insect, transmits the infection from the vector to a human. When a tick, the most common vector, bites someone, the tick, after attaching to the skin, sucks in some of that person's blood, and after a while, injects the contents of its stomach back into the person through the skin. "After a while" is an important phrase. Many physicians have been taught that there's a time lag of twenty-four hours or longer before the tick injects its stomach contents, so if a tick has not been attached for too long, you're safe from any possibility of Lyme disease. Unfortunately, there are many recorded cases of disease transmission within two hours of the bite, because the tick had partially fed on another animal previously, so spirochetes were already in the tick's salivary glands. Other tick-borne infections, such as the Powassan virus, can be transmitted within fifteen minutes of a tick bite; *rickettsia* infections can be transmitted within ten minutes, and relapsing-fever borrelia, *Borrelia hermsii*, can be transmitted within five minutes of a bite. Tick-transmitted infections can happen quickly, and physicians who believe that longer intervals are necessary for transmission of infection have contributed to inadequate treatment for some patients.

Studies of the bacterial content of tick stomachs show that in many states, up to 40%+ of ticks carry *Borrelia*, and in some states, 20% carry *Bartonella*. Smaller percentages (8–10%) carry the parasite *Babesia* or the bacteria *Ehrlichia*. Thus *Bartonella*, *Babesia*, and *Ehrlichia* are among the more common coinfections associated with Lyme disease, but other infections, like TBRF (tick-borne relapsing fever, *Borrelia miyamotoi*), have recently been increasing in number, especially in patients who live in the northeastern U.S. and in the San Francisco Bay Area.

Though most of the infections we've been discussing are from tick bites, some can be transmitted by blood transfusion (*Babesia*, *Borrelia miyamotoi*, *Ehrlichia*, and certain viruses); maternal-fetal transmission (Lyme, *Babesia*, *Bartonella*, Rocky Mountain spotted fever), and even—though rarely—by solid organ transplantation (*Babesia*). In the case of *Bartonella*, however, one can acquire it through the bite or scratch of a cat or from the bite of fleas, mosquitos, and spiders.

While these are fascinating aspects of understanding Lyme disease and its coinfections, I want to emphasize that *Bartonella* and Lyme are primarily responsible for creating an intense inflammatory response that will affect the limbic and vagal systems, triggering the possibility of sensitization. Once triggered, it will usually require treatment of the causative agent in order to truly heal that sensitization. Most important is that we can, with increasing accuracy and certainty, diagnose these infections and treat them effectively.

The sensitized individual should therefore make sure that mold toxicity and Lyme and *Bartonella* have been carefully looked for, or their sensitivities are likely to increase and worsen with time.

The Treatment of Lyme and *Bartonella*

First, the good news: For the majority of patients, we can effectively treat these infections so that our patients can resume normal activities and enjoy their lives.

Next comes the sobering news (not bad, just realistic): It can take a long time to bring these infections under control for some of the sickest individuals. Occasionally, a patient responds quickly to our treatment program, but more often than not we're talking at least a year, and often longer, for full recovery. In the past seven years, however, Dr Horowitz has published in the peer-reviewed literature on new treatments for Lyme disease and *Bartonella* that are proving much more effective and require less antibiotics than in years prior. For more information, see his work and articles on dapsone combination therapy.

A brief history of our understanding of these tick-borne infections may be helpful so you can see how our knowledge of treatment has evolved over the years. In the 1980s and 1990s, we were primarily aware of Lyme disease as an infection by the *Borrelia* spirochete. As such, as with all infections, we used what we'd always used to treat bacterial infections: antibiotics. We were able to help many patients with the use of these antibiotics, both oral, intramuscular, and intravenous, but many patients fell through the cracks.

Though the CDC and NIH did not provide the research funds required to get a handle on this infection, through the private efforts of several pioneering physicians and funding from Lyme organizations, it was slowly realized that *Borrelia* was a very advanced organism (called *pleomorphic*), meaning that when threatened with antibiotic annihilation, it could change its shape to make it less affected by the antibiotics. There are four main forms that *Borrelia* can assume:

- The classical spirochete form (it's a relative of syphilis, which has a similar form) with a cell wall;
- an L-form, also called a cell-wall deficient form or cystic form;
- an intracellular form; and
- a biofilm/persister form.

Each has a different response to antibiotics, so we learned that in order to treat Lyme disease properly we had to use multiple antibiotics in combination with biofilm agents that would address the different forms. That way, when *Borrelia* shifted into another form, we could effectively address its pleomorphic nature. We only learned about the biofilm/persister forms of Lyme about eight years ago, however, so it took trial and error and a variety of antibiotic combinations before we saw significant progress.

In the mid-1990s, when the parasite *Babesia* (similar to malaria) was discovered, adding treatments for this parasite improved our outcomes. Yet it wasn't enough. By the late 1990s, it was appreciated that *Bartonella* was another organism that created inflammation and chronic disease, and by incorporating new treatments, we had better outcomes treating chronic Lyme disease. The recognition of *Ehrlichia,* and more recently, Relapsing Fever organisms, has also added to our understanding.

By the early 2000s we realized that antibiotic treatment alone was insufficient for many patients, and that much more was going on than we had originally thought. A major issue for many patients was that these microbial organisms, when killed, released the toxins they carried, and until we improved our patients' ability to detoxify, those toxins remained in their bodies and created cytokine "storms," which added to the inflammatory burdens already created by the original infections.

We became increasingly aware that these toxins and infections directly impacted the pituitary (master) gland and interfered with the body's ability to make our most important hormones, especially adrenal, thyroid, and sex hormones, and that we needed to evaluate and treat these if our patients were going to get well.

The very nature of these infections, according to the Cell Danger Response model developed by Robert Naviaux, MD, was such that any threat to the body would result in a programmed series of biochemical shifts that the body required to deal with those threats. When the threats were not immediately neutralized, we needed to consider these biochemical deficiencies so that mitochondria could heal, and the accumulation of heavy metals, creating additional toxicity, could be recognized and dealt with.

These infections almost always affected our patients' ability to sleep, and without adequate rest, healing was difficult. Also, these infections nearly always affected our patients' livers, hepatic function (which need help with detoxification), and gastrointestinal tracts, causing leaky gut, SIBO, and intestinal dysbiosis in most.

Dr. Horowitz has synthesized this information in his books, *Why Can't I Get Better?* and *How Can I Get Better?* and created the Horowitz 16-Point Differential Diagnostic Map, which allows patients and physicians to comprehensively review all of our new findings about the complexities of Lyme disease by looking at all of these issues and bearing them in mind while we create a detailed treatment plan.

Most physicians are not aware of this information, and unless your doctor has had advanced training in Lyme disease to become what we call an LLMD (Lyme-Literate Medical Doctor), it's not likely you'll be able to get the comprehensive treatment you need.

Newer Developments in the Treatment of *Borrelia* and *Bartonella*

It is beyond the scope of this book to go into the details of the antibiotic and botanical treatments for these illnesses. What we're trying to do here is simply help the reader understand that these infectious illnesses can be key players in the creation of sensitivity, and they need to be looked for and then treated to reverse this sensitivity. I hope you now see that while this is indeed possible, it's also quite complicated; you need to work with health-care practitioners who are knowledgeable about all of these important details.

One of the most important new discoveries of the past few years is the recognition that *Borrelia* and *Bartonella* are two types of bacteria that are capable of changing into *persister cells,* meaning that despite appropriate antibiotic treatments that can kill off a majority of these bacteria, a few of them will become impervious to these treatments and *persist,* and grow, hiding under biofilms. This helps us understand why some patients may respond initially to our antibiotic treatments, but their symptoms may recur over time as they become less and less responsive to what we give them. Dr. Ying Zhang, at Johns Hopkins, has published several important papers on the persister cells of both *Borrelia* and *Bartonella,* along with laboratory cultures that show which antibiotics and botanicals might be able to deal with them effectively.

With this information, Dr. Horowitz has created treatment programs to make exciting improvements in our ability to treat those patients with infections who hadn't responded to their previous regimens as we'd hoped. His Double Dapsone Protocol, available on his website and published in several peer-reviewed journals, has revolutionized our treatment for Lyme and *Bartonella* patients, and gives us great hope for the future of treatment.

The bottom line: given how important Lyme and *Bartonella* are as major triggers of sensitivity, the most appropriate testing should be done for all unusually sensitive patients to evaluate the possibility that there might be another treatable component of their illness.

DR. RICHARD HOROWITZ is a board-certified internist and medical director of the Hudson Valley Healing Arts Center, an integrative medical center that combines both classical and complementary approaches in the treatment of Lyme disease and other tick-borne disorders. In the past thirty years, he has treated more than 13,000 patients from all over the U.S., Canada, and Europe. He is one of the founding members and a former president of ILADS, the International Lyme and Associated Diseases Society. Dr Horowitz was given the Humanitarian of the Year award by the Turn the Corner

Foundation, and received awards from Project Lyme for his treatment of Lyme disease. He has dedicated his life to helping those stricken with this devastating illness.

He is also the author of two best-selling books on Lyme disease: *Why Can't I Get Better? Solving the Mystery of Lyme and Chronic Disease* (St. Martin's Press, 2013); and *How Can I Get Better? An Action Plan for Treating Resistant Lyme and Chronic Disease* (St. Martin's Press, 2017). These books incorporate recent scientific advances and explain in detail how health-care providers can effectively diagnose and treat resistant chronic illness. In addition, he has co-authored peer-reviewed Lyme guidelines. From 2017 to 2019, Dr Horowitz was a member of the HHS Tick-borne Disease Working Group and Co-chair of the "Other Tick-borne Diseases and Coinfections" subcommittee, which provided recommendations to Congress to help the U.S. improve the care of those suffering tick-borne disorders. He recently served as a member of the HHS Babesia and Tick-borne Pathogen Subcommittee, and now serves as a member of the NYS DOH Tick-borne disease Working Group.

Dr Horowitz recently published several scientific articles on classical and integrative solutions for COVID-19, which have been effective in helping those with acute and chronic illness (see www.cangetbetter.com).He released his first novel, *Starseed R/evolution, The Awakening,* a cli-fi (science fiction/climate change) novel in March 2022, providing new solutions and hope for our climate crisis. For more information, please see https://starseed-revolution.com/

Chapter 9: EMFs – Electromagnetic Fields

Riina Bray, MD, and Magda Havas, PhD

Dr. Nathan's Introduction

In the early 1990s I had the privilege of working with Dr. C. Norman Shealy and becoming the medical director for The Shealy Institute, a nationally recognized pain clinic. Its founder, Dr. Shealy, was the inventor of the TENS unit and the implanted neural stimulator for the treatment of chronic pain. He is considered the "grandfather of holistic medicine," having also founded the American Holistic Medical Association. Dr. Shealy had identified a number of patients who complained that when they worked with computers and other electrical devices, they would suddenly develop profound brain fog and fatigue.

Using a medical technique called brain mapping, he studied these patients. Brain mapping is a device that measures the brain waves emanating from the brain. In simple terms, beta waves are the type of brainwaves associated with conscious and clear thinking, while alpha waves are associated with relaxation, theta waves with creative thoughts, and delta waves with absence of thought ("the lights are on, but no one's home.")

With the device in place, if he brought a simple electrical clock down toward the head of the patient who had these complaints, Dr. Shealy found a sudden, reproducible shift in the brain-wave pattern from normal beta waves to the dysfunctional delta waves. This gave scientific credence to the fact that electromagnetic frequencies could instantly affect a patient with this disorder, which he termed "Electromagnetic Dysthymia" in a published paper in 1992. We now call it ElectroHypersensitivity Syndrome (EHS).

Bear in mind that in those days we didn't have cellphones. Cell towers were only just being erected in various parts of the country. I—and all physicians on call—had to constantly wear a pager, which beeped when the answering service needed to get in touch with me about a patient in distress. Often, when away from home, I had to hurry to try to find a phone and respond to the beeper.

I suspect that our current generation of teenagers can't imagine not being able to message instantly. This reminiscence is simply to emphasize the profound change in our exposure to EMF from just twenty-five years ago. It was rare to see a patient who had been affected by EMF in this way then, but as time went on it became much more common. Among the sensitive patients who composed my practice, 25–30% of them now complained of EMF sensitivity at their first visit!

This is more common than you might think. To repeat a paragraph in this chapter, for emphasis:

> According to a study in the UK, approximately 0.65% of the population are so sensitive to electromagnetic pollution that they can't work; 1.5% are severely affected, 5% moderately affected, and 30% have mild symptoms. Those in the *severe/can't work* category are considered disabled and are unable to function in what has now become the *normal environment* in many countries around the globe.

Drs. Bray and Havas have been at the forefront of studying this sensitivity for more than a decade. Despite the phone-service providers' denial of any medical issues from EMFs, hundreds of published papers document the reality of this disability. With the dramatic increase in EMFs since the shift from 4G to 5G, we've seen a marked increase in the incidence and severity of sensitivity in our patients, especially in those who had already manifested other sensitivities.

We are honored to have Drs. Bray and Havas help us understand the entire field of EMFs as a health hazard, and to educate us on how to protect ourselves from this growing problem. The extensive references that accompany this chapter add a great deal of weight to their discussion.

✿ ✿ ✿

Introduction to EMFs and Life on Earth

Natural Abiotic Sources of Electromagnetic Energy

All life on earth evolved within an electromagnetic envelope or cocoon. The earth's magnetic field, Schumann resonance, solar radiation, and cosmic radiation are all natural sources of electromagnetic exposure that life on earth has adapted to. Some of the high-energy frequencies coming from the cosmos are partially blocked by the ionosphere, a protective layer around the globe that filters out most harmful ionizing radiation (Presman, 1970; Dubrov 1978; Erdmann et al. 2021).

Earth's Magnetic Field – The earth's natural magnetic field is due to the circulation of the molten core deep within the planet. The magnetic field ranges from 500 mG at the equator to approximately 700 mG at both poles. Just as we use a compass to establish our relative position within this magnetic field, migratory animals (bacteria, insects, honeybees, sea turtles, monarch butterflies, and migratory birds) have an internal compass consisting of magnetic crystals that helps them navigate. This field is considered to be direct current (DC), like a battery or a bar magnet, as opposed to alternating current (AC) like household electricity. The biological effects of DC are quite different from those of AC, so this information is important.

This magnetic field is "considered" to be DC but, in reality, it alternates (or flips), and based on fossil records, we know that during previous polar reversals a number of species became extinct. Prior to this flip, the strength of the magnetic field decreased substantially and, as it reestablished its strength, the magnetic poles were reversed. The earth's magnetic field is currently weakening; a reversal is long overdue but is unlikely to happen within our lifetime.

Schumann Resonance – The Schumann resonance, predicted by Dr. Winfried Otto Schumann in 1952, is considered the earth's heartbeat. Caused by thousands of daily lightning strikes across the globe, it has a fundamental frequency of 7.8 Hz (cycles per second) with weaker harmonics (multiples of the fundamental frequency) of approximately 15, 21, 30 Hz, etc. The Schumann resonance helps us maintain our circadian rhythm, which controls several physiological/biochemical functions in the human body. Disturbances or blocking of the Schumann frequencies can lead to disrupted circadian rhythm and possibly illness (Panagopoulos and Chrousos, 2019).

Solar Radiation – All life on earth is influenced by radiation from the sun. The light/dark (day/night) cycles help us maintain a normal circadian rhythm but artificial light at night can disturb that rhythm, as can computer monitors.

The sun emits all colors of the rainbow and appears as white light, especially at noon. At both sunrise and sunset, portions of the blue part of the spectrum are filtered out and the sky appears red. Exposure to different colors of light also has biological effects. Blue light at night interferes with melatonin production and interferes with sleep. Melatonin supplements can reverse this trend, and those who suffer from jet lag often use melatonin to help them reestablish their circadian rhythm for their current location. Melatonin has many other functions as well. One of these is to protect against cancers, but the beneficial effects against cancer are reduced in the presence of a high magnetic field.

The sun periodically (every eleven years) emits sunspots, high-energy particles that rush toward the earth. A subset of the population is sensitive to these sunspots, and, during these periods, viral infections increase, as do psychological disturbances and crime rates.

Cosmic Radiation – The intensity of the cosmic radiation reaching the earth's surface and consisting of radio waves and ionizing radiation is generally low (figure 1). Large radio telescopes are needed to monitor their intensity. Greenbank, West Virginia, is a research site where radio telescopes monitor the radiation that comes from outer space. The intensity of the signals coming from space is such that a cellphone or a wireless smart meter within a few miles of these telescopes interferes with the monitoring, hence this is a community where use of technology that emits radio/microwaves is forbidden. Consequently, this location attracts those who are sensitive to electromagnetic radiation since their exposures are significantly lower than in other similar size communities in the United States.

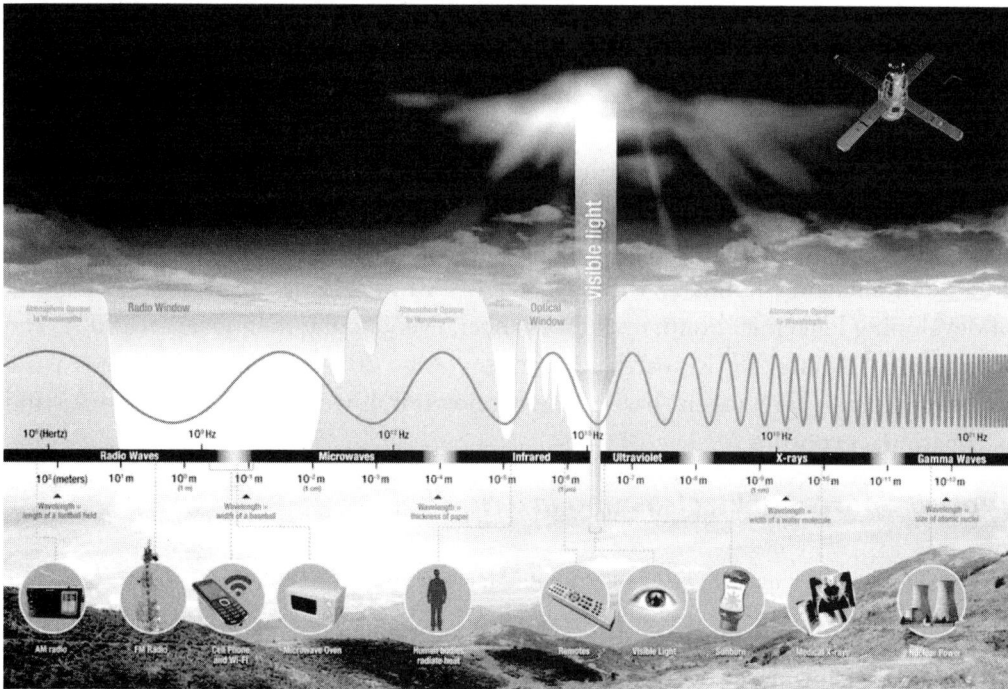

Natural sources of cosmic energies influence life on earth, so it shouldn't surprise any of us that anthropogenic (pollution or environmental change originating in human activity) sources are likely to also have biological effects.

Anthropogenic Sources of Electromagnetic Energy

Our exposure to anthropogenic sources of electromagnetic energy dates back to the turn of the last century when we began to use artificial light with Edison's light bulbs and Tesla's alternating current (AC). The rollout of this technology started in larger urban centers before it was adopted in rural communities. It wasn't until the middle of last century that electricity was available in most communities in North America.

Extremely Low-Frequency Electromagnetic Fields and Electricity – In North America the electricity that flows along wires from power plants to the final user consists of AC that has a frequency of 60 Hz (cycles per second) and a voltage of 120 V/240 V. The rest of world uses 50 Hz and 240 V. Initially, electricity was used for light bulbs and simple motors. Today, so many appliances use electricity that it would be difficult to live without it. Some electricity is DC and is supplied either by batteries or by DC power lines. It is possible to store electricity in batteries, as is done with solar energy, and to convert DC to AC.

Electricity falls within the realm classified as extremely low-frequency electromagnetic fields (ELF EMF), which consists of both an electric field and a magnetic field. An electric field can be easily blocked, but a magnetic field goes through walls, windows, and doors and is difficult to block or shield. An appliance plugged into a wall outlet has an electric field. When it's turned on and current is flowing there is also a magnetic field. Both fields are bioactive, which means they can affect living organisms. Early studies indicated that children living near power lines had a greater risk of developing childhood leukemia. Similarly, those exposed to ELF EMF at work had a greater risk of developing leukemia, brain, or breast cancer, even among men (Havas, 2000). The International Agency for Research on Cancer (IARC 2002) classified ELF EMFs as a "possible human carcinogen" based largely on research with childhood leukemia and occupational exposure.

Types & Sources of Electrosmog in a Nutshell!

1. *Extremely Low Frequency (ELF) Electric and Magnetic Fields (EMFs)*

   Sources: Transmission lines, distribution lines (above and below ground), substations, transformers, electric breaker panel, faulty wiring, knob and tube wiring in older homes, power supply cables, electric appliances especially those that generate heat (i.e. electric stove, toaster, hair dryer), computers, and grounded metal pipes (in some areas).

2. *Radio Frequency (RF) and Microwave (MW) Radiation*

   Sources: Cell phone, cordless phone, tablets, smart meters, wireless baby monitors, wireless computer games, microwave oven, Wi-Fi router, some wireless keyboards and wireless mouse, wireless wearables, wireless security systems, smart appliances, home wireless systems, cell phone antennas, radar, TV and radio broadcast antennas.

3. *Dirty Electricity (DE) (Intermediate Frequencies)*

   Sources: Computers, televisions, tube fluorescent lights, compact fluorescent light bulbs, dimmer switches, variable speed motors/tools, treadmills, vacuum cleaners, sewing machines, solar photovoltaic cells, wind turbines, smart meters and devices that require inverters. Dirty electricity flows along wires and can enter your home from neighbors through your electrical panel.

4. *Ground Current (GC) also known as "stray voltage"*

   Sources: distribution and transmission lines (power lines), transformers, substations, faulty wiring problems, insufficient capacity of neutral to return unbalanced loads, equipment in the home or on farm. Note: this is often an issue for the electric utility to resolve.

Radio Frequency Radiation

The next technological breakthrough was the radio developed by Tesla and capitalized on by Marconi. Radio uses higher frequencies that fall within the realm of "radio frequency radiation." This was called "radiation" because it radiates from a source, unlike electricity that has to travel along wires for its distribution and that generates a "field" around the conductor. The frequency signal from a radio is called the carrier wave and this can contain information in the form of sound. Sound frequencies are converted into electromagnetic frequencies and carried by the fundamental frequency of the radio station. At the user's end the EMFs are converted back into sound waves. Both television and the radio use radio frequency radiation (RFR) although at different frequencies so they do not interfere with one another. IARC (2013) classified RFR as a "possible human carcinogen" and they are currently reassessing this classification.

RADAR

During World War II, radar was invented to track enemy aircraft; this relied on microwave radiation (MWR). Microwaves are part of the radio frequency spectrum but at higher frequencies (above 300 MHz or millions of cycles per second). As the name implies, the microwave oven uses microwaves and was initially called the radar range. It is set at 2.45 GHz (billions of cycles per second), as this is a frequency optimally absorbed by water. Water molecules absorb the microwave energy and convert it into heat.

Cellphones and Cellular Antennas

The next set of inventions centered on the wireless phone or "cell" phone. Cellphones have now gone through at least five generations with higher frequencies that allow us to communicate around the world at the speed of light. The 5th generation, or 5G, has introduced millimeter waves (mmW), which are at even higher frequencies (above 30 GHz) but still within the radio frequency spectrum. These anthropogenic devices are shown in fig. 2.

The first generation of cellphones in the 1980s were large, powerful, and provided voice only. The second generation in the 1990s (2G) cellphones were smaller, faster (64 Kb/s), lighter, and enabled both voice and text transmissions. The third generation (3G) in 2001 included internet access in addition to voice and text messaging, and had speeds of 2Mb/s. The fourth generation (4G) cellphones in 2009 were smaller, faster, and lighter, with many more features including the ability to watch videos. Fifth generation (5G) and the Internet of things (IoT) promises even more possibilities. Upload speeds in excess of 1 Gb/s are now possible. Each time a new generation cellphone was introduced, slightly different frequency bands were engaged. With 5G, three frequency bands are used: those that are sub 1 GHz, sub 6 GHz, and millimeter waves (mmW).

Unfortunately, the bioactivity of these frequencies was not tested prior to the marketing of these cellphones. The same is the case for mmW. Scientists assumed they were safe, and only a thermal or heating effect of biological tissue was considered harmful. If there wasn't enough energy to heat tissue, scientists reasoned, the radiation should be safe. This turned out not to be the case.

While most of the scientific literature deals primarily with these two forms of non-ionizing radiation (ELF and RFR), there are two other forms that are also important: *dirty electricity* and *ground current pollution* (or stray voltage).

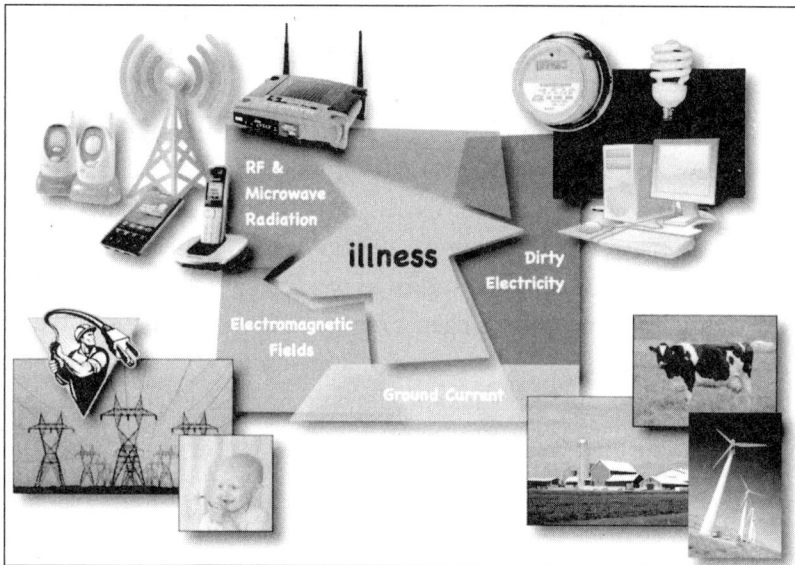

Figure 3: Types of Electrosmog

Dirty Electricity

Dirty electricity is a combination of ELF and RFR as it refers to higher frequencies, generally in the kHz–MHz range (thousands to millions of cycles per second) that ride along electrical wires. Another term used in the scientific literature is "high frequency voltage transients." Dirty electricity is generated by electronic devices that are not properly filtered, energy efficient technology, dimmer switches, on/off switching, switch mode power supply (DC to AC conversion), sparking on power lines from nearby vegetation, etc. Dirty electricity can damage sensitive electrical equipment and cause overheating so it isn't good for devices that consume electricity and it isn't good for our bodies. Dirty electricity flows along wires and also radiates from these wires. It can be "filtered" and various power conditioners/capacitors have been designed for this purpose. Dirty electricity is virtually ubiquitous but has received less attention than the other forms of electrosmog from the scientific community. This is now beginning to change (Havas and Stetzer, 2004).

Ground Current

Ground-current pollution, referred to as "stray voltage" in some of the older scientific literature, refers to electricity that flows along the ground. If this electricity (50/60 Hz) is contaminated by dirty electricity (kHz), it has a much greater biological effect. Above 2 kHz these frequencies penetrate deeply into the body.

Ground current pollution is a problem in some regions and is normally noticed on dairy farms as it affects milk production and herd health (Hillman et al., 2013). Since dairy cows are milked two to three times daily, the amount of milk *Daisy* produces is known; if her milk production changes, for whatever reason, the farmer will know within a day. Farmers and other farm animals (horses, pigs) are also affected, but it is most readily found on commercial dairy farms and in commercial hatcheries.

Each new technology contributes more electromagnetic energy to the environment at higher frequencies. With the contribution of satellites, there are few places on earth not exposed to some form of anthropogenic electromagnetic radiation. We haven't had time to evolve with these artificial frequencies, and some people are unable to tolerate the current levels of exposure, especially in densely populated areas. These people are classified as being electrohypersensitive (EHS).

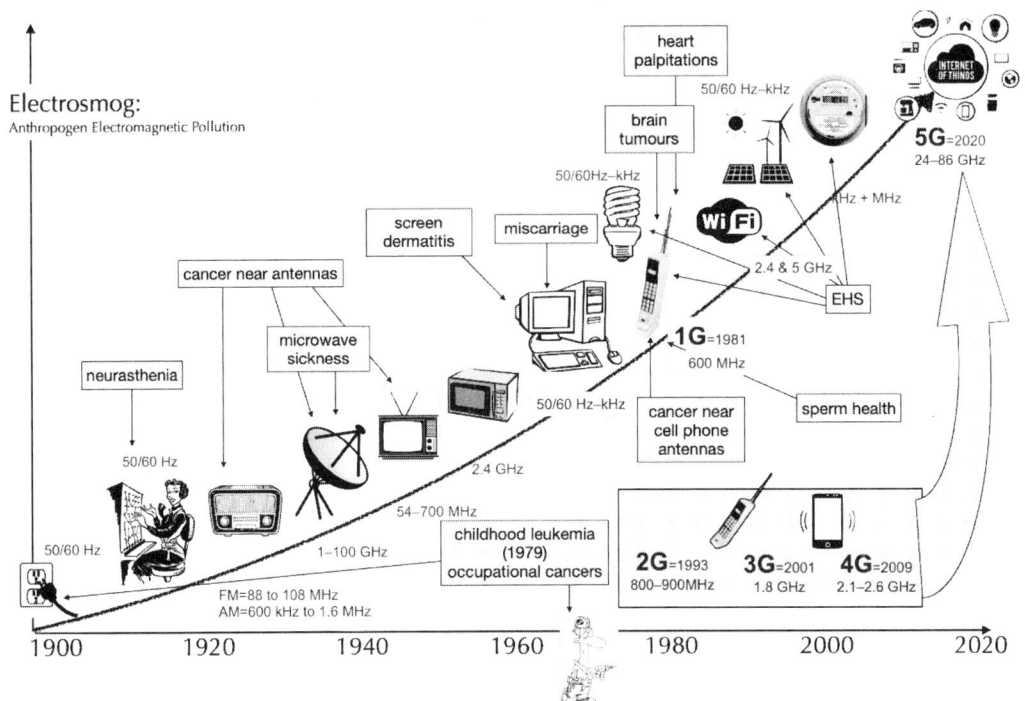

Figure 2: Devices that emit electrosmog.

Electrohypersensitivity: History, Symptoms, and Precursors

Over the past twenty years, doctors who have come to understand the impacts of electromagnetic field effects on health have seen a significant rise in those affected. It's no surprise that for years there was incredulity by those less informed that non-ionizing radiation actually had an impact on health. Think about it—our bodies were not meant to experience these foreign microwaves, which are subtle yet very potent and impact the delicate physiological systems of the body. EMF, in all its forms, causes a disturbance in the gentle currents created by ions flowing across cellular membranes in our bodies. Our exposure to non-ionizing radiation is at least 10 billion times higher than the exposure of our grandparents or great-grandparents!

The term "electrohypersensitivity" (EHS) refers to an individual who has an adverse reaction when exposed to even low levels of either electromagnetic fields (EMF) or electromagnetic radiation (EMR) (Belyae et al. 2016 and Belpomme and Irigaray 2022).

The definition of electromagnetic hypersensitivity is an awareness and/or adverse symptomatology in response to electromagnetic fields. There are multiple variations of the same theme. The incidence of EHS has been rising exponentially over the years. EHS is a functional impairment and a spectrum disorder; i.e., one can exhibit a variety of degrees of impairment. (Reported functional impairments of electrohypersensitive Japanese: A questionnaire survey. Kato Y. Johansson O. Pathophysiology. 2012; 19(2):95-100.)

Electromagnetic sensitivity follows the same criteria as those of multiple chemical sensitivities. Whereas genetic polymorphism and total body burdens are responsible for MCS, EHS is the same, except that there's ample evidence in the literature that all cells and physiological systems in the body are affected. Here's the officially accepted definition:

Multiple Chemical Sensitivity Case Criteria

Multiple Chemical Sensitivity: A 1999 Consensus (Bartha et al. Archives of Environmental Health, May/June 1999; 54(3): Based on: Nethercott JR., Davidoff LL, Curbow B., et al. Multiple chemical sensitivities syndrome: toward a working case definition. Arch Environ Health 1993;48:19-26).

The multiple chemical sensitivity is a chronic condition manifested by low levels of exposure (lower than previously or commonly tolerated). The symptoms are reproducible with repeated chemical exposure and improve or resolve with the removal of the incitants. The responses can occur to multiple chemically unrelated substances and involve multiple organ systems (added in 1999). This pattern of symptoms is also reported for sensitivities to electromagnetic phenomena.

Multiple Chemical Sensitivity Case Criteria

Multiple Chemical Sensitivity: A 1999 Consensus (Bartha et al. Archives of Environmental Health, May/June 1999; 54(3): Based on: Nethercott JR., Davidoff LL, Curbow B. et al. Multiple chemical sensitivities syndrome: toward a working case definition. Arch Environ Health 1993;48:19-26)

Multiple chemical sensitivity is a chronic condition manifested by low levels of exposure (lower than previously or commonly tolerated). The symptoms are reproducible with repeated chemical exposure and improve or resolve with the removal of the incitants. The responses can occur to multiple chemically unrelated substances and involve multiple organ systems. This pattern of symptoms is also reported for sensitivities to electromagnetic phenomena.

Those with electromagnetic hypersensitivity are affected by RF radiation, which ranges from 3 MHz to 300 GHz produced by Wi-Fi, routers, smartphones, tablets, cordless phones, and Bluetooth devices as well as ELE EF (electric fields) and MF (magnetic fields), which range from 3 kHz to 3 MHz and are produced by electrical wiring, lamps, and appliances. It is everywhere. ICNIRP (International Commission on Non-Ionizing Radiation Protection) only addresses ELF EMF and the thermal effects of RF radiation.

In 2004, the World Health Organization (WHO) held a meeting to discuss this issue and at that meeting they defined EHS as follows:

"...a phenomenon where individuals experience adverse health effects while using or being in the vicinity of devices emanating electric, magnetic, or electromagnetic fields (EMFs)."

"...EHS is a real and sometimes debilitating problem for the affected persons.... Their exposures are generally several orders of magnitude under the limits in internationally accepted standards."

They stated that they did not know what caused EHS and would prefer that the term *idiopathic environmental intolerance—attributed to electromagnetic fields* (IEI–EMF) be used instead.

History of Electrohypersensitivity

EHS is not a novel illness. It was first described as *neurasthenia* (weakening of the nervous system) at the turn of the last century; it affected switchboard operators in Toronto according to a Royal Commission Report in 1907.

During WWII, *microwave syndrome* or *radio wave sickness* was the term used to describe symptoms experienced by radar operators (Carpenter, 2015). Other terms in the literature used to describe this illness include electromagnetic intolerance, electromagnetic illness, and electromagnetic sensitivity.

EHS has genuine, pathological symptoms. There are no specific biomarkers, but genetic polymorphisms are associated with the condition. Under the influence of EMF and/or chemicals, a cerebral hypoperfusion/hypoxia-related neuroinflammation may occur and presents with symptoms of inadequate regulation (Belpomme, 2015).

Radiofrequency radiation causes oxidative stress in biological systems, and histamine release causes dermatological problems. It also causes peroxidation, DNA damage, changes to antioxidant enzymes, and voltage-gated calcium channel (VGCC) dysregulation affecting the cardiac and nervous systems. VGCCs are present at very high density in the nervous system and are responsible for releasing neurotransmitters and neuroendocrine hormones (Pall, 2015) [see chapter 10].

Radiofrequency radiation is also known to increase peroxynitrite formation, which causes chronic inflammation, damage to mitochondrial function and structure, reduction of ATP, and reduced glutathione and CoQ10, leading to fatigue and pain (Pall, 2018; De Luca, 2014). Clinical findings are not specific and create a multi-morbid picture in which various problems need to be delineated and addressed in order to overcome the symptom complex. All these classifications delineate degree of exposure to various sources of EMFs.

There are basic rules to help with diagnosis and management of this condition. Taking an exposure history is key, and other illnesses and diseases must be ruled out. Usually, a physical exam will reveal neurological, dermatological, or cardiac signs associated with it. Blood tests are expensive and not sensitive or specific but can help guide management if there are deficiencies or other disease states that must be corrected. There is no gold standard for EHS diagnosis; cases present symptoms within a wide spectrum. Also, it is referred to as "EMF sensitive" or "EMF susceptible" rather than "hyper."

Family members are the best litmus test. At times, lack of understanding of the sensitivity phenomenon leads to serious family conflict, child custody battles, labeling, and stigmatization. More often, spouses and children witness double-blind causal occurrences that persuade them that this is not the effect of a nocebo (a benign substance or treatment that may cause harmful side effects or worsened symptoms because the patient believes they may occur) as they watch their loved one react strongly to EMF exposures. Patients will feel anxious about potential exposures because they know how awful they feel when exposed. This gives the impression of paranoia, when in fact it is a reproducible reaction to exposure.

EHS Symptoms

Symptoms include: chronic fatigue; chronic pain; sleep disturbances; cognitive dysfunction with difficulty concentrating and poor short-term memory; anxiety and/or depression; dizziness; nausea; tinnitus; skin sensitivity; heart palpitations; increased night-time urination (bed wetting in children); nosebleeds (more common in children).

Symptoms may also include:

- Sensitivity to fluorescent lights
- Irritability, lack of appetite, memory problems, vertigo, visual, skin, and vascular problems
- Tinnitus, sleep disorders (disrupted stage-4 sleep with multiple shock-like wakening disruptions if there is any RFR > 10 µW/m2)
- Mood and personality changes (anxiety, depression, despair)
- Headache, weakness, pressure in the head, racing or fluttering heart
- Itching, pain, edema, erythema, Morgellons disease (crawling sensations on and under the skin, often compared to insects moving, stinging, or biting) secondary to transthyretin concentrations or mast-cell activation.
- Neurasthenic and vegetative symptoms (a state of consciousness in which a person is awake but is not aware of and cannot meaningfully respond to their surroundings), fatigue, tiredness, nausea, and digestive disturbances.

Other possible reactions include thermal (heat-related) effects. EMF may also prompt adverse biological effects. It can damage our DNA, suppress the immune system, cause thickening of the blood and leakage of the blood-brain barrier. It can have an effect on the cardiovascular, neurological, and endocrine systems as well. In those with electro-magnetic hypersensitivity, it can, as noted above, lead to cognitive problems, fatigue, tinnitus, headaches, dizziness, sleep disturbances, sensory upregulation, palpitations, pain in multiple sites, twitching, fatigue or hyperactivity, memory disturbances, and/or brain fog. These symptoms may resolve with withdrawal of the inciting electromagnetic frequency (Erica M Blythe, EHS a Summary, 2014). According to a study in the UK, approximately 0.65% of the population are so sensitive to electromagnetic pollution that they can't work; 1.5% are severely affected, 5% moderately affected and 30% have mild symptoms. Those in the *severe/can't work* category are considered disabled and are unable to function in what has now become the *normal environment* in many countries around the globe (Bevington, 2019).

What Causes EHS?

We know that electromagnetic energy triggers the symptoms of EHS, but what causes EHS? Though this is more difficult to answer, we *do* know that individuals with EHS have one or more of the following precursors: physical injury to the central nervous system (CNS) that may happen during a fall, athletic injury, or car accident leading to concussion or whiplash; exposure to toxic chemicals, especially those that are neurotoxins such as mercury, aluminum, and chlorinated hydrocarbon pesticides; excessive chronic or acute exposure to EMF/EMR, which could include multiple shocks as well as being struck by lightning; high load of parasites, unfriendly bacteria, yeast, as well as such illnesses as Lyme Disease and mold toxicity; and a weakened or overactive immune system attributed to age, illness, or medication. Most of these exposures are covered in other chapters in this book, and we provide more details below.

Predisposing co-morbid conditions include but are not limited to:

- Toxic metal/ metalloid body burden
- Mercury, due to the overconsumption of contaminated seafood in the form of methylmercury. Zinc/nickel/mercury dental amalgams also release elemental mercury vapor, which enters the brain. Patients can also present with cardiac and neurological manifestations.
- Inflammatory conditions of the nervous system

Patients fall into this category if they suffer from infectious diseases such as Lyme disease and its coinfections, other infections that affect the nervous system, as well as mold and other environmental toxins.

Traumatic Brain Injury and Brain Lesions

This category of patients suffer from lesions of the brain (including tumors such as pituitary adenomas), demyelination, microangiopathic changes, diffuse ischemia, inflammation (from neurotoxic pesticides or traumatic brain injury) and neurodegenerative diseases (multiple sclerosis and ALS, for example).

Heart-Rhythm Disturbances

These patients suffer tachycardic spells (elevated heart rate), especially at night, and may also experience premature ventricular contractions, premature atrial contractions, atrial flutter, and fibrillation. Those with Wolff Parkinson White syndrome are especially at risk for sudden cardiac death due to EMF exposures. Sleep time can also be particularly difficult.

Chronic Exposure to Stress/Exhaustion/Adrenal Fatigue

These patients include students and teachers. University, college, high school, and grade school students who may not have an optimum diet, are stressed, and likely sleep deprived, are all being exposed to high levels of radiation. They frequently work close to fluorescent lights.

Genetic Polymorphism (MCS)

Polymorphism refers to the presence of two or more variant forms of a specific DNA sequence that can occur among different individuals or populations. Many clinical similarities and overlapping comorbid conditions between EHS and multiple chemical sensitivities (MCS) are reflected in similar genetic polymorphism profiles. Inflammation resulting from impaired detoxification processes creates illness and functional impairment.

Chronic Mold Exposure

Mold mycotoxins can affect the immune system and worsen inflammation, leaving one vulnerable to EMF effects.

Diagnostic Tests

During diagnostic testing, biomarkers in combination would be helpful, but are largely unavailable or financially prohibitive for many patients. Of importance are markers of inflammation, mitochondrial dysfunction, oxidative stress, lipid peroxidation, o-myelin abs, nitric oxide production (nitrotyrosine), and lowered melatonin as possible indicators of EHS (Oberfeld 2016, Belpomme, 2015).

To further aid in diagnosis, the biomarkers for salivary cortisol, alpha-amylase, transthyretin, blood sugar levels after provocation, and live blood analysis showing rouleaux formation may be tested. The blood pressure and heart rhythm can be monitored for 24 hours (night-time changes) for heart-rate variability and heart-rate abnormalities (Havas, 2010). Histories gathering anecdotal evidence and data as well as questionnaires may also be used, such as the QEESI used for MCS evaluation. We refer to these as *precursors* because they precede EHS and might also play a causal role. This information is important because it will inform the doctor as to which treatments are required to help the patient heal. Someone with a concussion will require very different medical care than someone with mercury toxicity or Lyme disease. This focused care in combination with minimizing exposure can provide considerable relief to the patient.

Mitigating Electrosmog Exposure

If you are experiencing symptoms of EHS or if you simply don't want to be exposed unnecessarily to anthropogenic EMFs, here are some things you can do.

Distance Is Your Friend

The farther you are from an EMF/EMR-emitting device the lower your exposure. Ideally, cellphone-antenna base stations should be at least 500 yards from your home/school/

workplace. TV and radio broadcast antennas should be at least 1.25 miles away. These values are based on cancer research, which shows an association between chronic (constant) RF exposure and the risk of developing or dying from diverse types of cancers, leukemia being the most common. Some highly sensitive individuals may find these levels excessive.

Similarly, the farther you are from smart meters, cellphones, or other wireless devices the lower your exposure. Indeed, cellphone manufacturers provide a clause in their manuals for you to keep at minimum distance of at least an inch between a cellphone and your body. The same applies for laptop computers in Wi-Fi mode, though the recommended distance is closer to eight inches.

When it comes to power lines, the more current flowing along the wires the stronger the magnetic field. Consequently, power lines with multiple wires or thicker wires emit a more powerful magnetic field, all else being equal. Also, field strength varies with time of day. When more power is required, the magnetic field is higher. Field strength of approximately 3 mG has been linked to childhood cancers, and slightly higher fields have been linked to various adult cancers in occupational settings. Once again, a distance of approximately 500 yards from either a distribution or a transmission power line should be sufficient to ensure that the magnetic field is less than 3 mG.

Power lines also emit an electric field, and this is based on the line voltage set by the electric utility. Electric fields are also biologically active, though they don't penetrate buildings and hence are less of a concern inside a dwelling when the source is external to the building.

Finally, keeping at least an arm's length away from a handheld mobile device lowers your EMF/EMR exposure. Setting mobile devices down on a stand and using a stylus further increases your distance and reduces your exposure.

Electromagnetic Hygiene

Electromagnetic Hygiene is a novel concept that refers to creating an electromagnetically "clean" environment; i.e., keeping the levels of electromagnetic fields as low as possible.

Electromagnetic Hygiene at Work/School

Increase distance from electrical cords and electric equipment. Move the power bar at least one meter away from your feet. Use a wired extended keyboard and mouse to increase your distance from the computer screen. This will reduce the magnetic field.

Try to work with fluorescent lighting turned off. Remove CFLs (compact fluorescent light bulbs) from your work area; use incandescent bulbs or the specially designed LED bulbs that emit low radiation.

Use an Ethernet cable for internet access instead of Wi-Fi. You can also use broadband over powerline adaptors instead of Wi-Fi. If you need to use wireless, ensure that the router is as far as possible from your body; turn it off when not in use, or put it on a timer to shut it off at night. Ensure that you turn off the Wi-Fi on your computer and handheld devices, not just at the router.

Replace your cordless telephone with a corded landline phone. The new digital cordless phones in North America constantly emit microwave radiation, even when not in use. The older analog phones emitted microwave radiation only when used. The best option for reducing RF exposure is to use a wired landline phone.

Text instead of talk, use the "speaker phone" option when talking, and don't hold the phone next to your head. Do not keep your phone on your body—in a pocket, in your bra, or on a belt. When the signal is weak and/or the phone is searching for a carrier, it's transmitting at maximum power and should not be used at this time. When not using your cellphone, keep it in airplane mode (with Wi-Fi/Bluetooth turned off) so it doesn't radiate.

Ensure that workers or students are at least ten feet from an electric panel and are not adjacent to a utility room, as these generate high magnetic fields.

Note: Low-frequency magnetic fields (those that we use for electricity) can penetrate walls, windows, doors, ceilings and floors. Consequently, exposure in one room may be coming from an adjacent room. For this reason it's important to spend as little time as possible near such sources, even if they're on the other side of the wall. Radiofrequency radiation can also penetrate walls and is blocked or reflected by metal objects, generating potential hotspots. If you're in a location where there's a radio frequency (RF) source and metal objects (filing cabinet, fridge, stove, sink, etc.), your RF exposure might be higher or lower depending on the location of the source, the metal, and your body.

Recommendations

If uncertain, have a qualified technician measure your workplace for Electrosmog. In areas where people spend hours each day, levels should be less than the following values: 1 milligauss for power-frequency magnetic fields; 5 V/m for power-frequency electric fields; 40 GS units for dirty electricity; 0.01 microW/cm2 for wireless radiation; 0.5 V for ground current at 60 Hz; and 10 mV for kHz ground current.

Electromagnetic Hygiene in Your Bedroom

We spend a third of each day in our bedrooms, which is why it's important that the bedroom be electromagnetically clean. Reduce electrosmog in your bedroom by following the steps for your office as well as the steps below.

Remove wireless baby monitors or wireless sleeping pads. Wireless baby monitors constantly transmit microwave radiation. Infants should not be exposed to it. Sound-activated baby monitors are widely available. Do not use wireless baby pacifiers, or diapers that contain wireless chips.

Move your clock radio (and other electric equipment) at least 1 yard from your bed (clock radios emit electromagnetic fields that may affect sleep). Keep bedroom as dark as possible, as ambient light also affects sleep.

Unplug your computer at night if it's in your bedroom. Disconnect your Wi-Fi router and turn your cellphone off or keep it in airplane mode with Wi-Fi/Bluetooth turned off. This is especially important for children under the age of eighteen. Several national and international advisories are recommending that children under eighteen limit their cellphone use. Use iPods/iPads/smart tablets in airplane mode, with Wi-Fi/Bluetooth turned off, and use an Ethernet connection with wired adaptors for internet access. Most wireless devices can connect to Ethernet using wired adaptors.

Ask your utility provider to have your wireless smart meter wired or install an analog smart meter. If that's not possible, use GS filters or power conditioners to reduce the level of dirty electricity generated by smart meters. Do not sleep in a room adjacent to the smart meter. Shielding of the meter may be necessary if yours emits radiofrequency radiation. Wire-mesh baskets are commercially available. If you use one, check with an Electrosmog meter to ensure that you're reducing and not magnifying exposure.

Avoid using electric blankets and waterbeds. If you need to use an electric blanket, unplug it after it's warmed the bed. This eliminates the electric and magnetic fields these blankets generate. If you turn the electric blanket off but leave it plugged in, it will generate an electric field. Reducing exposure by unplugging the blanket is essential.

Consider turning off the power (at the electrical panel) to your bedroom (and adjacent rooms) while you sleep.

Shielding the radiation from external sources to the home is also possible with special paint, fabric for bed canopies and clothing, faraday cages, and shielding window film. Blocking the anthropogenic frequencies can, however, also reduce the natural earth frequencies that help us maintain our circadian rhythm. Paganopoulos and Chrousos (2019) recommend that shielding be done very carefully and that it be temporary rather than permanent. They also identify some problems that can produce hot spots if the shielding isn't done properly. (See resources list for shielding products and meters to measure exposure.)

Similarly, dirty electricity can be reduced with special power conditioners or filters/capacitors (see websites in resources list) that short circuit high-frequency transients. Audiophiles reply on power conditioners to reduce noise and improve sound quality;

at the same time, they are protecting their sensitive audio equipment and improving the electromagnetic environment in which they listen.

Management and Treatment Strategies

- CH2OPD2 mnemonic
- Community
- Home
- Hobby
- Occupation
- Personal habits
- Diet
- Drugs

Determine specific community, work, school, and home exposures to EMFs: proximity of cellphone towers, routers, DECT cordless phones, and any other wireless technology. Most important, determine whether the sleeping area is affected.

A helpful mnemonic to determine the parameters of exposure is FIND:

F – Frequency (Hertz)
I – Intensity (power in $\mu W/m^{2)}$
N – Nearness
D – Duration

Nutritional supplements and increased physical exercise should be introduced. Psychotherapy is not helpful for treatment (Hagstrom et al., 2012, 2013).

Treatment strategies can be applied using RIDE:

R – Reduce exposure
I – Immune system addressed
D – Detoxify by decreasing body burden
E – Emotional and psychological trauma needs attention for healing

(Havas, M., 2014. Electrosmog and Electrosensitivity: What Doctors Need to Know to Help their Patients Heal. Anti-Aging Therapeutics Volume XV.)

SEEDS of Health (Lynn Marshall)
S – Sleep
E – Exercise
E – Environment

D – Diet
S – Support (spiritual, family, social)

The best approach to management is to weed, seed, and feed. Weed out the EMF stressors from the environment—the poor diet, the body burden of other toxicants, the bad habits that lead to ill health, the unaddressed health issues—and seed our lives with positive behavioral changes, nourishing food and water, healing relationships, exercise, sleep, relaxation, and a clean environment.

Clean up your home and work environments to reduce exposure. Hardwire everything possible; use only corded phones, and create "white zones" that are clear of EMR. Stay clear of appliances, turn off all emitting devices at night, and consider using Stetzer filters to reduce dirty electricity.

Exposure can be reduced by increasing your distance from the source as much as possible (E=inverse square of distance). Use cellphones with the smallest SAR (specific absorption rate). Hard-wire or use fiber optics to transmit the signal (innovation). Protective gear or shielding for devices can be used to reduce long-term exposures (attenuation). Turn off Wi-Fi when not in use, and turn off all electronic devices that emit when you're sleeping. EHS is recognized as a disability under the Canadian Human Rights Code, and many patients are disabled with no accommodation, let alone validation of their illness. Accommodation would include shielding, hardwiring, prudent reduction of use, or remedial action by attenuation or removal of the source. Shielding from EMR can be provided by protective gear such as clothing with copper or silver. To shield a dwelling or workplace, foil or metal panels, metallic paints (all grounded to avoid the development of a magnetic field), and heavy foliage from trees can be used.

The exposure-reduction principles to decrease body burden aim to decrease input and increase output. Increasing metabolic conversion rates and enhancing antioxidant reserves by consuming fruits and vegetables increases mobilization (hydration and exercise) and assists in excretion of toxins (optimizes bowel and kidney function).

Natural detoxification and healing require getting your sleep in a relaxed, natural manner. Exercise daily in a way you enjoy; live, work, learn, and play in safe and healthy environments. Eat plenty of fruit and vegetables at every meal, and choose snacks with good-quality proteins and oils and high-fiber carbohydrates. Work toward a healthy, balanced nutrition with no food additives, sweeteners, or food coloring. Be sure to get adequate protein and micronutrients, and take a multivitamin daily. Drink plenty of water and other healthy drinks such as unsweetened juices and milks, avoiding energy drinks, soda pop, and concoctions. Have a daily prayer to give meaning and purpose to all you do. Finally, don't worry, be happy, and get and feel connected.

Reduce your body's burden of toxins by following CH2OPD2 (community, home, hobbies, occupation, personal habits, diet, and drugs) and reduce exposure to EMFs. Reduce oxidative stress through excellent nutrition and supplements. This will lessen the degree of gut dysbiosis, food allergy or intolerances, SIBO, IBS, celiac, and infectious diseases as well as (silent) inflammation. Improve mitochondrial function through the use of magnesium, D-ribose, L-carnitine, and CoQ10 (Oberfeld, 2016). Please see your medical practitioner to help you manage your doses of supplements.

Other ways to reduce the toxic load include detoxification of mercury, lead, and solvents, which can be done using ALA, NAC, glutathione, vitamin C, selenium, chelation with DMSA, DMPS, EDTA, depending on which toxins need to be treated. Sauna therapies, proper hydration, and daily exercise are important components of treatment. The correction of any dental work with toxic or immunoreactive materials such as mercury, lead oxide, gold, and titanium (zirconium dioxide is okay) will lower the toxic load, as will removing any dental amalgams. The use of chelation therapy may be necessary. Be aware that genetic polymorphisms are likely increasing the degree of vulnerability to these exposures (De Luca, 2014).

Natural detoxification can be enhanced by eating a diet rich in antioxidants, organic if possible. To decrease the body's burden of oxidative stress (peroxynitrite ONOO-) take antioxidants vitamins E and C, alpha-LA, NAC, B complex, zinc, resveratrol, CoQ10, selenium, and turmeric. Remove personal care products, cleaning products, amalgams, and unnecessary medications, and avoid all harmful substances (e.g., alcohol or tobacco). Herbs and adrenal hormone replacement can be useful in the management of adrenal fatigue. For those with sensitivities, homeopathic treatments may be useful.

It is important to receive psychological support and remove stress triggers. Cognitive behavioral therapy and/or mindfulness-based stress reduction methods as the cornerstone for dealing with stress. Therapies for limbic dysfunction (see chapters 1 and 2) are especially helpful for treating EHS. Your symptoms are real, and there's a reason for feeling so unwell. How do you cope without panicking? Decrease sympathetic stress overdrive with GABA, magnesium, or B complex. For heart arrhythmias take beta blockers until sources of exposure can be eliminated. Correct any sleep disorders using magnesium, melatonin, or fish oil. Try grounding by going barefoot outdoors where you know there are no grounded powerlines; use special grounding sheets at night, or spend time in natural bodies of water such as lakes and oceans. Take Epsom salt baths to help replenish lost electrons. Make positive lifestyle changes at home, work, and school. Join a support group.

Case Study (a particularly poignant example of how EHS can profoundly affect a patient's health):

In Our Patient's Own Words

"I try to be a positive, solutions-oriented person, and am grateful to have recovered from severe, disabling migraines and chronic Lyme disease with the help of physicians trained in functional and environmental medicine. I sought out the best care I could, including the Cleveland Clinic's Center for Functional Medicine. I wanted to be healthy, able to finish raising my five children, and work in a career I love.

Even with the best care, a seemingly innocuous wireless utility meter, commonly known as a smart meter, quickly reversed all this and caused me severe medical problems, disability, and even homelessness. My father worked for the electric company, and I have fond memories of company baseball games and family gatherings. I was shocked to have to leave my husband, children, and home, a painful experience for my family that some of my children still don't understand. After three days of being unable to be in my house, I accepted an invitation for a temporary stay with a kindhearted woman disabled by EMS who had remediated her home to have safe levels of electromagnetic radiation. I quickly returned to normal there and could soon run a half-mile.

Two months later, upon my return home, the medical problems returned with a vengeance. Though I had completed my doctorate using a laptop connected to Wi-Fi, I became unable to tolerate wireless devices or even be in a house with a smart meter, Wi-Fi, or smart phones. I could no longer go to church and sit where I wanted to, and I couldn't sit in the middle of a group of people with cellphones. I developed what is known in the U.S. as electromagnetic sensitivity (EMS, also referred to as EHS), a disability recognized by the U.S. Access Board. I developed cardiac and neurological problems I'd never expected in light of my healthy lifestyle, which included a diet prescribed by the dietician from the CCCFM (Cleveland Clinic Center for Functional Medicine). Chest pain, arrhythmias, headaches, near syncope, and other disabling problems kept me from my work as a medical professional, and even from accessing medical care, including cardiac care. The very high levels of microwave radiation used for medical and communications equipment in hospitals not only creates a barrier to those disabled by EMS but also creates oxidative stress in 90% of those exposed to it. Hospitals do not realize they are harming their staff as well as their patients. People with EMS often experience an exacerbation of their condition with these high exposures, which in some cases can be permanent. Worse, there is a tendency to misdiagnose a person with EMS as having a psychiatric disorder. People with EMS have been involuntarily committed to psychiatry, even those with a diagnosis of EMS. This failure of the medical community to address this condition properly contributes to difficulties in the rest of society and can lead to a lack of support from family, friends, and others. These people who face tremendous challenges are not given the support they need or even the right to basic medical care, even in an emergency.

I developed a clear understanding of the risk of an unaccommodated emergency-care visit when one of my children needed a thirty-minute visit to an Urgent Care facility. The nurse on duty did not understand the disability accommodation in place; i.e., that I was to be put in the X-ray room. I toughed it out, but ten minutes after leaving, I developed a left hemiparesis (weakness or inability to move on one side of the body) with increasing fatigue and malaise. Fortunately, the hemiparesis was transient, but it took me two days to recover from the severe fatigue, and my EMS had worsened.

I recently experienced a stroke after working for two days in a school with Wi-Fi; other significant exposures followed that I wasn't aware of until it was too late. Several times, I had difficulty articulating words. Initially, I thought my carpal tunnel was returning, until my entire left hand went numb and I had trouble opening it. I went to an Urgent Care familiar with EMS. The doctor thought I needed to go to a hospital and have a CAT scan to rule out a stroke. I tried to do so, first calling the medical director of the other Urgent Care that usually accommodates my disability. I hoped he could call ahead to the hospital for me; however, he told me that the hospital would not assist me, even to try to get me in and out quickly. He apologized and told me he wished he were in charge. I am grateful for his kindness, though he could not help. The experience of the transient hemiparesis following the unaccommodated Urgent Care visit remained clear in my memory. I hoped for a good outcome and chose to stay home in my shielded house and rest, understanding the risk involved with an unaccommodated hospital visit. I know of two people who died in hospitals when not accommodated for their disabilities. Fortunately, I have regained most of my hand function, though I still at times have dysarthria (difficult or unclear articulation of speech). I still have not had any care from a cardiologist or neurologist.

An attorney is working with the local hospital system to encourage them to provide a safe area and a plan to treat people who have EMS, including both in-patient and out-patient cardiac and stroke care. Currently, people with EMS who seek cardiac care are told to find a cardiologist who specializes in treating people with EMS. These specialists do not exist, and people need local care in the event of a heart attack or stroke when minutes count. We are hoping that all hospitals will provide this necessary care before someone has a poor or even fatal outcome."

Dr. Bray Comments

To find further help for her EMF sensitivity, the patient decided to look at functional genomic testing to see if there might be any clues. Functional genomics is looking at how the body functions, not what is typically considered disease-related genomics, which is given by a professional geneticist. Functional genomics looks at how the body may be handling iron, making free radicals, potentially not making enough antioxidants, which may lead to inflammation from environmental factors such as mycotoxins, virus, *Borrelia,* or EMFS Upon examination of her functional genomics it was found that the patient had two SNPS (single nucleotide polymorphisms) on a gene called HFE, which may cause her to absorb more iron. If not transported properly through the body, iron can be inflammatory. Additionally, there is a proinflammatory cytokine called TNF-α that creates inflammation when the body is faced with a pathogen; however, the patient also had a genetic mutation that caused the TNF-α to be overreactive. As it turns out, iron stimulates TNF-α. The patient has the proverbial perfect storm—two genetic markers that would cause her to over-absorb iron, stimulating the tumor necrosis factor, and the tumor necrosis factor being overactive. As Bob Miller wrote in chapter 19, the heme oxygenase enzyme can be critical in holding back the inflammation created by TNF-α. However, the patient has weakness in the genes that make the HEME that supports the heme oxygenase enzyme, thus further allowing this inflammation to increase in cascade throughout her body. The TNF-α and the iron will stimulate an enzyme called NADPH oxidase that may stimulate mast cells and histamine, which are all very inflammatory and account for her discomfort when exposed to EMF.

Electromagnetic fields also stimulate the NOX enzyme that creates more inflammation. As you now understand, the patient already had NADPH oxidase stimulated by genetic predispositions, and the additional stimulation from EMF was creating this perfect storm.

The patient reported feeling better when therapies were introduced that helped her break down histamine, calm the NADPH oxidase enzyme, and more physiologically process the iron. In addition to the TNF-α causing the production of mast cells and histamine, it also stimulates an enzyme called PLA2 that will pull arachidonic acid out of the cell membrane, whereupon the arachidonic acid can stimulate another inflammation-creating molecule called leukotriene B4. The patient also had a mutation in the ALOX5 enzyme, a gain of function that would cause her to make more leukotriene B4; and she also had homozygous mutation on GPX4, which also causes overactivation of ALOX5. Consequently, she has another perfect storm of the arachidonic acid turning into leukotriene B4; additionally, excess iron will also stimulate the leukotriene B4.

It appears that this combination of environmental factors along with her genetic predisposition contributed to the development in this patient of becoming sensitive to EMFs. Fortunately, by targeted nutrition to calm these overactive enzymes, the patient is now getting some relief and some of the most recent findings based upon the excess leukotriene B4 should help her even more as that is addressed. (This discussion, as in depth as it is, will help you to appreciate the information in chapter 19 on genomics).

Recommendations

More research, public health initiatives, and healthcare-provider guidance is needed. Cardiac and central nervous system impacts are the most serious and range from mild to debilitating. Cardiologists and neurologists should be doing exposure histories in that regard. A neurocognitive assessment should be done on all patients with suspected EHS. Valid screening tools need to be developed, and sentinel biomarkers should be chosen as the strongest. Physician education in this area is critical. An individual's susceptibility and environmental factors cannot be neglected, and intrinsic and extrinsic predisposing and precipitating factors always need to be considered and reported. Gaps in the knowledge and understanding of the medical community and general public about how our current technology works need to be addressed, and the reality of EHS and how many people are affected by this technology needs to be brought to light.

We are energetic beings. When the electricity in our body stops flowing in our nervous system, which keeps everything running, including our heart, we die. Every organ and system in our body gives off natural frequencies that impact one another. How can we possibly deal with the technological onslaught of non-ionizing radiation, electrical and magnetic fields, electrosmog, and dirty electricity? Our bodies are made of water, with ions and electric microcurrents flowing across all of our membranes facilitated by natural electric potential gradients. These include those in the mitochondria, whose membranes respond to currents created by this ionic flow. Our bodies are a symphony of electrochemistry, of chemical reactions predominantly based on the movement of electrons, and so we cannot escape this onslaught of electromagnetic exposure. We are at great risk of having the biological balance of life processes significantly disturbed by our lack of appreciation of what we call "progress." After all, we are not robots, and even *they* would be affected by this electromagnetic exposure.

Medical doctors require guidance in managing patients with electromagnetic field hypersensitivity. After twenty years of observations, assessments, and management of patients at the environmental health clinic, preliminary guidelines have been developed to help doctors navigate this new medical illness. Internationally, experts in this field have published guidelines that have been of great assistance. Here is the Canadian version:

Preliminary Clinical Practice Guidelines in the Diagnosis and Management of Electromagnetic Field Hypersensitivity (EHS), Dr. Riina Ines Bray, BASc, MSc, MD, FCFP, MHSc

Preliminary-Clinical-Guidelines-for-EHS.pdf (womenscollegehospital.ca)

Resources

Websites

mdsafetech.orgphysicians for safe technology

www.electrosensitivesociety.cominformation for those with EHS and for doctors

www.emf-portal.org/en scientific literature

www.globalemf.netRFR monitoring by citizen scientists

www.lessemf.com products to mitigate and measure EMF/EMR

www.magdahavas.comharmful effects of electrosmog

www.microwavenews.comnew about microwave radiation

www.powerwatch.org.ukresearch, products, etc.

www.saferemr.comscientific research on electrosmog effects

www.shieldyourbody.comproducts to mitigate EMR

www.slt.coproducts to mitigate and measure EMF/EMR

www.strayvoltage.comground current & dirty electricity

www.zoryglaser.com> 4000 archival references, free downloads

Videos

Discussing the 5G Experiment. https://www.youtube.com/watch?v=Vh8DNKmDGk0&t=11s

Electrosmog and Electrohypersensitivity https://www.youtube.com/watch?v=fqMCjEs9oxE

Wi-Fi in Schools is Safe. True or False? https://www.youtube.com/watch?v=6v75sKAUFdc&list=UUxs1UgZ6DivWUfG1dX-3TELw&index=28

Cellphone Towers, Are they Safe? https://www.youtube.com/watch?v=AEOcB7Svhvw&t=176s

Microwave radiation affects the heart https://www.youtube.com/watch?v=p-mw_nCJWs4&list=UUxs1UgZ6DivWUfG1dX3TELw&index=26

Microwave radiation affects the blood https://www.youtube.com/watch?v=L7E36zGHxRw&list=UUxs1UgZ6DivWUfG1dX3TELw&index=39 19)

Diabetes and dirty electricity https://www.youtube.com/watch?v=gJcM6RZwyfA&list=UUxs1UgZ6DivWUfG1dX3TELw&index=40

Multiple Sclerosis and dirty electricity https://www.youtube.com/watch?v=xdtIPb3Veuw&list=UUxs1UgZ6DivWUfG1dX3TELw&index=31

Rapid Aging Syndrome https://www.youtube.com/watch?v=_fzmmjtHQUw&t=2s

Ground Current on Farms https://www.youtube.com/watch?v=AhIPgdOt3SE

Scientific Publications

Natural Earth Electromagnetic Frequencies

Paganopoulos, DJ and GP Chrousos, 2019. Shielding methods and products against man-made Electromagnetic Fields: Protection versus risk Science of the Total Environment 667 (2019) 255–262. PMID: 30831365 DOI: 10.1016/j.scitotenv.2019.02.344

Presman AS: Electromagnetic Fields and Life. Springer: New York; 1970.

Dubrov AP: The Geomagnetic Field and Life: Geomagnetobiology. Plenum Press: New York; 1978.

Erdmann W, Kmita H, Kosicki JZ, Kaczmarek L. How the geomagnetic field influences life on earth - An integrated approach to geomagnetobiology. Orig Life Evol Biosph 2021;51:231–57.

Electrohypersensitivity

Carpenter, DO. 2015. The microwave syndrome or electro-hypersensitivity: historical background. November 2015 Reviews on Environmental Health 30(4) DOI: 10.1515/reveh-2015-0016 https://www.researchgate.net/publication/283718065_The_microwave_syndrome_or_electro-hypersensitivity_historical_background

Belyaev et al. 2016. EUROPAEM EMF Guideline 2016 for the prevention, diagnosis and treatment of EMF-related health problems and illnesses. https://pubmed.ncbi.nlm.nih.gov/27454111/

Belpomme, D and P. Irigaray. 2022. Why electrohypersensitivity and related symptoms are caused by non-ionizing man-made electromagnetic fields: An overview and medical assessment. Environmental Research 212 113374, 15 pp.

Bevington, M. 2019. The Prevalence of People With Restricted Access to Work in Man-Made Electromagnetic Environments, J.Env Health Sci. 5(1):1-12. DOI: 10.15436/2378-6841.19.2402

ELF EMFs

Havas, M. 2000. Biological effects of non-ionizing electromagnetic energy: A critical review of the reports by the US National Research Council and the US National Institute of Environmental Health Sciences as they relate to the broad realm of EMF bioeffects. Environ. Rev. 8: 173–253. https://cdnsciencepub.com/doi/10.1139/a00-004

IARC 2002. Non-ionizing Radiation, Part 1: Static and Extremely low-frequency (ELF) Electric and Magnetic Fields. IARC Monographs on the Evaluation of Carcinogenic Risks to Humans Volume 80

https://publications.iarc.fr/Book-And-Report-Series/Iarc-Monographs-On-The-Identification-Of-Carcinogenic-Hazards-To-Humans/Non-ionizing-Radiation-Part-1-Static-And-Extremely-Low-frequency-ELF-Electric-And-Magnetic-Fields-2002

Radiofrequency Radiation

IARC 2013. Non-ionizing Radiation, Part 2: Radiofrequency Electromagnetic Fields IARC Monographs on the Evaluation of Carcinogenic Risks to Humans Volume 102. https://publications.iarc.fr/Book-And-Report-Series/Iarc-Monographs-On-The-Identification-Of-Carcinogenic-Hazards-To-Humans/Non-ionizing-Radiation-Part-2-Radiofrequency-Electromagnetic-Fields-2013

Intermediate Frequencies (Dirty Electricity)

Havas, M. and D. Stetzer. 2004. Dirty Electricity and Electrical Hypersensitivity: Five Case Studies, Presented at the WHO EHS Meeting, Prague, https://www.researchgate.net/publication/228978746_Dirty_electricity_and_electrical_hypersensitivity_Five_case_studies

Ground Current

Hillman, D. et al. Relationship of Electric Power Quality to Milk Production of Dairy Herds. Science of the Total Environment 447 (2013) 500–514

References

Baliatsas C, Van Kamp I, Lebret E, et al. Idiopathic environmental intolerance attributed to electromagnetic fields (IEI-EMF): A systematic review of identifying criteria. BMC Public Health. 2012;12(1).

Belpomme, Dominique, Christine Campagnac, and Philippe Irigaray. "Reliable disease biomarkers characterizing and identifying electrohypersensitivity and multiple chemical sensitivity as two etiopathogenic aspects of a unique pathological disorder." Reviews on environmental health 30.4 (2015): 251-271.

Belpomme D, Irigaray P. Electrohypersensitivity as a Newly Identified and Characterized Neurologic Pathological Disorder: How to Diagnose, Treat, and Prevent It. International Journal of Molecular Sciences. 2020 Jan;21(6):1915.

Belpomme D, Irigaray P. Why electrohypersensitivity and related symptoms are caused by non-ionizing man-made electromagnetic fields: An overview and medical assessment. Environ Res. 2022 Sep;212(Pt A):113374. doi: 10.1016/j.envres.2022.113374. Epub 2022 May 7. PMID: 35537497.

Bray RI, Fancy DH. Clinical Practice Guidelines for EHS - Proceedings of a Symposium of the Impacts of Wireless Technology on Health. Environmental Health Clinic, Women's College Hospital, University of Toronto. October, 2020.

Bray RI, Marshall LM Total Toxic Load. Teaching Tool.

Canadian Human Rights Commission. Environmental sensitivity and scent-free policies. https://www.chrc-ccdp.gc.ca/eng/content/policy-environmental-sensitivities. 2019.

De Luca C, Thai JC, Raskovic D, et al. Metabolic and genetic screening of electromagnetic hypersensitive subjects as a feasible tool for diagnostics and intervention. Mediators Inflamm. 2014;2014:924184. doi:10.1155/2014/924184

EUROPAEM Guideline 2015 for the prevention, diagnosis and treatment of EMF-related health problems and illnesses. Belyaev I. Dean A. Eger H. Hubmann G. Jandrisovits R. et al. Rev Environ Health. 2015; 30(4):337-371.

Genuis SJ, Lipp CT. Electromagnetic hypersensitivity: fact or fiction? Sci Total Environ. 2012;414:103-12.

Havas, M. (2014). Electrosmog and Electrosensitivity: What Doctors Need to Know to Help their Patients Heal. Anti-Aging Therapeutics Volume XV.

Havas M. Radiation from wireless technology affects the blood, the heart, and the autonomic nervous system. Reviews on Environmental Health. 2013 Nov 1;28(2-3):75-84.

Johansson O. Disturbance of the immune system by electromagnetic fields—A potentially underlying cause for cellular damage and tissue repair reduction which could lead to disease and impairment. Volume 16. Issue 2-3. August 2009.

Johansson O. Electrohypersensitivity: a functional impairment due to an inaccessible environment. Reviews on environmental health. 2015 Dec 1;30(4):311-21.

Marshall LM, Bray RI Assessment Questionnaire and Exposure History https://static1. squarespace.com/static/593f8894e3df288fc64b6cf0/t/598bbabdf14aa18c52a6dcce/ 1502329836033/Environmental+Health+Clinic+Pre-Visit+Questionnaire.pdf

Marshall L, Weir E, Abelsohn A, Sanborn MD. Identifying and managing adverse environmental health effects: 1. Taking an exposure history. Cmaj. 2002 Apr 16;166(8):1049-55.

Pall ML. How to approach the challenge of minimizing non-thermal health effects of microwave radiation from electrical devices. Int. J. Innov. Res Eng. Manag (IJIREM). 2015 Sep;2(5):71-6.

Pall ML. Microwave frequency electromagnetic fields (EMFs) produce widespread neuropsychiatric effects including depression. Journal of Chemical Neuroanatomy. 2016 Sep 1;75:43-51.

Pall ML. Wi-Fi is an important threat to human health. Environmental research. 2018 Jul 1;164:405-16.

Rea WJ. Chemical Sensitivity. Vol 1. Boca Raton. Lewis Publishers. 1992.

Right to Know, CCOHS https://www.ccohs.ca/oshanswers/legisl/responsi.html

Sanborn M, Grierson L, Upshur R, Marshall L, Vakil C, Griffith L, Scott F, Benusic M, Cole D. Family medicine residents' knowledge of, attitudes toward, and clinical practices related to environmental health: Multi-program survey. Canadian Family Physician. 2019 Jun 1;65(6):e269-77.

Sears ME. Chelation: harnessing and enhancing heavy metal detoxification—a review. The Scientific World Journal. 2013 Jan 1;2013.

WHO, Electromagnetic Fields and Public Health, December 2005

https://static1.squarespace.com/static/593f8894e3df288fc64b6cf0/t/598bbabd-f14aa18c52a6dcce/1502329836033/Environmental+Health+Clinic+Pre-Visit+Questionnaire.pdf

RIINA BRAY is an assistant professor in the Department of Family and Community Medicine at the University of Toronto and is cross appointed to the Dalla Lana School of Public Health. She graduated with a medical degree from The University of Toronto in 1994 and prior to that, attained a bachelor's degree (Hons) in Chemical Engineering and a master's in Pharmacology/Toxicology in drug addiction and neurotoxicology. She did her residency in Family Practice at the University of British Columbia and then a Fellowship in Environmental Health at University of Toronto, followed by a Master's in Health Sciences with a focus on Public Health, Occupational and Environmental Health. She was chair of the Environmental Health Committee at the Ontario College of Family Physicians for ten years and has been Medical Director of the Environmental Health Clinic at Women's College Hospital for eighteen years. She is founder of the Well Earth Collaborative, an organization which aims to provide comprehensive care to those suffering from environmentally-linked chronic complex conditions.

Riina Bray, BASc, MSc, MD, FCFP, MHSc
Human Health and the Environment
13069 Keele St.
King City, ON
L78 1G1
Email: riina.bray@rogers.com

Magda Havas is Professor Emerita at Trent University. During the past twenty-five years, her research has focused on the biological effects of electromagnetic pollution and pulsed electromagnetic field (PEMF) therapy. She works with those who have developed sensitivity to electrosmog, and has documented several objective markers that can be used to help diagnose this illness. She has published more than 200 articles and has given 360 lectures in thirty countries about environmental pollution and the need to practice electromagnetic hygiene. Dr. Havas has provided expert testimony in Canada and abroad. She serves as a science advisor to various government and non-government organizations in Canada and internationally.

Magda Havas, B.Sc., Ph.D., Professor Emerita,
Trent University School of the Environment,
1600 West Bank Drive, Peterborough, ON, Canada, K9L 0G2
email: drmagdahavas@gmail.com
websites: electromagnetic pollution www.magdahavas.com
electromagnetic therapy www.theroselab.com
historical research on microwaves: www.zoryglaser.com

Chapter 10: The Biochemistry and Physiology of EMFs

Martin L. Pall, PhD

Dr. Nathan's Introduction

The subject of EMFs and its relevance to sensitivity is so important, yet has not reached those who most need to be aware of it, that I feel it's important to add a second chapter on this subject. My hope is that this will dispel the myth that EMF sensitivity is essentially a psychological aberration, and not the reality that it has come to be. Dr. Martin Pall has been working for decades on verifying the biochemical details of the chronic conditions we're discussing in this book, and his many published papers testify to that passion. We are honored to have him write this chapter, which will make it clear that a growing body of information demonstrates the biochemical—not psychological—reality of biochemical changes that EMFs provoke in our bodies. Becoming aware of this information provides us tools to treat it more effectively. This chapter is somewhat more technical than some of our others, but I encourage lay readers to get from it what they can and health professionals to study it for the pearls it contains. As you read the first few sentences, hang in there, as Dr. Pall will explain as he proceeds.

✿ ✿ ✿

Preface

The primary target of EMFs in the body is the voltage sensor that controls the activation of voltage-controlled calcium channels (VGCCs) in the plasma membrane of cells, with low-intensity EMFs producing large increases in $[Ca^{2+}]i$. EHS is a genuine sensitivity condition produced via hypersensitivity of the VGCCs to activation. That hypersensitivity is thought to be produced via three calcium stimulated protein kinases which increase the sensitivity of the VGCCs. Chronic elevation of EHS is also thought to involve activity of the NO/ONOO(-) cycle. Two simple specific tests for EHS are proposed here as are six different therapeutic approaches for EHS treatment.

Biology, including medicine, is incredibly complex. Consequently, one can often come up with many explanations of complex findings such as EHS, but with no fundamental understanding of what biological mechanisms are involved, it's often difficult if not impossible to determine whether such an explanation has any merit. Consequently, an understanding of the mechanism of action of electromagnetic fields (EMFs) in the body, and how that mechanism can impact those affected by EHS to produce this hypersensitivity, is essential in helping us treat those patients. Accordingly, this chapter is outlined as follows:

1. How electronically generated EMFs impact the cells of our bodies.
2. EHS studies showing that it is a genuine physiological sensitivity impacting the brain, other parts of the nervous system, and other tissues, including the heart and immune system.
3. EMFs cause EHS and trigger symptoms via VGCC activation; EHS appears to be caused by hypersensitivity of the VGCCs to activation.
4. Role of the NO/ONOO(-) cycle in producing chronic effects.
5. Two approaches toward developing a specific test for EHS and why such tests are so important.
6. Six proposed approaches to EHS therapy and prevention.

How Electronically Generated EMFs Impact Our Bodies' Cells

Electronically generated EMFs are distinctly different from most natural EMFs in that they're coherent, being emitted with a particular frequency, vector direction, polarity, and phase and are for those reasons produce strong electric forces and time-varying magnetic forces (Pall 2021a and b). It is those forces, placed on electrically charged chemical groups in the cells of our bodies, that produce biological effects. Chapter 7 of Purcell (1985), entitled "Electromagnetic Induction," focuses on the fact that electric currents induce EMFs in the space around them. Most natural EMFs are composed of astronomical numbers of photons, each produced by a single quantum event, where the photons are emitted in different vector directions, with different polarities and phases, often but not always with different frequencies, and are therefore incoherent. As a consequence, most natural EMFs produce only miniscule electric forces, typically no greater than twenty times the forces produced by single photons. The EMFs I am referring to in this article are all electronically generated coherent EMFs. These are the types of EMFs that are used in all wireless communication because wireless communication always involves both emitting and receiving antennae where the emitting antenna produces a coherent EMF that acts by placing forces on mobile electrons in the receiving antenna.

Let me make clear that I am not the first scientist to discuss the importance of coherence of electronically generated EMFs. In Pall 2021a I cited ten papers, each of which discussed the importance of coherence in various contexts; however, the central importance of coherence in generating the electric and time-varying magnetic forces that in turn produce biological effects has not been widely recognized in the EMF literature. Further, because the ICNIRP and other international and national "safety guidelines" are based on thermal (heating) effects rather than electric and magnetic forces, they are simply misleading.

Pall 2013a cited twenty-four studies, each showing that low-intensity EMF effects could be blocked or greatly lowered by voltage-gated calcium channel (VGCC) blockers. I have since published on six additional studies showing similar findings. Each study shows that EMFs act predominantly by activating the VGCCs. Those findings have been widely recognized in the scientific literature, as shown by the fact that 477 studies have cited Pall 2013a. The VGCCs are each controlled by a structure called the voltage sensor. The voltage sensor structure is discussed below and the electric charges on the voltage sensor are thought to the primary targets of the electric forces and time-varying magnetic forces produced by coherent EMFs (Pall 2021a and b).

There are eleven different known voltage-controlled channels, each controlled by a similar voltage sensor (table 1) and each is activated by low-intensity EMFs; however, the calcium channels produce most of the EMF effects both in animals and in plants, so that to a first approximation, other ion channel effects can be ignored.

Table 1: Voltage-Regulated Ion Channels in Animal and Plant Cells Each of Which Is Regulated by a Voltage Sensor and Activated By Low-Intensity EMFs

Channels	Citation
L-type, T-type, N-type, P/Q-type voltage-gated calcium channels (VGCCs)	Pall, 2013
Voltage-gated sodium, potassium, and chloride (anion) channels	Pall, 2018
Calcium-activated potassium channels (BKCa)	Pall, 2021a
TPC, GLR3.3, GLR 3.6 (in plants)	Pall, 2016b; unpublished

EMF-induced forces act on the structure of the voltage sensor modeled below:

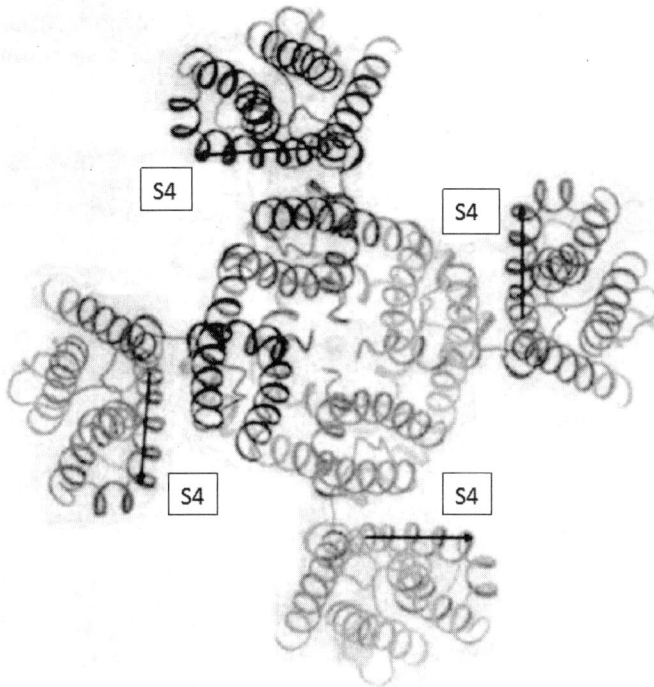

Figure 1. The portion of the voltage-regulated channels have a four-domain structure; each domain contains six alpha helixes, designated S1 to S6. The S4 helixes in the VGCCs and other channels each contain circa 5 positive charges on arginine-residue side chains. When EMFs or other forces activate these channels, they cause the S4 helixes to ratchet in the direction of the black arrows. Ratcheting involves at least three steps and may involve as many as five steps in the direction of the arrows. In my opinion, the EMFs that are most effective in channel activation are approximately perpendicular to the plasma membrane where the channel is located, because perpendicular EMFs will produce similar forces on each S4 helix, and each of them needs to ratchet out to activate the channel. When all four S4 helixes ratchet in the arrow direction, each will pull on the S5 and S6 helixes away from the center of the structure, and after a period of a few microseconds, a conformational change can occur, opening the channel in the center and allowing ions to flow. Below the structure shown (toward the cellular side of the plasma membrane) is a contained aqueous phase, and below that is another structure called the specificity filter, which will determine which ions flow into the cell. The voltage sensor acts, therefore, independently of the ion specificity.

So why are the calcium channels the primary ones producing biological effects? Probably for two reasons: Intracellular calcium $[Ca^{2+}]i$ levels are usually maintained at levels circa 10^{-4} of the extracellular calcium levels, such that there is often a 10,000-fold concentration gradient driving calcium into the cell, and circa a million-fold electrochemical gradient driving calcium into the cell. The second reason is because of the great importance of calcium-influenced effects, as can be seen in figure 2, next page.

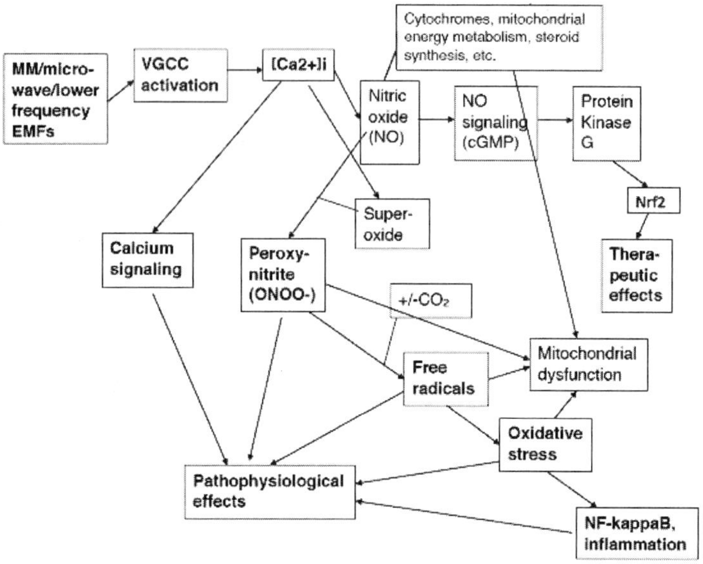

Figure 2. The figure and discussion here are from Pall 2022 and earlier papers (used with permission). As shown (upper left), various frequencies of EMFs produce VGCC activation, which produces increases in $[Ca^{2+}]i$ levels. Higher such increases produce pathophysiological effects, largely through excessive calcium signaling and through the peroxynitrite/free radical/oxidative stress/NF-kappa B/inflammation pathway. Modest increases in $[Ca^{2+}]i$ levels act via nitric oxide (NO) signaling and increases in Nrf2 to produce therapeutic effects; NO increases are, however, *not* an unmixed blessing. NO is not only a precursor for peroxynitrite but also binds to and inhibits cytochromes, including cytochrome oxidase and cytochrome P450s, all important enzymes (see top of figure).

As can be seen from figure 2, the two main pathophysiological pathways of action following electronically generated EMF exposure are the excessive calcium signaling pathway and the peroxynitrite/free radical/oxidative stress/NF-kappa B/inflammation pathway. Both are involved in many but not all pathophysiological EMF effects. In contrast, relatively modest increases in $[Ca^{2+}]i$, act via nitric oxide (NO) signaling, cGMP, and elevated Nrf2 to produce therapeutic effects. The therapeutic pathway and the peroxynitrite/oxidative stress/inflammation pathway produce opposite effects and, as shown in Pall 2022, each of these pathways inhibits the other. One way of interpreting EHS is that it shifts the EMFs needed to move from the therapeutic pathway to the pathophysiological pathway to much lower exposure levels. Each of the findings discussed above is essential for understanding EHS. Studies show that EHS is a genuine physiological sensitivity that impacts the brain, other parts of the nervous system, and other tissues, including the heart and immune system.

I'll discuss a number of studies, each of which provided clear evidence that EHS clearly occurs in some individuals who have reported that they react to EMF exposure.

I'll start with the first published of these, the 1991 Rea et al. study. In that study Dr. William Rea and his colleagues initially started with a group of 100 possible EHS patients and did preliminary studies on them using 3 min. low-intensity, non-pulsed microwave EMFs. They measured five different objectively measurable potential response to exposure: Blood pressure, pulse rate, body temperature (thermoregulation), pupillary constriction, and electrical resistance (measured by a polygraph). They identified twenty-five patients who showed highly consistent responses, and compared them with normal controls in blinded studies. Each of these endpoints was objectively measurable. They found very highly consistent differences between the two groups. With EMF exposure, EHS people showed highly consistent changes in each of these five parameters, but not otherwise, whereas normals showed no changes with exposure.

Havas published three studies that were methodologically similar to Rea (1991) but looked at very different biological endpoints. Havas (2006) showed that both diabetes and multiple sclerosis effects were produced in EMF-exposed patients. Havas (2008) followed up on the diabetes findings of her previous paper, showing that brittle diabetes was produced by EMF exposures from dirty electricity. Havas (2010) added cardiac effects to the experimentally demonstrated EMF effects in EHS patients, showing that cordless phone radiation could produce instantaneous tachycardia when the phone was turned on, responses that instantaneously turned off when the cordless phone radiation was turned off. Each of these studies involved objectively measured responses and blinded radiation exposures, responses that did not occur in normal controls.

In some ways, the Heuser & Heuser study (2017) was the most important of these. It showed that in a series of ten EHS patients, blinded low-intensity EMF exposures produced hypersensitive activation of certain neural circuits in the brain, as measured by fMRI, responses that were missing in normal controls. This directly showed hypersensitivity in the brains of EHS patients but not in controls.

The McCarty (2011) paper was done using a specific EHS patient who had highly consistent perceived responses to low-intensity EMFs. Unlike the other five studies discussed above, each of which measured objectively measurable EMF responses in the body, the McCarty paper looked only at perceived responses. It was done, as it had to be, using double-blinded conditions so that neither the experimenter nor the patient knew when EMF exposure were occurring. McCarty (2011) also showed that this specific patient was a genuine EHS sufferer, responding with high-level consistency when EMF exposed, but not otherwise.

These six studies clearly show that EHS is a genuine EMF sensitivity whereby, unlike normal controls, EHS people respond to low-intensity EMF exposures, but not otherwise.

There are three other papers that I want to discuss in this section. The Greco (2020) study showed that using a method called ultrasonic cerebral tomosphygmography, there were large regions of the brains in EHS and multiple chemical sensitivity (MCS) patients that differed with extremely high levels of statistical significance from those same brain regions in normal controls. These findings clearly show that large regions of the brain in these two sensitivity conditions differ from normal controls.

The Belpomme meta review (2021) showed that in addition to the specific changes described above, there were many nonspecific physiological/biochemical changes that occurred as well. Such nonspecific changes are of great importance because they show the large diversity of measurable changes that occur in EHS.

The Puri paper (2020) was preceded by other studies showing that lymphocytes isolated from EHS patients showed substantial increases in $[Ca^{2+}]i$ when exposed to low-intensity EMFs, whereas lymphocytes from normals showed much lower increases. Puri showed that when patients were treated with low-dose immunotherapy ascertained by provocation neutralization, this decreased the increases in $[Ca^{2+}]i$. These findings show that lymphocyte responses to EMFs in EHS patients become hypersensitive to EMFs, that EHS hypersensitivity may be produced by hypersensitivity of the VGCCs, and that these measured responses may be useful in assessing patient response to a therapy.

Evidence that EHS is Caused by EMF Exposure and Possibly by Chemicals

Is EHS caused by EMF exposure? There were several important studies suggested in the very important EUROPAEM EMF review (Belyaev et al., 2016) suggesting EMF causation. Belyaev (2016) cited five studies involving DECT phone or Wi-Fi exposures. The Molla-Djafari review summarized thirty different studies of mobile-phone base-station exposures, including several reporting EHS-like effects. Havas (2019) describes the long history of EHS, starting with telephone operators in the early 20th century and later in radar operators in the 1940s. Subsequently, these effects began to be seen much more widely as diverse electronically generated EMFs spread almost like wildfire worldwide. Her paper, titled "Electrohypersensitivity (EHS) is an Environmentally-Induced Disability that Requires Immediate Attention," cites a NASA study (Petrov, 1970) that documents much of the early history.

Carpenter (2015) described a series of healthy people who were exposed to a single high-level EMF exposure and developed EHS. Symptoms included chronic headaches, irritability, emotional lability, decreased libido, and memory dysfunction often lasting for years. Hedendahl (2015) described somewhat similar EHS-like symptoms in two fifteen-year old male students and a forty-seven-year-old female teacher exposed to Wi-Fi radiation.

Lebedeva & Sulimova (1994) showed in an experimental human study that low-intensity millimeter-wave EMFs produced long-term stress-like changes in the human brain. The neurological effects of these changes are very similar to those widely reported to occur in EHS patients exposed to EMFs.

The most extensive reviews of the epidemiological literature on EMF causation of EHS are the two studies of Professor Emeritus Karl Hecht (2001, 2016). Both reviewed the Eastern European studies, written mostly in Russian, of occupational exposure studies dating from around 1970 through 1990. These were all done during a period when there were no problematic EMF exposures in the general population, such that effects of occupational exposures could be studied cleanly. What those extremely extensive studies showed is that EHS (and EHS was originally called *microwave syndrome,* see Carpenter, 2015) developed over months and years of occupational exposures, becoming more severe with time and with less spontaneous recovery with increased time of exposure when people were later removed from their EMF exposures.

The last epidemiological studies I will discuss here are the Conrad (2011) and Lamech (2014) research into smart-meter radiation. Both studies, despite using quite different methodologies, found large increases in EHS following smart-meter installation. Conrad (2011) also found that people who had mild EHS symptoms before the smart meters were installed often reported much more severe symptoms following smart-meter radiation exposure.

There are also experimental studies of EMFs producing EHS-like changes in animals, and again, the experimental basis of these studies is important. Burachas and Mascoliunas (1989) described sensitivity changes in the compound action potential (CAP) in the frog sciatic nerve following MM-wave exposures.

A second study by Chernyakov et al. [53] also reported sensitivity changes using a different frog nerve using different MM-wave exposure protocols.

A fourth MM-wave animal study, discussed above, also suggests possible EHS-like effects in animals. This is the Potekhina [54] study in the rat, which found that non-pulsed MM-wave exposures produced rapid changes in the heartbeat of animals. Exposures of three hours or more started to produce apparent sudden cardiac death in these exposed rats. I cited four reviews on EHS in Pall (2021a), each reporting that among the most common sensitivities in EHS patients are neurological/neuropsychiatric sensitivity and cardiac sensitivity. Given that Havas (2010) found that EMFs cause almost instantaneous changes in the heartbeat in some EHS patients, the Potekhina rat study shows that low-intensity EMFs cause EHS-like cardiac effects.

Pall (2021a) reviewed studies showing that EMF impact on the heartbeat were mediated by their impact on the pacemaker cells in the sinoatrial node of the heart and concluded, "The reason the pacemaker cells of the sinoatrial node may be particularly sensitive to EMFs is because they contain particularly high densities of T-type VGCCs, with both T-type and L-type VGCCs having essential roles in producing the pace-making activity."

Akoev (1995) found EHS-like effects following low-intensity MM-wave exposures on the activity of electroreceptors of sea skates (the article cited here is an English-language study, published in an international journal that appears to be similar or identical to the Russian-language article also discussed in Pall 2021a).

Bellono [60] showed that the electroreceptor is the VGCC Ca(V)1.3. What the studies done by Akoev and Bellono clearly show is that EHS-like effects can be produced via sensitization of the VGCCs following previous VGCC activation following EMF exposure.

Waldmann-Selsam (2019) showed that a very sensitive EHS patient, who also had a parathyroid deficiency, when exposed to extremely low EMF levels had a very large drop in extracellular levels, including plasma levels, of calcium. These drops must then be produced by hyperactivation of a plasma-membrane calcium channel, because the only place the extracellular calcium can go so quickly is into the cells of the body. The parathyroid deficiency means that this EHS patient is unable to control extracellular calcium levels because that control is the central function of the parathyroid gland. In principle, it might be possible that some channel other than the VGCCs could be involved here. The fact that we know that EMFs activate VGCCs in mammalian (including human) cells and that EMFs cause the VGCCs in the electroreceptor of the skate to become hypersensitive to activation,, argues against another channel being involved. So does Occam's razor.

The next section asks the question: How do EMF exposures produce hypersensitivity of the VGCCs?

EHS is caused by sensitization of the VGCCs. The increased VGCC sensitization will act in multiple situations to produce EHS, but the most important of these is likely to be via increased long-term potentiation and decreased long-term depression, making many synaptic connections in the central nervous system more sensitive, which is called *neural sensitization*. Consequently, one approach to EHS treatment, which is discussed elsewhere in this volume, is to decrease neural sensitization (see chapters 1, 2, and 3). I will also discuss one possible therapeutic approach to accomplish this below.

One additional point here: De Luca (2011) showed that a genetic polymorphism producing lower enzymatic activity of an enzyme involved in chemical detoxification was associated with higher incidence of EHS. This finding strongly suggests that chemicals too can cause EHS, not just EMFs. This is not surprising. Many chemicals act to produce higher activity of the NMDA receptors, and the first thing that occurs on such NMDA receptor activation is increased $[Ca^{2+}]i$.

Probable Roles of the NO/ONOO (-) Cycle in EHS

It is rare for biological models to include all the complexities of the biology. Consequently, the model of EHS outlined here, while it clearly makes very useful predictions—notably how previous EMF exposures (and possibly chemical exposures) can cause EHS and how, subsequently, low-intensity EMF exposures produce various EMF-sensitivity responses (see figure 3).

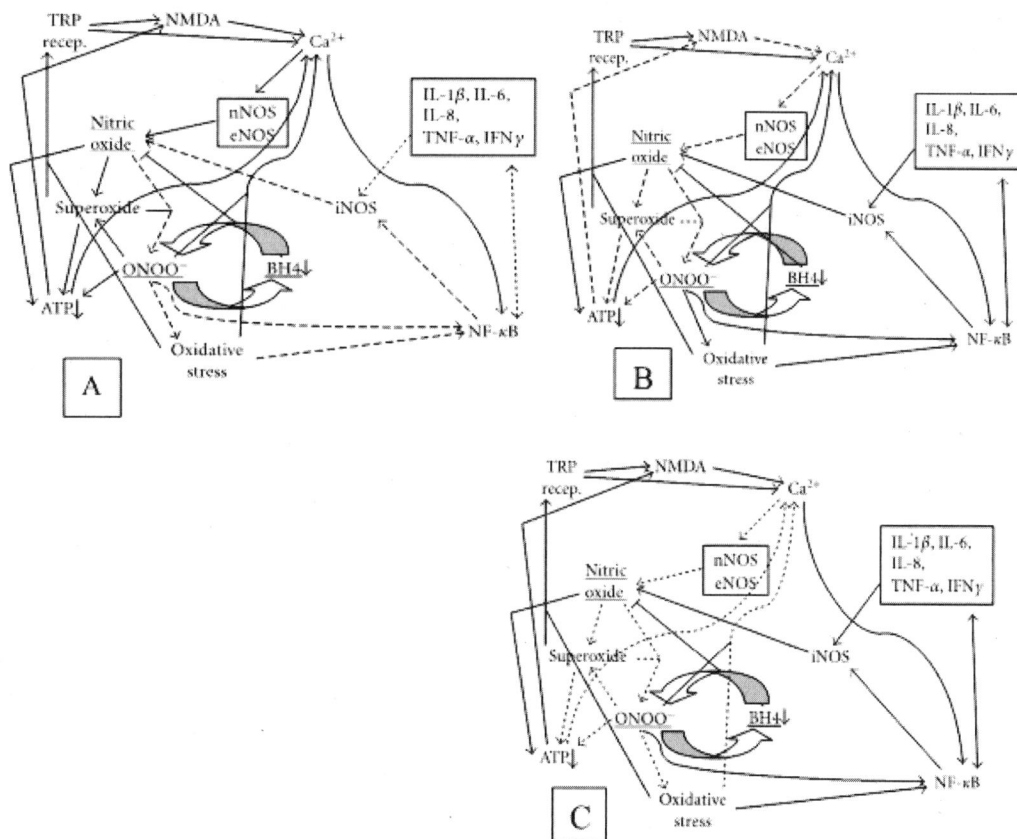

Figure 3 A, B, C. Three underlying cycles of the NO/ONOO (-) cycle. The dashed or dotted arrows are the ones to pay closest attention to for the individual sub-cycles. A is focused peroxynitrite, free radicals, oxidative stress, NF-kappa B inflammation, and

consequences of inflammation. B and C are each focused on Ca^{2+} (actually $[Ca^{2+}]i$) and various other cycle elements. These are from Pall 2013b&c (used with permission). Additional information on the cycle can be obtained from each of those papers. One point needs to be emphasized: everything in a vicious cycle is both a cause and effect of the cycle, but that doesn't mean this model is complete. In my opinion, what is called the NO/ONOO (-) cycle is likely to have an important role in generating the chronic nature of EHS. The NO/ONOO (-) cycle is a primarily local biochemical vicious cycle made up of five underlying cycles, each of which is described in Pall 2013b&c. The only element in common in each of those five cycles is elevated peroxynitrite levels. Three of the five cycles most relevant here are shown in fig. 3.

The most important evidence that the NO/ONOO (-) cycle is involved in EHS is that both Igaray (2018) and Belyaev (2016) have shown that both 3-nitrotyrosine (a specific biomarker of peroxynitrite) and oxidative stress are elevated in EHS. Because peroxynitrite is the common element in all five cycles, its chronic elevation in EHS is strong evidence for NO/ONOO (-) cycle involvement.

Two Possible Simple, Specific Tests for EHS

We've already discussed three possible specific tests for EHS or possibly EHS and/or MCS. These are the tomosphygmography test of Greco (2020), the fMRI study of Heuser & Heuser (2017), and the lymphocyte $[Ca^{2+}]i$ of Puri (2020). The problem is that each of these tests is very expensive to do, requires specialized equipment to do it, and each cannot be done simply by sending one or a few blood-derived samples to a clinical lab. Belpomme and his colleagues have shown that there are other physiological/biochemical changes that occur in EHS patients, as has Belyaev (2016) in the EUROPAEM review, and while most of these are nonspecific, they do show that EHS is a disease of pathophysiology. Some of them might be found to be more EHS-specific if they were measured before and after EMF provocation. I'm going to suggest two possible simple, inexpensive EHS tests.

Waldmann-Selsam (2019) showed that a very sensitive EHS patient, who developed a parathyroid deficiency when exposed to extremely low EMF levels, had a very large drop in extracellular (including plasma) levels of calcium. These drops must then be produced by hyperactivation of the VGCCs in the cells of the body, produced by EMF exposures. EHS patients with normal parathyroid function would be predicted to release large amounts of parathyroid hormone following EMF exposure in order to maintain extracellular calcium levels within or close to the normal range. My guess is that parathyroid hormone levels will increase within about ten minutes of EMF exposure, but the timing of such increases needs to be established experimentally. Because parathyroid levels can be measured by a readily available commercial blood test, it may be possible to test large numbers of people for EHS simply by taking blood samples before and after EMF provocation. This might serve as a means of assessing EHS severity.

The origin for a second possible EHS test will no doubt sound peculiar. I was with my female partner at the Shakespeare festival in Ashland, Oregon, and we went to a bank there to get some cash. I was talking to a woman who apparently knew that she had EHS. She was diagnosed, according to her, by someone who showed that the electrical resistance of her body was very low. She told me that this was common knowledge in the low-EMF zone in West Virginia. Unfortunately, I got neither her contact information nor contact information of the person who diagnosed her. I called my scientific contact in West Virginia, Dr. Bertil "Bert" Schou, who told me that he had not heard about this but that EHS people served as much better antennae than do normals. Because antenna function is strongly related to electrical conductivity, that observation is consistent with the claim I heard in Ashland. Furthermore, I found this claim to be credible based on the fact that most of the electrical resistance of the body is produced by the high electrical resistance of the plasma membranes in the body's cells, resistance that is greatly lowered by the activation of VGCCs or other voltage-gated ion channels. Is there any published evidence that supports this interpretation? The answer is yes, and it comes from the Rea (1991) study of EHS. Dr. Rea showed that patients with EHS had a significant decrease in electrical resistance in their bodies following EMF exposure, as measured by polygraph testing.

One can buy ohm meters for about $30, and by connecting each of the two electrodes to a short section of copper pipe, one can measure body electrical resistance between one hand and the other. I suggest putting both hands into salted water to avoid any possible effect of perspiration.

The development of such a test might be of great importance in helping to determine whether a specific patient has EHS and how severe it might be.

Examining groups of people suspected of having EHS because of EMF exposure or other possible triggers, I suggest we look at each of the following groups as being at risk for having or developing EHS, and I encourage readers to consider expanding this list.

- Airline personnel and frequent flyers
- Air traffic controllers
- People living near cell-phone towers (mobile-phone base stations).
- Police who have high EMF exposures in police cars
- People with Havana syndrome
- The Unhomed
- Drug addicts

- Migraine sufferers with and without aura
- Athletes who have been saved from apparent sudden cardiac death
- Those who work in the IT field
- Those with digital dementia

Assessing the efficacy of possible treatments through a quantitative measure of EHS sensitivity was shown to be promising in the Puri 2019 paper. Given the challenge of quantifying the severity of EHS, such a simple test for EHS will be invaluable in assessing the effectiveness of possible EHS treatments.

It is clear that we need a simple, inexpensive test for EHS as essential for assessing EHS incidences in groups of people and for developing and evaluating effective EHS therapies.

EHS Therapy – Various Approaches

I refer the reader to Puri, 2020 to access the literature on the use of neutralization/potentiation in the treatment of EHS. (For those who are interested, this is taught by the AAEM.)

1. Correct Three Common Deficiencies

In human populations, two common deficiencies might be predicted to exacerbate EHS—magnesium and vitamin D deficiencies. These should therefore be measured and corrected to the extent possible. Magnesium deficiency raises the activity of the NMDA receptors and raises the synthesis of the VGCCs. Each of these effects raises $[Ca^{2+}]i$. I suggest magnesium citrate or malate, and perhaps magnesium taurate in the evening. Magnesium oxide should be avoided because of poor absorption.

Vitamin D deficiencies greatly exacerbate much of the pathophysiology produced by EMFs. These are also common in our societies because we spend so much time indoors, away from the UV light in sunlight. These problems are still much more serious in dark-skinned people. Doses on the order of 5000 IU per day are recommended for most patients, with vitamin D levels monitored by blood tests.

EMFs themselves produce deficiencies in nocturnal melatonin which act, in turn, to exacerbate EMF-induced pathophysiology. It follows that melatonin supplements could be helpful taken just before bedtime.

2. EMF Avoidance and Use of Shielding

EMF avoidance is of course becoming increasingly difficult as the telecom industry puts out more devices as well as more pulse-modulated "smart" devices, producing ever-increasing human EMF impacts. Somewhat similarly, we have ever-increasing amounts of dirty electricity in our power wiring, producing even greater biological impacts, so our challenge for avoidance becomes ever greater.

Let me mention a few things I've done to minimize my personal exposure. I use a wired connection to the internet with Wi-Fi turned off both on my computer and my modem; you can use a cable modem where there is no Wi-Fi. I use a wired keyboard, mouse, and printer. Wired connections are always much better, faster, and more secure in addition to the human health advantages.

I have a smart meter on my house, but I use particularly good shielding on the inner wall adjacent to the meter to protect myself (more about shielding later).

I have neither a cell phone nor cordless phone because each of these is problematic. I use an old-fashioned corded phone. With the exception of a phone available in Europe, all cordless phone bases irradiate twenty-four hours per day. This is an unnecessarily horrible design because the bases don't *need* to irradiate except when sending or receiving a call. If you must have a cordless phone, keep the base far away from where you sleep—and preferably anywhere else you spend a lot of time.

If you must carry a cellphone, you can buy cases that are shielded on one side but not the other. Carrying your cellphone in such a case, with the shielding toward your body, helps shield your body but not the bodies of others around you. Cellphones are continually sending off pulses to locate the nearest cell tower (mobile-phone base station), so where you carry your cell phone influences human biological effects. These are reported to include such effects as male fertility, breast cancer, cardiac effects, and rectal cancer. If you don't need your cellphone to be active all the time, the best thing to do is to have it in airplane mode and carry it fully shielded; take it out and check it when needed. There are air-tube earbuds that can be used to lower head EMF exposures when on a cellphone call; my understanding is that different cellphones often require different air-tube earbuds.

The telecom industry often assures us that cellphones cannot produce human biological effects; however, studies show that there are selective effects: the ipsilateral side of the head (where people use their cellphones) is much more affected than the opposite (contralateral) side of the head. These include brain cancer, long cellphone call-associated headaches, changes in blood flow in the brain, cellular DNA damage, and tinnitus.

Let's talk about EMF shielding. In my opinion, the most important effect of shielding is to disrupt the coherence of the EMFs; the tiny metal fibers in shielding cloth materials and much tinier graphite fibers and metal flecks in shielding paint act in this way. Aluminum foil has been used, but it reflects the EMFs such that areas receiving such reflective EMFs may have high exposures. I suggest crumpling aluminum foil used in this way, so reflections will have lower coherence.

Dr. Panagopoulos has argued that we should not be doing shielding because it prevents our bodies from being exposed to the Schumann resonance of the earth (frequency circa 7.8 Hz.) I agree with his concern but not with his conclusion. I believe that earthing, the favorable effects produced when people walk barefooted on the earth or otherwise ground their bodies, is due to the Schumann Resonance as suggested by Sinatra et al., 2017. Elhalel (2019) showed that very low intensity EMFs near the Schumann resonance frequency, 7 to 9 Hz, lowered the peak VGCC-dependent calcium transients in the heart by about 40%, producing cardiac protection. I know of health care providers who have claimed that devices emitting the Schumann resonance are helpful in the treatment of EHS and the EUROPAEM guidelines suggest using the Schumann resonance in EHS treatment (Belyaev, 2016). There is a simple technological fix for the Panagopoulos concerns: use inexpensive electronic devices that emit the Schumann resonance for EHS treatment. Such devices may also be useful in many other situations to lower EMF effects.

3. Use of VGCC Calcium-Channel Blockers for Treatment of EHS

With the beautiful mechanism discussed above, where VGCC sensitization can be produced as described, you'd think there would be a lot of evidence showing that VGCC calcium-channel blockers act to lower EHS effects, but there is actually very little. I've been contacted by two people with apparent EHS, each of whom reported that they had been treated for hypertension with one of the VGCC calcium-channel blockers and experienced substantial lowering of their EHS symptoms and their hypertension symptoms. The blocker used in the first case was diltiazem. I don't know which blocker was used in the second. We clearly need some studies on effects of VGCC channel blockers on EHS patients, preferably using a test of EHS severity to monitor effectiveness. I suggest starting with diltiazem and with nitrendipine, the latter being the most effective such blocker in Alzheimer's treatment (Pall, 2022). It's possible that nitrendipine may be more active than the other dihydropyridine blockers in treating Alzheimer's because nitrendipine blocking may be less affected by phosphorylation near the bonding site. In any use of VGCC calcium-channel blockers, it is essential to avoid excessive hypotensive effects, so low doses might be preferable. It may be predicted that EHS brains might be especially sensitive to lowered oxygen availability.

There's one common food that contains calcium-channel blockers and might therefore be useful for EHS treatment: Garlic contains substantial amounts of two calcium-channel blockers (Neuhaus-Carlisle et al., 1997), allicin and trans-ajoene; garlic is also active in raising the levels of Nrf2. Consequently, there may be two reasons why eating garlic could be useful. Allicin is also found in green onions, shallots, and Chinese garlic chives, but not in bulb onions. Because garlic is reported to lower hypertension in a systematic review (Xiong et al., 2015), these findings suggest that the VGCC calcium-channel blocking by garlic may occur at substantial levels in humans.

4. Raising Nrf2 in EHS Therapy

The NO/ONOO (-) cycle has a highly probable role in maintain the chronicity of EHS. The complexity of the cycle makes lowering the cycle a challenging process. It has, however, been argued that raising the level of Nrf2 is nature's way of preventing or treating NO/ONOO (-) cycle diseases because many of the elements in the cycle, including the most central one, peroxynitrite, are lowered by raising Nrf2 (Pall & Levine, 2015). There are many health-promoting factors that raise Nrf2, as shown in figure 4, each of which may be useful in therapy. For those who are limited to conventional pharmaceuticals for raising Nrf2, you may consider off-label use of methylene blue, which has been shown to raise Nrf2.

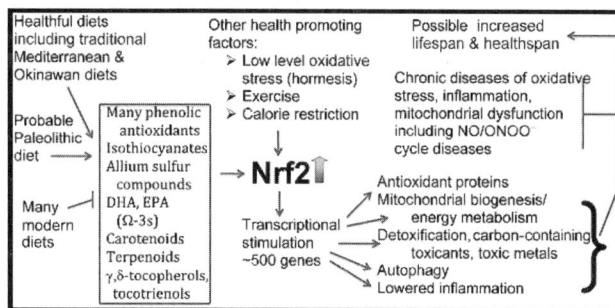

Figure 4. From Pall & Levine, 2015 (used with permission).

Some months ago, I read a book by Eric Kandel, a Nobel laureate, entitled *The Disordered Mind: What Unusual Brains Tell Us About Ourselves*. In the context of PTSD, Kandel noted that when an event occurs that brings to the surface the symptoms recalling a much earlier stressful event, the synaptic connections that produce those symptoms are weakened such that they can become disrupted by the beta blocker propranolol. In researching this, I found there was a much larger scientific literature on this than Kandel cited. It might be possible to disrupt specific synaptic connections previously strengthened by long-term potentiation, when they are active (see Brunet, 2018). There is no reason to think that the role of the beta-adrenergic receptors in learning and memory is PTSD-specific (O'Dell, 2015). It might be possible, therefore, to *selectively unlearn* the long-term potentiation that leads to neural sensitization following EMF exposure (and for that matter, chemical exposure in MCS) by using a beta blocker before an exposure of a sensitive individual to EMFs or chemicals. Studies on this could be done either in conjunction with a series of provocations, as were the Brunet PTSD studies (2018) or by allowing EHS patients to use propranolol or other beta blockers when the individual knows from previous experience that they need to go to a location where a particular exposure is likely to produce a sensitivity response. This, of course, would be an off-label drug usage. Beta blockers such as propranolol have substantial side effects and they should only be used, in my opinion, shortly before an EHS patient will be exposed to an EMF.

A number of products on the market claim to help protect us from EMF effects. Some of them produce an EMF of their own, but more commonly, these products apparently have within them crystals or other highly structured materials that may reflect incoming EMFs, producing other, much weaker, EMFs coming toward our bodies from a different direction. The voltage sensor must have all four S4 helixes ratcheting away from the center of the closed channel in order to activate the channel. I believe that these devices may work by producing another EMF that causes one or more of the helixes to ratchet back toward the center of the closed channel, thus blocking the opening of the channel. I have neither time nor space here to document this, and I'm not endorsing any of these devices, but in my opinion they may be worth trying in EHS therapy.

This paper is dedicated to the memory of
Dr. Peter Ohnsorge, a great man and wonderful friend.

Citations

Akoev GN, Avelev VD, Semenjkov PG. 1995. Reception of low-intensity millimeter-wave electromagnetic radiation by electroreceptors in skates. Neuroscience 66:15-17.

Burachas G, Mascoliunis R. 1989. Suppression of nerve action potential under the influence of millimeter waves. In Devyatkov ND (ed): "Millimeter Waves in Medicine and Biology." Moscow: Radioelectronica, 1989;168–175 (in Russian).

Bellono NW, Leitch NW, Julius D. 2017. Molecular basis of ancestral vertebrate electroreception. Nature 2017;543:391-396. doi: 10.1038/nature21401.

Belpomme D. et al., 2021. The Critical Importance of Molecular Biomarkers and Imaging in the Study of Electrohypersensitivity. A Scientific Consensus International Report. Int. J. Mol. Sci. 2021, 22(14), 7321.

Belyaev I, et al. 2016. EUROPAEM EMF Guideline 2016 for the prevention, diagnosis and treatment of EMF-related health problems and illnesses. Rev Environ Health 3: 363–397.

Brand-Schieber E, Werner P. 2004. Calcium channel blockers ameliorate disease in a mouse model of multiple sclerosis. Exp Neurol 189:5-9.

Brunet A, et al. 2018. Reduction of PTSD Symptoms With Pre-Reactivation Propranolol Therapy: A Randomized Controlled Trial. Am J Psychiatry 175:427-433.

Burachas G, Mascoliunis R. 1989. Suppression of nerve action potential under the influence of millimeter waves. In Devyatkov ND (ed): "Millimeter Waves in Medicine and Biology." Moscow: Radioelectronica, 1989;168–75 (in Russian).

Carpenter DO. 2015. The microwave syndrome or electro-hypersensitivity: historical background. Rev Environ Health 30:217-222.

Chernyakov GM, Korochkin VL, Babenko AP, Bigdai EV. 1989. Reactions of biological systems of various complexity to the action of low-level EHF radiation. In Detyakov ND (ed): "Millimeter Waves in Medicine and Biology." Moscow: Radioelectronica, 1989:141-67 (in Russian).

Conrad, Richard. 2011. PRE-FILED TESTIMONY OF RICHARD CONRAD, PhD, MPUC Docket No. 2011-00262, 1-124. http://www.mainecoalitiontostopsmartmeters.org/wp-content/uploads/2013/01/Exhibit-9-Conrad-Web.pdf.

De Luca C, Raskovic D, Pacifico V, Thai JC, Korkina L. 2011 The search for reliable biomarkers of disease in multiple chemical sensitivity and other environmental intolerances. Int J Environ Res Public Health. 2011 Jul;8(7):2770-97. doi: 10.3390/ijerph8072770.

Elhalel G, et al., 2019 Cardioprotection from stress conditions by weak magnetic fields in the Schumann Resonance band. Sci Rep 9, 1645 (2019).

Greco F. 2020. Technical Assessment of Ultrasonic Cerebral Tomosphygmography and New Scientific Evaluation of Its Clinical Interest for the Diagnosis of Electrohypersensitivity and Multiple Chemical Sensitivity Diagnostics 2020, 10(6), 42.

Grueter CE, Abiria SA, Wu Y, Anderson ME. 2008. Differential regulated interactions of calcium/calmodulin-dependent protein kinase II with isoforms of voltage-gated calcium channel β subunits. Biochemistry 47:1760-1767.

Havas M. 2006. Electromagnetic hypersensitivity: biological effects of dirty electricity with emphasis on diabetes and multiple sclerosis. Electromagn Biol Med. 25:259–268.

Havas M. 2008. Dirty Electricity Elevates Blood Sugar Among Electrically Sensitive Diabetics and May Explain Brittle Diabetes. Electromagn Biol Med 27:135-146.

Havas M. et al., 2010. In: Giuliani L, Soffritti M, editors. "Non-thermal Effects and Mechanisms of Interaction Between Electromagnetic Fields and Living Matter," European J Oncology — Library. National Institute for the Study and Control of Cancer and Environmental Disease Bologna: Mattioli; 2010. p. 273–300.

Havas M. 2019. Electrohypersensitivity (EHS) is an environmentally-induced disability that requires immediate attention. J Sci Discov (2019),3(1)jsd18020.

Hecht K. 2001. [Effects of electromagnetic fields: A review of Russian study results 1960-1996]. Umwelt-Medizin-Gesellschaft 14: 222-231.

Hecht K. 2016 Health Implications of Long-Term Exposures to Electrosmog. Brochure 6 of A Brochure Series of the Competence Initiative for the Protection of Humanity, the Environment and Democracy. http://kompetenzinitiative.net/KIT/wp-content/uploads/2016/07/KI_Brochure-6_K_Hecht_web.pdf (accessed Feb. 11, 2018).

Hedendahl L, Carlberg M, Hardell L. 2015. Electromagnetic hypersensitivity – an increasing challenge to the medical profession. 30:209-215.

Heuser G, Heuser SA. 2017. Functional brain MRI in patients complaining of electrohypersensitivity after long term exposure to electromagnetic fields Rev Environ.Health 2:291-299.

Irigaray P, Caccamo D, Belpomme D. 2018. Oxidative stress in electrohypersensitivity self-reporting patients: Results of a prospective *in vivo* investigation with comprehensive molecular analysis. Int J Mol Sci 42: 1885-1898.

Jahn H, et al. 1988. Site-specific phosphorylation of the purified receptor for calcium-channel blockers by CAMP-and cGMP-dependent protein kinases, protein kinase C, calmodulin-dependent protein kinase I1 and casein kinase I1. Eur J Biochem 178:535-542.

Kamp TJ, Hell, JW. 2000. Regulation of cardiac L-type calcium channels by protein kinase A and protein kinase C. - Circulation research; 87:1095 1102.

Lamech F. 2014. Self-Reporting of Symptom Development From Exposure to Radiofrequency Fields of Wireless Smart Meters in Victoria, Australia: A Case Series. Alt Ther 20:28-39.

McCarty DE, Carrubba S, Chesson AL, et al. 2011. Electromagnetic hypersensitivity: evidence for a novel neurological syndrome. Int J Neuroscience 121:670-676.

Lebedeva NN, Sulimova OP. 1994. [MM-waves modifying effect on human central nervous system functional state under stress]. Zh Millimetroye Volny v biologii i medicine 3:16-21 (in Russian).

Liu YQ, Gao YB, Dong J, Yao BW, Zhao L, Peng RY. 2015 Pathological changes in the sinoatrial node of the heart caused by pulsed microwave exposure. Biomed Environ Sci 28:72-75.

McCarron JG, et al. 1992 Calcium-dependent enhancement of calcium current in smooth muscle by calmodulin-dependent protein kinase II. Nature 357: 74-77.

McCarty DE, et al. 2011 Electromagnetic hypersensitivity: evidence for a novel neurological syndrome. Int J Neurosci. www.ncbi.nlm.nih.gov/pubmed/21793784. 2011 Sep 5.

Molla-Djafari H, Witke J, Poinstingl G, Brezansky A, Hutter HP, et al. Leitfaden Senderbau -Vorsorgeprinzip bei Errichtung, Betrieb, Um- und Ausbau von ortsfesten Sendeanlagen. Wien (AT): Ärztinnen und Ärzte für eine gesunde Umwelt e.V. (Hrsg.), 2014 Oct. 2. Auflage, 42 p, Available at: www.aegu.net/pdf/ Leitfaden.pdf.

O'Dell TJ, Connor SA, Guglietta R, Nguyen PV. 2015. β-Adrenergic receptor signaling and modulation of long-term potentiation in the mammalian hippocampus. Learn Mem 22:461-471.

Pakhomov AG, Akyel Y, Pakhomova ON, Stuck BE, Murphy MR. 1998. Current state and implications of research on biological effects of millimeter waves: a review of the literature. Bioelectromagnetics 19:393-413.

Pall ML. 2013a. Electromagnetic fields act via activation of voltage-gated calcium channels to produce beneficial or adverse effects. J Cell Mol Med. Aug; 2013;17(8):958–65. Published online 2013 Jun 26. doi: 10.1111/jcmm.12088.

Pall ML. 2013b. Pulmonary hypertension is a probable NO/ONOO disease: A review. ISRN Hyperten 2013, Article ID 742418, 27 pages.

Pall ML. 2013c. The NO/ONOO- cycle as the central cause of heart failure. Int. J. Mol. Sci. 2013;14(11), 22274-22330; https://doi.org/10.3390/ijms141122274.

Pall ML. 2016a. Microwave frequency electromagnetic fields (EMFs) produce widespread neuropsychiatric effects including depression. J Chem Neuroanat 75(part B):43-51.

Pall ML. 2016b. Electromagnetic fields act similarly in plants as in animals: Probable activation of calcium channels via their voltage sensor. Curr Chem Biol10:74-82.

Pall ML. 2021a. Millimeter (MM) wave and microwave frequency radiation produce deeply penetrating effects: the biology and the physics. Rev Environ Health 37:247-258.

Pall ML. 2021b. Coherent MM-wave EMFs produce penetrating effects via time-varying magnetic fields: response to Foster & Balzano. Rev Environ Health 2021.https://doi.org/10.1515/reveh-2021-0125.

Pall ML. 2022. Low intensity electromagnetic fields act via voltage gated calcium channel activation to cause very early onset Alzheimer's disease: 18 distinct types of evidence. Curr Alzheim Res 19:119-132.

Pall ML, Levine S. 2015. Nrf2, a master regulator of detoxification and also antioxidant, anti-inflammatory and other cytoprotective mechanisms, is raised by health promoting factors. Acta Physiologica Sinica (Sheng Li Xue Bao) 67: 1-18.

Petrov IR (ed). 1970. Influence of Microwave Radiation on the Organism of Man and Animals. National Aeronautics and Space Administration Technical Translation (NASA TT F-708), Springfield, Virginia. 1970; 229 pp.

Puri BK, Segal DR, Monro JA. 2020. The effect of successful low-dose immunotherapy ascertained by provocation neutralization on lymphocytic calcium ion influx following electric field exposure. Complementary and Integrative Medicine, vol. 17, no. 1, 2020, pp. 20170156. https://doi.org/10.1515/jcim-2017-0156.

Rea WR. et al. 1991. Electromagnetic field sensitivity. J Bioelectr 10:241-256.

Sculptoreanu A, Rotman E, Takaharashi M, Catterall WA. 1993. Voltage-dependent potentiation of the activity of cardiac L-type calcium channel alpha 1 subunits due to phosphorylation by cAMP-dependent protein kinase. Proc Natl Acad Sci US 90: 10135-10139.

Sinatra ST, et al. 2017. Electric Nutrition: The Surprising Health and Healing Benefits of Biological Grounding (Earthing). Altern Ther Sep/Oct 2017, 23:8-16.

Waldmann-Selsam C. 2019. Hochfrequenzinduzierte Hypokalzämie mit Rezidivierenden Tetanien Umwelt Med Gesel 2019;32:30-4.

Welsby PJ, et al. 2003. A Mechanism for the Direct Regulation of T-Type Calcium Channels by Ca2+/Calmodulin-Dependent Kinase II. J Neurosci 23:10116-10121.

Purcell EM. 1985. Electricity and Magnetism, 2nd edition (Berkeley Physics Course, vol 2) (New York: McGraw-Hill). Neuhaus-Carlisle K, Vierling W, Wagner H. 1997. Screening of plant extracts and plant constituents for calcium channel blocking activity. Phytomedicine 4:67-69.

Xiong XJ, Wang PQ, Li SJ, Li XK, Zhang YQ, Wang J. 2015. Garlic for hypertension: A systematic review and meta-analysis of randomized controlled trials. Phytomedicine 22:352-361. https://doi.org/10.1016/j.phymed.2014.12.013

MARTIN L. PALL, PhD: Bachelor's degree in physics, Johns Hopkins University, Phi Beta Kappa with Honors, 1962; graduated with 180 semester hours of credit in four years. Ph.D. degree in Biochemistry and Genetics, Caltech, 1968. Asst. Prof., Reed College, 1967–72. Asst., Assoc., and Full Professor, Genetics and Cell Biology and Biochemistry/Biophysics, later Professor of Biochemistry and Basic Medical Sciences, Washington State University, 1972–2008. Professor Emeritus of Biochemistry and Basic Medical Sciences, Washington State University, 2008. Received nine international honors for research in Environmental Medicine. Author of 108 professional publications. Since 1998 his research has focused on mechanisms of chronic disease; oxidative/nitrosative stress; inflammation, mitochondrial dysfunction, other mechanisms; environmental stressors causing chronic disease; regulatory systems acting to prevent chronic disease; and chemicals acting to trigger chronic disease via excessive NMDA activity. Since 2013, his research has focused primarily on how electronically generated coherent electromagnetic fields place forces on the voltage sensor controlling the voltage-gated calcium channels to activate mechanism of action of electromagnetic fields (EMFs) via activation of voltage-gated calcium channels (VGCCs). His latest paper is on how such EMFs cause very-early-ly-onset Alzheimer's in animals and humans.

Martin L. Pall, Professor Emeritus of Biochemistry and Basic Medical Sciences,
Washington State University,
638 NE 41st Ave.
Portland, OR 97232
martin_pall@wsu.edu

Chapter 11: Other Environmental Toxins

Lyn Patrick, ND

Dr. Nathan's Introduction

While mold toxicity is the single most common cause of sensitization, it would be a serious mistake to underestimate the effects of other environmental toxins on sensitization. We're honored to have Dr. Patrick, truly an expert in this area, share with us her knowledge about this subject. Every time I've had the opportunity to learn from Lyn, her presentations have left me increasingly concerned about the toxicity of our world, and this chapter is no exception. I urge you to hang in there, as this information might be crucial to you or your loved ones or your patients in understanding what you're being exposed to and how to treat it successfully.

Note: I refer to non-biologic toxins as toxicants because that is how they are defined in toxicology and how they're differentiated from biologic toxins like mycotoxins, etc. Also, toxic metals are referred to as such, not as "heavy metals," because toxic metals like aluminum are not "heavy"; their molecular weight on the periodic chart does not denote them as such. It seems more precise to call them what they are, neither heavy nor light but definitely toxic.

✧ ✧ ✧

The History of Recognizing Multiple Chemical Sensitivity

To understand the specific chemicals that can cause chemical sensitivity or multiple chemical sensitivity, we must look back in history at the doctors who were decades ahead of their time in understanding how these toxicants caused disease, what kinds of health problems could be traced back to specific chemical exposures, and how to treat them.

Often called the "father of environmental medicine," Theron Randolph, MD, was the first physician to identify chemicals in air, water, food, and soil that he believed led to physical and psychological symptoms in his patients. As an allergist on staff at Northwestern University Medical School in Chicago in the early 1940s, he began to identify food allergies that were responsible for his patients' medical conditions. He later started to identify the connection between a wide variety of symptoms and everyday chemical exposures: fragrances, pesticides, petrochemicals (gasoline and natural gas), and cleaning products. In contrast to the standard blood IgE allergy testing of his day, he developed a method of diagnosis whereby he put these patients in rooms with clean air and chemical-free furnishings, gave them only uncontaminated spring water to drink, and observed that their symptoms improved. He then introduced a variety of chemicals, foods, etc., to see if the symptoms returned. He called his field Clinical Ecology, and his chemical-free rooms "clinical ecology units."

Today, clinical ecology units, now called "environmental control units," are accepted in conventional medicine, and the avoidance and reintroduction of foods shows this to be an effective method of food-allergy diagnosis.

Doctor Randolph worked with two other pioneering allergists, Herbert Rinkel and Arthur Coca, to use other methods of identifying reactions to foods and chemicals: pulse testing and intradermal injections. The second, intradermal provocation and neutralization (IDPN), is a technique for both identification and treatment of food, pollens, and chemical allergies and sensitivity. It is used today by doctors around the globe who practice "clinical environmental medicine," the new term for clinical ecology.

Dr. William Rea, the father of one of Randolph's patients, was a heart surgeon who had a sick son, later identified as having an illness caused by pesticide exposure. Bill Rea became so convinced of Randolph's theories and methods of treatment that he himself developed a practice centered around identifying toxic exposures in patients. He opened a clinic in Dallas, Texas, to treat chemically sensitive individuals. He was able to set up environments similar to Randolph's environmentally clean units, and created a room where patients could be re-exposed to small amounts of specific toxicants (pesticides, components of indoor and outdoor air pollution, solvents, etc.) to see if they reacted to these individual exposures.

At the same time, across the country in Buffalo, New York, Dr. Kalpana Patel, MD, a young pediatrician at the time, started to see patients from a housing development called Love Canal, outside of Niagara Falls, New York. Love Canal was a neighborhood built on a toxic waste dump whose contents literally started to surface in 1978 as a result of heavy rains. The Environmental Protection Agency named Love Canal "one of the most appalling environmental tragedies in American history." The neighborhood was eventually evacuated. and the soil of the homes and yards was hauled away as hazardous waste.

Dr. Patel sought help from Theron Randolph and eventually met William Rea who was also seeing very sick patients who had been exposed to myriad chemicals. They started to collaborate on finding a way to treat these individuals, and the rest is modern history—both of their environmental health centers have treated tens of thousands of patients, and they have written a five-volume series of medical textbooks on the subject.[1]

Many other allergists, pediatricians, internists, researchers, and family doctors became students of Randolph's approaches, and many are members of the American Academy of Environmental Medicine (www.aaemonline.org), an organization that Dr. Rea and Patel helped create.

Here's a simple explanation of how chemicals can cause very diverse reactions that include Mast Cell Activation Syndrome (MCAS). Most of the references to the following environmental medicine concepts originally came from Theron Randolph, but are referenced in the textbook series by Rea and Patel. They have also been further developed by a brilliant researcher, Cynthia Miller, MD; we'll talk about her groundbreaking studies further on.

Basic Theories of Environmental Medicine

Total Body Burden

The concept of total body burden is that chemical toxicant and toxin exposure leads to signs and symptoms only when pollutants in the body reach a certain level, at which point an individual who may have previously been able to metabolize and get rid of them no longer can. Dr. Rea referred to the idea of a water barrel full of a variety of pollutants and chemicals to explain total body burden, a barrel that everyone is exposed to daily. He was very specific about identifying these pollutants as he tested for them in his patients' blood, urine, and fat tissues: pesticides, herbicides, solvents, chlorine and chlorine byproducts, gasoline (and gasoline additives like MTBE), electromagnetic frequencies, solvents such as benzene and formaldehyde, carpets, glues, radon, ozone, toxic metals such as mercury and lead, molds, toxic algae in food or water, air pollutants (polycyclic aromatic hydrocarbons, nitrous and sulfur dioxides), carbon monoxide, food additives (dyes, artificial colors, and flavors), biological toxins (molds, viruses, bacteria, parasites) and naturally occurring food toxins like solinine and other glycoalkyloids found in the nightshade food family. Since the opening of his practice, his team gathered a database of 60,000 patients, which has formed the basis for much of what we know about how pollutants affect the body and cause disease.

Dr. Rea found that when the amount of these chemical exposures (plus the degree of toxicity of all the exposures) increases to a certain point, the barrel becomes full and begins to spill over. At this point, signs of the body's inability to cope with the burden of chemicals will start to show up. Again, Dr. Rea was very specific about these—you'll see MCAS symptoms among them:

- sensitivity to odors, smelling odors when others in the immediate environment can't (a common symptom of those who have been chemically exposed)
- ringing in ears
- swelling, pain, sinus infection
- runny nose, postnasal drip
- blood-vessel spasms that cause flushing, burning, heat intolerance, cold intolerance, clotting problems
- pain
- itching
- weakness
- fatigue
- transient anxiety
- depression
- heart palpitations
- faster- or slower-than-normal heartbeat
- breathlessness, shakiness, ravenous desire to eat or drink (often misinterpreted as hypoglycemia or low blood sugar)
- cough, wheezing
- dry mouth
- bloating, cramping, nausea, constipation, diarrhea, loss of appetite
- headache
- lightheadedness
- numbness/tingling in any part of the body
- high/low blood pressure
- urinary urgency and frequency, vaginal discharge, premenstrual syndrome
- muscle and joint pain
- edema (swelling) around the eyes or in hands, feet, or any other part of the body

Symptoms resulting from chemical exposure are by no means limited to the list above; those are just the most common problems seen in patients with chemical exposure.

How Do You Know You Have Chemical Sensitivity?

In the past fifteen years, the number of people diagnosed with multiple chemical sensitivity, or MCS, has tripled, and self-reported chemical sensitivity has more than doubled.

Among a population of US adults surveyed in 2016, 13% reported medically diagnosed MCS and 26% had symptoms of chemical sensitivity. A similar survey of 1,027 individuals in North Carolina identified 33% of that population with chemical sensitivity.[2]

Of those with MCS, 86% experienced health problems such as migraine headaches when exposed to fragranced consumer products; 71% were asthmatic; 70% could not go into places that use fragranced products such as air fresheners; and 61% had lost workdays or a job in the past year due to fragranced products in the workplace.

A brilliant allergist and researcher from the University of Texas in San Antonio, Dr. Claudia Miller, noticed that her patients seemed to react to a broad range of chemicals in the environment that were possibly causing their allergies. In order to find out if chemicals or foods were related to her patients' symptoms, she created a series of questionnaires (the BREESI and the QEESI), as well as an intake form that has been used in hundreds of studies in the last forty years.

She found that if her patients answered yes to at least one of the following questions, there was a good chance they were reacting to a food or chemical in their environment. This is called the BREESI (Brief Environmental Exposure and Sensitivity Inventory).

1. Do you feel sick when you are exposed to tobacco smoke, certain fragrances, nail polish/remover, engine exhaust, gasoline, air fresheners, pesticides, paint/thinner, fresh tar/asphalt, cleaning supplies, new carpet, or furnishings? By sick, we mean headaches, difficulty thinking, difficulty breathing, weakness, dizziness, upset stomach, etc.

2. Are you unable to tolerate or do you have adverse or allergic reactions to any drugs or medications (such as antibiotics, anesthetics, pain relievers, x-ray contrast dye, vaccines or birth control pills), or to an implant, prosthesis, contraceptive chemical or device, or other medical/surgical/dental material or procedure?

3. Are you unable to tolerate or do you have adverse reactions to any foods such as dairy products, wheat, corn, eggs, caffeine, alcoholic beverages, or food additives (such as MSG, food dye)?

A yes answer to any of the above would be followed by the patient's taking the longer assessment, called the QEESI (Quick Environmental Exposure and Sensitivity Inventory) available free online: https://tiltresearch.org/qeesi-2/.

The QEESI has four scales: Symptom Severity, Chemical Intolerances, Other Intolerances, and Life Impact. Each is scored from 0 to 10 (0 = "not a problem" to 10 = "severe or disabling problem"). Total scores range from 0 to 100.

There is also a 10-item Masking Index, which gauges any intake of caffeine, tobacco, or drugs that can reduce or mask an individual's awareness of their intolerances.

Those with QEESI scores of 40 or greater on both the Symptom Severity and Chemical Intolerance scales may be suffering from chemical intolerance. More than sixty studies globally have looked at the ability of this questionnaire to accurately identify those who are made sick by environmental/dietary exposures.

Dr. Miller identified chemical sensitivity as a cause of illness and called it "toxicant-induced loss of tolerance," or TILT. The conditions she has identified that can result from chemical exposure and sensitivity include fibromyalgia, chronic fatigue syndrome, depression, irritable bowel syndrome, asthma, eczema, attention deficit/ hyperactivity disorder (ADHD), and autism spectrum disorder.

That's not the only groundbreaking research Dr. Miller has done. She worked extensively with Gulf War veterans with Gulf War Illness, a debilitating and somewhat mysterious chronic condition brought on by their many exposures in the Gulf War: oil-well smoke, pesticides, and solvents.

Dr. Miller is clear that the chemical exposure that started the problem isn't always the same as the chemical or chemicals that the individual ends up reacting to. Drs. Randolph and Rea also identified this and called it "spreading," meaning that the initial exposure that caused the damage can lead to chemical intolerance to new and different chemicals or foods. A common example is someone who had an original pesticide exposure that made them sick leading to an inability to be around solvents (fabric softener, cleaning products, air fresheners, nail polish, nail polish remover, car exhaust, gasoline, gas stoves or furnaces, etc.) or made them react when eating specific foods such as dairy products or eggs.

Dr. Miller has published several medical journal articles on TILT; they can all be found at https://tiltresearch.org/tilt-program/research/. In her research looking at large groups of individuals who had known chemical exposures and then became sick, she was able to identify many of these initiating exposures. These groups included the 9/11 workers in New York City, veterans who were diagnosed with Gulf War Illness, and 2,000 EPA employees who moved into a new headquarters with brand-new carpeting and furnishings.

Many of the initial exposures were solvents (known as volatile organic compounds or VOCs) from carpeting, gasoline fumes, the wreckage of buildings (9/11), and burning oil and garbage pits (the Gulf War). Pesticide exposure was also a common initiator for both Gulf War Illness and for workers in a casino whose common area had been sprayed for pests.[3]

Why Doesn't Everyone Become Ill From Chemical Exposure?

Why aren't we all sick from everyday exposure to that list of common indoor and outdoor chemicals? There are several reasons that some individuals become chemically sensitive. Dr. Rea found them consistently in his chemically sensitive patients:

1. They were significantly lacking in specific nutrients. After evaluating both blood and intracellular levels (inside white blood cells) of vitamins and minerals, he found that environmentally ill patients tended to have very low levels of magnesium, vitamin B6, B1, B2, niacin, vitamin C, taurine, and glutathione.[4] These low levels were either the result of dietary deficiencies or because nutritional deficiencies were created by using these nutrients in metabolizing and excreting chemical pollutant exposures. It just so happens that all of the above nutrients are needed for the body to break down and eliminate many toxicants such as metals, pesticides, and solvents.

2. They had inherited small alterations (called "SNPs"—single nucleotide polymorphisms) in how specific genes were constructed, that make it harder for them to detoxify certain pollutants. These changes are common in everyone, and testing for them has become commonplace in medicine, especially in pregnancy and cardiovascular disease. Testing for these SNPs is available directly through companies like 23andMe; however, the results need to be interpreted carefully by trained healthcare providers, as the wrong supplementation can be harmful rather than helpful.

Dr Rea found that chemically sensitive patients commonly had gene variants (a substitution of one amino acid for another) in the n-acetyltranserase (NAT2) genes, as well as the glutathione-s-transferase (GSTM1 and GSTT1) gene variants. The importance of this information is that it takes the early warning concept and backs it up with hard science. There is good research to show that these individuals are challenged in being able to detoxify chemicals and more vulnerable to pollutant exposure.[5]

3. They were unable to get sufficient oxygen to their tissues. Dr. Rea studied the research of Dr. Von Ardenne, a Belgian physician who had been able to identify problems with tissue oxygenation in certain individuals. Rea concluded that chemical exposures cause inflammation in blood vessels that makes it difficult for oxygen to move from the capillaries into the tissues. The capillaries are the smallest blood vessels leading into tissues (the kidney, liver, brain, etc.), and even red blood cells have to bend to enter these small tubes. Dr. Rea found that using oxygen at high pressure for a few hours a day opened up these capillaries and increased blood supply to all the organs, making it easier for patients to detoxify and recover. Oxygen therapy—tanks or bags that supply oxygen through the nose at a certain pressure for specific amounts of time—is used in environmental health centers today to help correct this problem in those with mold and chemical exposure.

4. Toxic exposures have an effect on the nervous systems of chemically sensitive people through a specific mechanism involving the NMDA receptor, a "docking station" on the surface of nerve cells that controls the activity of the cells and allow messages to go from one nerve cell to the next. Chemicals and electromagnetic frequencies (such as those emitted from cellphones, smart meters, Wi-Fi, etc.) can affect these receptors and make them more sensitive to chemicals or other environmental triggers and can lead to an increased reaction to the presence of both chemicals and other inputs such as temperature and pressure.

When NMDA receptor function is altered by chemical exposure, the nerve itself can become 1,000 times more sensitive to a variety of stimuli (pressure, temperature, other chemical exposures). This may explain the experience of chemically sensitive individuals who say they can smell odors like cigarette smoke on entering a room when others can't smell anything, or who react to a building where mold is present by feeling sick when they enter but no one else reacts.[6,7,8]

Why Is Avoidance Important?

Drs. Randolph, Patel, and Rea showed that patients improved by avoiding specific chemical exposures. This is a crucial concept in environmental medicine. Many individuals with chemical sensitivity cannot handle the exposures commonly found in commercial buildings, homes, and urban environments. Dr. Rea found that after a period of avoidance, patients would get better, and by being re-exposed in "environmental control chambers" (special rooms where exposures were controlled), their symptoms returned. (These people did not know what they were being exposed to—whether just filtered air or a chemical they might react to.)

Although individuals did not respond to tests of filtered air, they always reacted to specific toxicant exposures with altered heart rates, blood-pressure changes, ringing in the ears, headaches, irritability, severe fatigue, and even fainting. Dr. Rea performed this test in more than 1,000 patients.

He also tested for food and mold allergies using intradermal testing, injecting tiny amounts of a food or chemical under the skin to check for local reactions of swelling or redness. He tested a total of 20,000 individuals this way and found that chemically sensitive patients would react to very small amounts of chemicals or foods sometimes immediately, not only by skin changes but reactions that would often include sleepiness, irritability, confusion, delirium, and sometimes fainting.[9] Sadly, intradermal testing did not make it to conventional allergy practice; this method of testing is currently only available through environmental medicine providers.

Which Exposures Make Most Environmentally Ill and Chemically Sensitive Patients Sick?

Mold, EMFs, and Lyme disease and its coinfections are addressed in separate chapters in this book. This chapter deals with other environmental pollutant exposures that have been connected to chemical sensitivity, allergy, mast-cell syndrome, and chronic illness.

First, it's important to know that our environment is full of chemical exposures that our bodies are not evolutionarily equipped to handle. The number is overwhelming: in 2019 a new study was published that found there are 350,000 synthetic chemicals currently in commerce (this was about two to three times the previous estimates), and there are about 1,500 new chemicals being added every year in the U.S. alone.[10]

Of these 350,000 chemicals, 50,000 are "confidential" (proprietary formulas that are kept secret), and 70,000 are not described clearly enough to be understood, so fully one third of this cornucopia of chemicals is a secret. Since the enactment of the Frank R. Lautenberg Chemical Safety for the 21st Century Act, meant to enforce stronger chemical safety regulations, a total of only 700 chemicals have been tested and deemed safe; 707 others were "possibly unsafe," which could mean anything, and that's no guarantee that the remaining 348,600 are safe.

Fortunately for all of us, Drs. Rea and Patel have identified the major chemicals their patients were exposed to that actually made them sick. These exposures were seen in breath-testing levels in patients, indoor air analysis of their homes, *and* reactions to the same chemicals in the environmental control chambers. Here are the chemicals he identified and their major sources of exposure. Be prepared—*most* of them come from inside your home.

Natural Gas Fumes

Even though natural gas is often an inexpensive source of both heating and cooking fuel, it is anything but "clean." Natural gas always contains some level of by-products from the process of refining natural gas. These pollutants include the solvents (also called VOCs or volatile organic compounds): benzene, toluene, hexane, ethylbenzene, and xylene (benzene and xylene are carcinogenic) as well as methane, carbon monoxide, nitrous oxide, formaldehyde (another solvent that is a carcinogen and neurotoxic) and radon (a radioactive element). All of these are commonly found in homes from the use of natural gas as a heating and cooking fuel.[11,12]

A study by the Lawrence Berkeley National Laboratory and Stanford University involved a team of scientists that went into a group of homes in Southern California to study emissions from gas cooking stoves. Based on the homes they tested that did *not* have vented gas ranges, they estimated that during the winter, an estimated 1.7 million Californians could be exposed to gas stovetop pollutants in their homes that would exceed both federal and state allowable levels for outdoor air.

This study did not monitor levels of other gases from these stoves, but it's clear that having emissions that exceed EPA standards for outdoor clean air inside a home is never a good thing and probably involves elevated levels of other pollutants found in natural gas.[13]

Exposure to gas appliances (cookstoves, furnaces, water heaters) without the use of ventilation has been linked to asthma, impaired lung function, and respiratory illnesses.[14] Children who grow up in a home with a gas stove are twice as likely to be diagnosed with asthma compared to children who grow up in homes with electric stoves.[15]

Dr. Cynthia Miller, whose research is discussed below, has identified unvented gas stoves as a significant risk for chemical sensitivity; an article on her clinical research site explains why these appliances are so harmful for those with chemically sensitivity: https://tiltresearch.org/2022/08/15/hidden-dangers-of-gas-stoves/.

Dr. Rea tested the indoor air in the homes of patients and found high levels of volatile organic compounds (solvents). Often these homes had no ventilation, no hoods over the stove, and sometimes leaky furnaces, water heaters, or cookstoves. He identified natural gas (along with pesticide exposure) as the main causes of chemical sensitivity and allergy in his patients. Natural gas and all of the contaminants in it act as "sensitizing agents"—something that can cause reactions (rashes, asthma, allergies, etc.) and lead to sensitivity to other chemicals or substances in the person's environment. With the advent of EMF exposure from smart meters and Wi-Fi, Rea later added that EMF exposure would be as much of a cause of chemical sensitivity and chronic illness as natural gas. More information on EMF exposure can be found in chapters 12 and 13 in this book.

How Do I Know If I'm Exposed to Natural-Gas Fumes?

A study published in 2022 by the Harvard School of Public Health found significant levels of volatile organic compound contaminants in indoor kitchen air from natural gas in the seventy homes they tested. Benzene, probably the most dangerous because it's a carcinogen and considered a hazardous air pollutant, was found in 95% of the homes sampled. There were 296 contaminants identified—all components of natural gas and targeted for removal in the refining process. The study found, however, that these contaminants were still in the fuel that entered homes and were released during the process of cooking.

Customers of natural-gas utility providers can call the company and have a technician come to the home to check for levels of carbon monoxide and methane. The tech cannot, however, check for levels of benzene, toluene, ethylbenzene, xylene, and hexane that have been identified in indoor environments and that Rea, Miller, and others have found related to many sensitivity reactions. If you want information about what solvents and other pollutants are in your indoor environment, an assessment by an indoor environmental professional (https://iseai.org/finding-the-right-indoor-environmental-professional-to-assess-your-home/) may be necessary.

You can add an exhaust vent to your cookstove if you don't already have one. According to a study at the Lawrence Berkeley National Lab, exhaust fan effectiveness at capturing gas fumes and cooking fumes varies widely, from 15% to 98%, so make sure the vent actually covers both front and rear burners and has a strong fan. The fans usually make a lot of noise if they're working well, but that's a small price to pay for protection from 296 toxicants.

The Berkeley Lab researchers also found that cross-ventilation, opening windows while cooking, was effective at lowering indoor levels of natural-gas pollutants. Air filtration with an effective air filter will also lower exposure.

A note of caution: Dr. Rea's clinical experience showed that patients with severe chemical sensitivity had to switch to electric appliances because they continued to react to even small amounts of the volatile organic compounds emitted from gas appliances, even with air filtration.

Pesticides

The second group of environmental exposures that contribute to chemical sensitivity is pesticides. Blood and urine testing at both EHC-Dallas and EHC-Buffalo have found significant levels of pesticides in the chemically sensitive. The term "pesticides" is a general umbrella for all chemicals used to treat unwanted insects and/or plants. This section addresses problems with exposure to herbicides, insecticides, and fungicides as one group and refers to all of them as pesticides.

Pesticides are truly an American experiment: According to the USDA, about 400 different agricultural pesticides, totaling >1 billion pounds, were used in the United States in 2017, the latest year for which data is available. Sixty percent were considered hazardous to human health, according to the World Health Organization's data. Twenty-five of these pesticides are banned in more than thirty other countries. Phorate, the most used "extremely hazardous" insecticide in the U.S., is banned in thirty-eight other countries, including China, Brazil, and India. None of the "extremely hazardous" pesticides we use here in the U.S. can be used in the twenty-seven nations of the European Union.[16]

A large study done by the Centers for Disease Control showed that more than 50% of children and adults in the U.S. have measurable levels of an entire group of organophosphate pesticides in their urine. For some individual pesticides, like chlorpyrifos, levels were detectable in 93% of those tested.[17]

Organochlorine pesticides still show up in our blood, though most were banned in the 1970s. These compounds do not break down easily and can be stored in our fat tissue for up to fifty years. DDT was banned in 1972, but DDT metabolites, which are also toxic, have been found in 98% of the child and adult population in the U.S.[18]—no, that's not a typo; most of us still carry these toxic pesticides in our bodies.

A 2021 study showed that higher levels of a DDT metabolite in the bodies of grandmothers can predict obesity and early onset of menstrual periods in their granddaughters. This is possible because these chemicals are passed from mother to child and act to alter the way hormones work even two generations away.[19] Drs. Rea and Patel found significant levels of these pesticides in the blood of their patients as recently as 2020, and though levels of organochlorine pesticides have gone down in the American population significantly in the last twenty years, *there are some pesticides that can still be very problematic and contribute to chemical sensitivity.* They are:

Pentachlorophenol – The Gift That Keeps On Giving

Pentachlorophenol (PCP) is an organochlorine restricted-use pesticide (herbicide, fungicide, and insecticide) that is being phased out of production starting in 2022 due to its classification as a "probable" human carcinogen and its known toxicity in many organs of the body. Homes and commercial buildings historically used PCP as a wood preservative from 1936–1984 when it was banned for residential and commercial use. However, it is currently approved for structural wood in non-residential buildings like barns or stables to prevent wood rot and won't be totally phased out until 2027.

As recently as 2003–2004 (the last time the CDC measured levels of this pesticide in the US population), PCP was found in at least 25% of children and adults. Because it's a chlorinated pesticide (like DDT) it accumulates in the body—not just in the fat, muscle, and organs (liver) of humans and the animals we eat but in buildings too. PCP levels were elevated in both the residents of homes with old wood paneling and in the dust of the homes whose builders had used PCP many decades earlier.[20]

The reason for this special mention of PCP is that Drs. Rea and Patel identified many families who had become severely chemically sensitive and ill after living in log homes treated with PCP. They strongly advocated for the banning of all PCPs from building materials.

Chlordane – The Invisible Toxicant

The other pesticide that needs mention is chlordane (also called "technical chlordane," heptachlor, cis-chlordane, trans-chlordane, and trans-Nonachlor). It's another organochlorine pesticide (like DDT) that was used as a termiticide in foundations and basements of approximately 30 million homes in the southeastern and southwestern United States. Its use was banned in 1988 because it was identified as a human carcinogen as well as toxic to animals, and it was banned from crop and garden use five years earlier. Chlordane is long-lived in both the foundations and the basements of homes and commercial buildings. Studies as recent as 2003 (it had been banned at that point for twenty-five years) found elevated levels of chlordane in the air of more than half the homes tested. In these homes, the air levels of this pesticide were between four and forty times the EPA allowable levels. Blood levels of chlordane in residents of these homes were about twenty-five times higher than they would have been from eating produce sprayed with chlordane.[21] Individuals with elevated levels of chlordane in their blood have a two to three times higher risk of diabetes and a significantly increased risk of certain cancers.[22]

Can pesticides cause sensitivity reactions? The following case is a dramatic but clear example of the effects of chlordane:

A fifty-five-year old woman complained of chronic fatigue, muscle pain, memory loss, insomnia, hyperactivity and repeated lung infections. She had positive food allergy reactions to thirty-six foods. The insomnia started after major pelvic surgery and the removal of her appendix. Post-surgically, she had a high fever that was believed to be a reaction to anesthesia.

Two years after the surgery she had not improved. Testing for chemical exposure showed elevated levels of chlordane in her blood. The Texas Department of Health tested her home carpet and found high levels of chlordane, heptachlor, DDT, and diazinon (an organophosphate pesticide). She had had the home treated for pests and termites many years prior, and these pesticides were still measurable in both the home air and carpet. On the advice of her physician, she had the carpeting removed and the crawlspace ventilated. The ground in the crawlspace and around the foundation, which had been impregnated with chlordane for termite control, was sealed off so it could no longer off-gas. Her recurrent lung infections stopped, as did the rest of her symptoms, within a month of these interventions, and she was able to continue living in her home environment without health issues.

Carpeting, new or old, has its own "body burden" of toxicants. New carpeting collects and then off-gases multiple toxicants, mostly solvents. Synthetic carpets are made from nylon fibers with a polypropylene backing. The glue that sticks to the backing is made of styrene and 4-phenylcyclohexane (4-PC), a toxic solvent that is an eye and sinus/lung irritant found in 95% of carpets. It may also be a brain and nervous-system toxicant. Dr. Cynthia Miller's research into what made so many employees of the EPA sick when they moved into brand-new headquarters was the new carpeting off-gassing high levels of 4-PC. The "new-carpet aroma" is the odor of 4-PC off-gassing. The adhesive used to affix the carpet to the floor typically contains benzene and toluene, additional harmful chemicals. Older carpeting, especially in homes that are water-damaged, becomes a sink for mycotoxins.[23]

Triclosan – The Antibacterial Pesticide

The FDA removed Triclosan from "antiseptic" antibacterial soaps in 2016, but it's still found in many consumer products that are not labeled ANTISEPTIC: liquid soaps, deodorants, toothpaste, shaving cream, mouthwash, cleaning supplies, sports clothing (as Microban), as an intentional additive in grapefruit-seed extract, and added to cutting boards and other kitchen items as an "antimicrobial." Triclosan is actually registered with the EPA as a pesticide and is undergoing a review based on a call by several consumer groups to ban it.[24]

Young people with elevated urinary levels of triclosan are more likely to have inhalant allergies and hay fever, and children with higher urinary triclosan levels are at increased risk of developing food allergies.[25]

Triclosan is also linked to thyroid and sex-hormone disruption in animals, and, like pyrethroids, it may increase risk for contact dermatitis (think eczema). Triclosan also interferes with a pathway for detoxification called glucuronidation. This pathway is also necessary for specific mycotoxins and hormones. Exposure to both triclosan and BPA (the plastic lining in canned food and major plastic in hard water bottles) makes glucuronidation potentially more difficult for other toxicants. And as Drs. Rea and Patel consistently stated, total body burden, especially when it overloads major detoxification pathways, leads to chemical sensitivity.

Pyrethroid Insecticides – Progress?

Pyrethroid insecticides have historically been considered safer than other insecticides and are currently replacing them in homes and office buildings as well as in sprays for outside insects such as mosquitos. Unfortunately, there is growing evidence that these "cleaner, safer" pesticides are toxic to the nervous system and brain, and are related to asthma and skin problems.[26]

Pyrethroid pesticides have also been linked to learning problems in children and cognition and memory problems in older adults.[27] Pyrethroids are known as "sensitizers" by allergists because they can initiate allergic reactions to further pyrethroid exposure from other sources. The following case is a good example of how this insecticide can lead to severe allergic reactions:

A twenty-nine-year-old woman took her first trip to Africa, flying from Brussels, Belgium, to the Democratic Republic of the Congo. She was returning to Brussels on her way home when, after closing the doors, the cabin crew sprayed insecticides as part of their routine procedure for flights originating in many countries in Africa and South Asia. Because these countries have endemic malaria, yellow fever, and other insect vector-borne diseases, international health regulations specify that all the inhabitants (humans) in the cabin have to be sprayed prior to takeoff. Shortly after the cabin spraying, the woman's lips and eyelids became swollen, and she developed diarrhea, shortness of breath, and dizziness. A doctor on the flight found her with a red face, and swollen eyes and lips. She appeared to be suffocating, though her pulse rate and blood pressure were normal. He gave her albuterol inhalation and oral steroids, which he carried in his luggage, since the flight crew brought only a first-aid kit containing bandages, but no emergency medical kit containing epinephrine. Once in Kinshasa, the woman suffered persistent mild wheezing, which she had never experienced before. The wheezing stopped after she turned off an electric anti-mosquito vaporizer.

Three months after the airplane incident, the woman developed a severely itchy, swollen eyelid after contact with a neighborhood dog whose fur had just been treated with flea powder. Her allergist, comparing the ingredients of the flight-cabin insecticide spray, the electric anti-mosquito vaporizer, and the flea powder, found one common ingredient: pyrethroids. The woman was able to endure future flights only with asthma medication and by using a face covering for breathing. Two years later she was diagnosed with asthma.[28]

Pyrethroid insecticides, specifically one called permethrin, are used in fabric for clothing intended to repel ticks and mosquitos. Known as "Insect Shield," it has historically been used in clothing for the military and forestry workers. Permethrin has been shown to penetrate skin and end up in the urine of individuals after only eight hours of wearing the clothing. It may very well have the ability to act as a sensitizing agent, just as the permethrin spray does.[29]

Organophosphate Pesticides

Organophosphate (OP) pesticides are among the most commonly used pesticides in the United States, sprayed on 65% of food crops and used widely for home lawn and garden weed and insect treatment.

OP pesticides are neurotoxins, which is how they work to kill pests. Sadly, recent research has shown that they also cause inflammation and act as endocrine disruptors—altering how hormones are produced and how they act in the body. We now realize that they are not very different from their toxic predecessors, the organochlorine pesticides (DDT and others). They also increase risk for asthma in children and adults and cause mast-cell release.[30,31,32]

Many organophosphate pesticides have been shown to damage cell membranes in ways that allow calcium and sodium to have access to the inside of the cells. This process increases the cells' vulnerability and may be one of the ways that pesticides initiate chemical sensitivity. This damage to membranes can also cause damage to the nerves in the olfactory system, contributing to the increased sensitivity to odors that many chemically sensitive individuals develop. This membrane damage can also increase vulnerability to molds and mycotoxins, cause food intolerance, chronic infections, and damage to mitochondria (the powerhouse of the cell), leading to fatigue and brain fog.[33] Other pesticides: atrazine, carbamates, glyphosate, pyrethroids, and fungicides, can also trigger chemical sensitivity through these pathways.[34]

Pesticide exposure-caused chemical sensitivity can masquerade as many other illnesses. Claudia Miller's published studies showed that patients with pesticide-exposure histories had significant problems in addition to chemical sensitivity: digestive issues, difficulty breathing, altered heart rate, depressed mood, and chronic muscle pain.[35] Dr. Rea also reported that 93% of 2,000 chemically sensitive patients he treated had classic symptoms of organophosphate nervous-system damage: episodes of blurred vision, headache, followed by nausea, cramping, chest tightness, muscle twitching, difficulty with attention span, and impaired thinking—commonly known as brain fog.[36]

Glyphosate

Glyphosate is the most widely used herbicide in human history. Eighteen billion pounds of glyphosate-based herbicides have been sprayed worldwide since 1974. Glyphosate use has increased fifteenfold since 1996 when it began to be used on Roundup-resistant GMO crops like soy, sugar beets, canola and corn.

In 2015 the International Agency for Research on Cancer classified glyphosate as a "probable human carcinogen" and glyphosate became a household word. In August 2018, when a groundskeeper in his mid-forties recovered a $289 million verdict against Monsanto, the controversy around glyphosate mushroomed. In his job, the man had used Roundup, a glyphosate-based herbicide, regularly, and two years after an episode where he was soaked in the chemical, he was diagnosed with non-Hodgkin's lymphoma. Another court case that followed awarded $55 million to a couple who had both contracted non-Hodgkin's lymphoma after years of using a glyphosate-based herbicide. The jury fined Monsanto another $2 billion. According to Bayer, who purchased Monsanto, they have paid out about $411 billion to settle cases pending against them for damages allegedly resulting from glyphosate exposure.

Can Glyphosate Cause Chemical Sensitivity?

Pesticides of all classes can cause cancer, and the mechanisms are largely unknown. We know very little about glyphosate's effects on the body because, like most pesticides, we have only limited animal research.

We do know that glyphosate can accumulate in our tissues for hours to months before we eliminate it. From animal research, we also know that glyphosate can alter the microbial balance in the gut and damage the intestinal tract, and lead to breast and liver tumors in rodents. In humans, there is a proven association between higher levels of glyphosate in the urine and increased risk for advanced fatty liver disease.[37]

Higher-dose exposures of glyphosate-containing herbicides have been associated with memory loss and anxiety in mice.[38] Though it is dangerous to assume effects in mice will translate to humans, there was a clear signal in these studies that glyphosate suppressed levels of a critical brain and body nervous system-control mechanism, an enzyme called acetylcholinesterase, which breaks down nerve-signaling compounds. This same mechanism can occur in OP poisoning and can lead to serious problems.

Other brain and body nervous-system effects of glyphosate in animals are also concerning. Short-term treatment of mice with significant doses of glyphosate resulted in suppression of dopamine and serotonin markers in the brain, which can lead to significant mood changes. It appears that glyphosate has an array of effects on the nervous system that alters NMDA receptors too. Glyphosate damages nerves in the same way that organophosphate pesticides do, allowing large quantities of sodium and calcium inside the cells to alter the sensitivity of the nerves.[39] Though there are no good human studies on glyphosate toxicity and chemical sensitivity, there are some red flags in the animal research.

Avoiding Glyphosate Exposure

Glyphosate has been detected in streams and rivers near farmland, on school playgrounds (where it is routinely used for weed control), on many crops post-harvest for fungus control (wheat, oats, beans), and has literally made its way into every corner of our food chain: breastmilk, infant foods, meat (beef, pork), breakfast cereals, and hidden sources like soy sauce and honey. It has even been detected in organically grown food where it is not supposed to be, and, of course, it has been found in human blood and in the urine of 80% of the US population.[40] The best way to avoid glyphosate is not to eat it. USDA-certified organic foods cannot be grown with glyphosate-containing herbicides, and in general, have significantly lower levels or undetectable levels of glyphosate compared to conventionally grown food.

How Do I Know If I'm Exposed to Pesticides Or Whether I React to Them?

Pesticides can be measured in the blood and urine through lab testing, which has to be ordered by a medical provider. Air levels or dust levels of pesticides can be measured by indoor environmental professionals (IEPs).

Formaldehyde

Formaldehyde is another solvent, a chemical that exists as a gas and a liquid, has an odor, and is found commonly in both indoor and outdoor spaces. According to Dr. Rea, formaldehyde is the third most common environmental trigger of disease in indoor air after natural gas and pesticides.

Formaldehyde is included in a group called "hazardous air pollutants"—a classification of the most dangerous chemicals in outdoor air. The EPA has identified formaldehyde as the most dangerous of all of these hazardous pollutants because it causes cancer and lung damage, even when the level of exposure is low, like that found in schools, homes, and retail stores.[41]

Even though formaldehyde is found in outdoor air from car exhaust and industrial activity, studies show global levels indoors are higher than in the outdoor environment,[42] so cleaning up the indoor spaces you inhabit is more important than not exposing yourself to outdoor air like smoke and smog. New homes (those built after 1990), and especially new carpet, pressboard furniture, and laminate flooring are sources of formaldehyde in indoor air.

Studies following office workers through their day found that that while only about 2% of their formaldehyde exposure was due to outdoor air, 24% was due to the workplace air, 12% was due to cigarette smoke exposure, and the majority, 61%, was due to their home air.[43]

Elevated levels of formaldehyde in the body are damaging to the brain and have been linked to memory loss and Alzheimer's disease. Exposure to formaldehyde can lead to irritation of the eyes, nose, sinuses, skin, and throat. Exposure has also been linked to allergies, thirst, dizziness, fatigue, brain fog, insomnia, irritability, respiratory problems, and reproductive problems.

Long-term exposure to significant levels of formaldehyde, such as living in a mobile home for years, can be linked to other problems as well. Out of the approximately 5,000 patients Drs. Rea and Patel have seen with formaldehyde exposure, those with prolonged exposure were found to develop not only allergies but also arthritis, vasculitis (inflammation of blood vessels), and digestive and/or urinary diseases.[44]

Mast-cell activation and histamine release due to formaldehyde exposure has been a long-recognized cause of the allergic response to this toxicant. Though formaldehyde has other damaging effects in the body, immediate mast-cell release (which can take less than a second) is responsible for the eye, nose, throat, and lung irritation that can happen on exposure, leading to not just allergies but chronic runny nose, eczema, asthma, and other respiratory issues.[45]

Formaldehyde levels in home air can be directly responsible for a variety of reactions, and the higher the exposure levels the worse the effect. An Australian study of children, allergies, and formaldehyde levels in the home showed that higher formaldehyde levels in indoor air were associated with more severe allergic reactions, including skin rashes and hives.[46]

Where Does All That Formaldehyde Come From?

Formaldehyde is found naturally in the body as part of the breakdown of DNA, RNA, and protein, but it is damaging to the brain as well as our genes, so it's metabolized quickly to a benign compound called formate or formic acid. Our capacity to detoxify formaldehyde, however, is limited, and exposure to larger amounts from external sources like indoor and outdoor air can deplete the compounds necessary to break it down. The body uses its main antioxidant, glutathione, as a detoxifying protein to break down formaldehyde.[47] Glutathione is also used in the detoxification of metals, other solvents, pesticides, plastics, and many other pollutants, so this crucial compound is in short supply in those of us who are exposed to any of these common pollutants.

Formaldehyde is used in glues that make up particleboard (new furniture and new construction materials) and is part of the production of many household items: paints, cleaning products, pesticides, adhesives, flooring and new carpets, home-fragrance products, incense, scented candles, plug-in air fresheners, permanent-press fabrics, chewing tobacco, cigarettes, and cosmetics. Formaldehyde is also released from natural gas and from using unvented gas-burning appliances like gas stoves and furnaces.[48]

Cancer of the nasopharynx (nose, sinuses, and throat] is a known occupational exposure of salon workers where "Brazilian blow-outs" are performed. The solutions used in these hair-volumizing treatments contain formaldehyde, the cause of the cancer. Even if those products are labeled FORMALDEHYDE-FREE, they may contain up to 12% formaldehyde and pose a risk in salon workers and those who receive the treatments.

Some of the highest levels of formaldehyde released from consumer products has been found in floor finishes, fingernail hardener, pressboard, and nail polish. The floor finish was by far the highest level of off-gassing formaldehyde: 1,050,000 mcg/m³/hr. For a comparison: allowable levels for formaldehyde in outdoor air, according to the California EPA, are 33 mcg/m³.[49]

How Do I Know If I'm Exposed To Formaldehyde and Whether I React To It?

Environmental control units as used by Dr. Miller and Dr. Rea are not common in hospitals or clinics, and insurance doesn't reimburse for them, so the avoidance and reintroduction testing Dr. Randolph developed and Dr. Rea used in their environmental health centers is not available for most people. There are, however, common blood tests for antibodies to formaldehyde. Any antibody production to chemicals is an indication of exposure and the binding of the chemical to human tissue, resulting in a chemical body burden. Functional medicine providers can order these tests to see if immune reactions have occurred to formaldehyde, indicating a loss of tolerance and increased sensitivity to formaldehyde exposure. Industrial hygienists, building biologists, and indoor evaluation professionals can test home air levels of formaldehyde.

Toxic Metals

Toxic metals such as mercury, lead, and many others are directly damaging to the immune system and organs as well as muscle, nerve, and bone tissue, and can lead to autoimmune disease, kidney disease, damage to the brain and nervous system, and cardiovascular events such as stroke and heart attack.

But metals can also act as allergens—a very different reaction than the direct toxic effects of metals. Metal toxicity is determined by the amount of exposure: one tuna sandwich you ate last week vs. eleven silver-amalgam fillings placed when you were fifteen years old, for example. The sandwich does not contain enough mercury to do any damage as long as that's your only exposure; however, having eleven silver-amalgam fillings may have long-lasting effects on your body.

Metal allergies are different: They are the result of exposure that the immune system reacts to and are not necessarily dependent on the amount of the metal you're exposed to, but more a result of how your immune system is programmed to respond.

The response is varied: such metals as gold, silver, and nickel can cause mast-cell release, but others, such as tin, copper, and zinc which are also used in dental amalgams, can initiate allergic reactions through other pathways.[50]

Other metals used in dental materials (implants, bridges, crowns, etc.) and orthopedic implants such as hip and shoulder implants can contain beryllium, copper, cobalt, chromium, iridium, mercury, palladium, platinum, rhodium, and titanium, all of which can also cause metal sensitivity. Recent research has also identified a chronic reaction that can develop from gadolinium, a metal used as an enhancer in MRI scans.[51]

Exposure to metals can occur from either inside the body, such as amalgam silver fillings, implants, IUDs, vaccines, and piercings, or from outside the body, such as cigarette smoke, jewelry, cosmetics, or even tattoo ink.

Of all the metals we're exposed to, nickel is the most allergenic and is found everywhere in our environment: stainless steel, jewelry, belt buckles, buttons, glasses, coins, keys, and even mobile phones, laptop computers, and video-game controllers. Most people will know if they have a nickel allergy due to the rash, swelling, and discomfort that a stainless-steel earring will cause, but some metal allergies aren't as easy to identify. Nickel is used in many alloys, like titanium, the main metal in dental implants. Dental implant failure due to metal sensitivity is a growing problem.

There are a variety of ways metals can damage our bodies: they can alter the function of the intestinal lining, disturb the bacteria in the gut, drive stress hormones like cortisol up or down, and interfere with the production and activity of thyroid hormones. The metals that are most concerning, though, are the ones implanted in our bodies through various medical devices or materials: intraocular lenses, stents, dental implants, and orthopedic devices such as hip replacements or the pins and screws used to stabilize broken bones. These metals can corrode inside the body over time, as the recent problems with cobalt/chromium hip replacements have shown, and almost any metal can act as a sensitizing agent.

Metal allergy or hypersensitivity can cause problems with the skin, mouth and throat, heart, joints, brain, thyroid gland, and the immune system. These reactions are not always immediately obvious, as the following case makes clear:

In November 2006, while in Argentina, a twenty-three-year-old woman developed a fever of 104 degrees, extreme fatigue, and swollen lymph nodes. At the time, she was diagnosed with dengue fever, but was later told she didn't have dengue fever and that there was no other cause of her symptoms.

In May 2007 she had another episode of high fever, extreme fatigue and weakness, swollen lymph nodes in her neck, and a swollen liver and spleen. All tests for viral infections were negative, and another biopsy of her lymph nodes showed that she was reacting to something but the cause wasn't clear.

She was diagnosed with adult-onset Still's disease, an inflammatory disease of unknown cause. She was put on steroids, but when she tried to go off, once in 2008 and again in 2010, she had the same reaction: high fever, anemia, muscle and joint pain, and extreme fatigue.

Unfortunately, her history of prior surgeries had not been taken into account when her doctors attempted to figure out the cause of her condition. At age twenty-two, she had a nickel–titanium chin implant put in for cosmetic reasons. Taking this into consideration, in January 2010, at the urging of her allergist, she decided to have the implant removed. All of the symptoms of joint pain and fatigue went away, and in three months she was off of all medication, symptom-free, with normal bloodwork, and she remained well as of the last follow-up in June 2012.[52]

How Do I Know If I'm Reacting to A Metal Inside or Outside My Body?

Mercury amalgams are a common source of problems for chemically sensitive individuals, and must be removed by a competent and trained dentist. Appropriate protection for both the patient and the dental personnel, as well as air filtration during the procedure, is necessary to protect everyone from exposure to mercury as the fillings are drilled out. The International Academy of Oral Medicine and Toxicology offers a protocol dedicated to the safe removal of amalgams available at: https://iaomt.org/resources/safe-removal-amalgam-fillings/.

There are lab tests for metal allergies; some are used by orthopedic surgeons who test their patients prior to implanting metal devices. These tests must be ordered by a licensed healthcare provider. Here are the main labs that do metal-sensitivity testing:

- LTT-MELISA: (Lymphocyte Transformation Testing) – This test is only available from the MELISA labs in the EU, but some providers here in the U.S. do send blood to these labs. https://melisa.org/melisa-laboratories/
- Orthopedics Analysis Lab in United States: lymphocyte transformation testing https://www.orthopedicanalysis.com/health-faqs.
- PATCH testing is a standard skin test done by allergists; it compares well with the MELISA test. It can be done for nine metals but not for titanium.
- ELISA/ACT Laboratories also does a lymphocyte transformation test using their own technology and includes metals and dental materials (test formerly done by Clifford Laboratories) https://www.elisaact.com/.

Treating Chemical Hypersensitivity – What Works?

Improving Indoor Air Quality

Claudia Miller looked at the effect of cleaning up indoor air on chemical sensitivity symptoms in thirty-seven individuals who had been part of a medical home visit from her team. These individuals had chemical sensitivities and high scores on the QEESI evaluation.[53]

After the team looked at exposures in the home and tested the indoor air, the chemically sensitive individuals and their families were educated about chemicals in the home that added to indoor air pollution. This included identifying volatile organic compounds (solvents, fragrances), personal care products, air fresheners, fabric softener, vinyl shower curtains, new carpeting, and other sources of indoor air toxicants. The medical team measured the VOC air levels after those in the home cleaned up their environment and got rid of products that contributed to VOC exposure.

The medical team identified specific items in the home that contributed to poor indoor air quality, and gave the participants an individualized action plan, including recipes for safer cleaning products. Note: There was one similarity in all the homes the teams visited. This indoor air exposure is best to hear about in the medical team's own words: "Our team observed near-universal use of potent cleaning chemicals, personal care products, and commercial fragrance products like air fresheners, incense, scented candles, or plug-in scents—as many as ten of these in a single home." These VOCs and fragrances contributed to poor indoor air quality, and the team identified them as exposures that needed to be eliminated.

Six to ten months after making suggested changes, the participants repeated the QESSI. Those in the study who had the greatest improvement in their indoor air quality (the largest drop in indoor air VOC levels) had the greatest improvement in their QEESI symptom scores, meaning the greatest improvement in their chemical sensitivity. Below is the table that identifies sources of VOC in standard indoor air and suggested substitutions.

The personal precautionary principle	
Instead of using:	Try using:
Pesticides indoors or on lawns, or mothballs	Baits or traps to control bugs indoors (Avoid attracting bugs by tightly sealing foods, including pet foods)
Paints, varnishes, glues, and polishes with high solvent content	Low-solvent-content paints, water-based finishes and glues (Have these applied when you are away from home)
Bleach, ammonia, disinfectants, and strong cleaning products	'Elbow grease', soap and water, baking soda and vinegar
Scented products, perfumes, air fresheners and incense	Unscented cleansers, laundry detergent, fabric softeners,, and cosmetics
Hair coloring, permanents, hair spray, or any aerosol product	New haircut and hair gel or styling products that are unscented and do not require spraying
Dry cleaning, odorous soft plastic toys, or mattress covers	Washable toys, bedding, and clothes
Odorous flooring, such as vinyl, pressed wood or particle board, or carpeting which can also trap allergens	Ceramic, stone tile, or hardwood floors
Commercial foods that may contain pesticides or other questionable ingredients	Organic foods and foods without additives or artificial colors

From Perales RB, Palmer RF, Rincon R, Viramontes JN, Walker T, Jaén CR, Miller CS. Does improving indoor air quality lessen symptoms associated with chemical intolerance? Prim Health Care Res Dev. 2022 Jan 12;23:e3. Pg.9.

Eating Organically Grown Food

Adopting a diet of only organically grown food can be challenging; however, it may be worth it. Dr. Rea and his colleagues found that patients who adhered to consuming only organic food improved faster. He actually called it "less contaminated" food rather than organically grown because USDA-certified organic food contains about 75% less pesticide residue than conventionally grown food.

Pesticide residue on conventionally grown (non-organic) food is very common. In a national survey, at least 73% of USDA's conventionally grown fruit and vegetable samples had pesticide residues. For five crops (apples, peaches, pears, strawberries, and celery) more than 90% of samples had residues.[54]

Some of the pesticide residue can be eliminated by soaking fruits and vegetables in a solution of vinegar, but some pesticides are absorbed through the skin of the plant and cannot be washed off.

Another important reason to eat "less contaminated," organically-grown food has to do with mold residue. Probably because pesticides, especially glyphosate-containing herbicides, encourage fungal overgrowth in the soil and plant roots, organically grown grains like barley, oats, and wheat have significantly lower levels of molds like Fusarium.

They also have lower levels of mycotoxins, like toxic trichothecenes. Two trichothecenes, HT-2 and T-2 toxin, were significantly lower in organic oats and barley compared to conventionally grown grains. Organically grown wheat has also been shown to have lower concentrations of the mycotoxins deoxynivalenol and moniliformin.[55,56]

Depuration Therapy

Heat depuration is a medical term for exposure to elevated temperatures that induce sweating. Dr. Rea had several medical saunas in his facility; they're still in operation in EHC-Dallas. Patients are prescribed one or two sessions daily. A medical sauna is different from a sauna in a gym or a fancy infra-red sauna that some companies market as necessary for "detox." A medical sauna has a controlled temperature that can be adjusted for the individual's needs, meaning it can be kept as low as 95 degrees if necessary. It also has an exhaust fan to eliminate the airborne pollutants, such as solvents, that come out of the fat tissue and are eliminated in sweat through the skin.

Published medical studies on saunas and cardiovascular disease in Finland use temperatures as high as 170 degrees, and found that the sauna effect is better at this high temperature. As long as the individual is comfortable and able to sweat for twenty minutes, there is evidence that both sweat and urine levels of toxicants increase. Many people with POTS (postural orthostatic tachycardia syndrome—an autonomic nervous-system problem that affects the heart and pulse rate) have difficulty sweating and have low tolerance for heat. A slow and gradual exposure to low-heat sauna (95–100 degrees) for even five minutes will eventually increase their tolerance for both the temperature and the amount of time they can stay in the sauna. Research shows that after twenty minutes of sweating, the gain from staying in the sauna plateaus, so twenty to thirty minutes is the prescribed time for medical sauna.

Contrary to popular marketing claims, an infra-red sauna, though popular, is unnecessary. Dr. Stephen Genuis conducted a pilot study with individuals who either worked out on an exercise bike to sweat, sat in an infra-red sauna, or sat in a dry heat sauna without infra-red radiation. He found that equal amounts of pesticides, solvents, plastics, and metals came out in the participants' urine and sweat no matter which sauna they used. Those on the exercise bike, no matter how much they were sweating, did not release as many toxicants.

Conclusion

Our modern indoor and outdoor environment contains a significant amount of exposures that can make us sick and sensitive. Eliminating those exposures, what environmental medicine providers call "avoidance," is a first step in addressing chemical sensitivity. Other simple interventions, like dietary changes that include eliminating pesticide exposure as much as possible and using appropriate sauna therapy, can also contribute to minimizing chemical reactions. They certainly couldn't hurt.

LYN PATRICK, ND, graduated from Bastyr University in 1984 with a doctorate in naturopathic medicine and has been in private practice in Arizona and Colorado for thirty-five years. She is a published author of numerous articles in peer-reviewed medical journals, a past contributing editor for Alternative Medicine Review, and recently authored a chapter in the newly released textbook *Clinical Environmental Medicine.*

She speaks internationally on environmental medicine, nonalcoholic fatty liver disease, endocrine disruption, metal toxicology, and other topics. She is currently faculty for the Metabolic Medicine Institute Fellowship in collaboration with George Washington School of Medicine and Health Sciences. She is also a founding partner and presenter at the Environmental Health Symposium, an annual international environmental medicine conference based in the United States. After the passing of her longtime colleague and mentor, Dr. Walter Crinnion, she continues to educate primary care providers in the area of environmental medicine through the EMEI Global platform and the EMEI Review podcast (emeiglobal.com).

Notes

1 Rea WJ, Patel K. *Reversibility of Chronic Degenerative Disease and Hypersensitivity Vol. 1-5.* Boca Raton FL, CRC Press; 2010.

2 Steinemann A. National Prevalence and Effects of Multiple Chemical Sensitivities. J Occup Environ Med. 2018 Mar;60(3):e152-e156. doi: 10.1097/JOM.0000000000001272. PMID: 29329146.

3 Masri, S., Miller, C.S., Palmer, R.F. *et al.* Toxicant-induced loss of tolerance for chemicals, foods, and drugs: assessing patterns of exposure behind a global phenomenon. *Environ Sci Eur* 33, 65 (2021). https://doi.org/10.1186/s12302-021-00504-z.

4 Rea WJ, Patel K. *Reversibility of Chronic Degenerative Disease and Hypersensitivity Vol. 2.* Boca Raton FL, CRC Press; 2015. Pg 464-469.

5 Schnakenberg E, Fabig KR, Stanulla M, Strobl N, Lustig M, Fabig N, Schloot W. A cross-sectional study of self-reported chemical-related sensitivity is associated with gene variants of drug-metabolizing enzymes. Environ Health. 2007 Feb 10;6:6. doi: 10.1186/1476-069X-6-6. PMID: 17291352.

6 Pall ML, Anderson JH. The vanilloid receptor as a putative target of diverse chemicals in multiple chemical sensitivity. Arch Environ Health. 2004 Jul;59(7):363-75. doi: 10.3200/AEOH.59.7.363-375. PMID: 16241041.

7 Pall ML. NMDA sensitization and stimulation by peroxynitrite, nitric oxide, and organic solvents as the mechanism of chemical sensitivity in multiple chemical sensitivity. FASEB J. 2002 Sep;16(11):1407-17. doi: 10.1096/fj.01-0861hyp. PMID: 12205032.

8 Bell IR, Baldwin CM, Fernandez M, Schwartz GE. Neural sensitization model for multiple chemical sensitivity: overview of theory and empirical evidence. Toxicol Ind Health. 1999 Apr-Jun;15(3-4):295-304. doi: 10.1177/074823379901500303. PMID: 10416281.

9 Rea WJ. History of chemical sensitivity and diagnosis. Rev Environ Health. 2016 Sep 1;31(3):353-61. PMID: 27383867.

10 Wang Z, Walker GW, Muir DCG, Nagatani-Yoshida K. Toward a Global Understanding of Chemical Pollution: A First Comprehensive Analysis of National and Regional Chemical Inventories. Environ Sci Technol. 2020 Mar 3;54(5):2575-2584. PMID: 31968937.

11 Vardoulakis S, Giagloglou E, Steinle S, Davis A, Sleeuwenhoek A, Galea KS, Dixon K, Crawford JO. Indoor Exposure to Selected Air Pollutants in the Home Environment: A Systematic Review. Int J Environ Res Public Health. 2020 Dec 2;17(23):8972. PMID: 33276576.

12 Michanowicz DR, Dayalu A, Nordgaard CL, Buonocore JJ, Fairchild MW, Ackley R, Schiff JE, Liu A, Phillips NG, Schulman A, Magavi Z, Spengler JD. Home is Where the Pipeline Ends: Characterization of Volatile Organic Compounds Present in Natural Gas at the Point of the Residential End User. Environ Sci Technol. 2022 Jul 19;56(14):10258-10268. PMID: 35762409.

13 Logue JM, et al. Pollutant exposures from natural gas cooking burners: a simulation-based assessment for Southern California. Environ Health Perspect 122(1):43–50 (2013); http://dx.doi.org/10.1289/ehp.1306673.

14 Franklin PJ, Loveday J, Cook A. Unflued gas heaters and respiratory symptoms in older people with asthma. Thorax. 2012 Apr;67(4):315-20. PMID: 22250101.

15 Phoa LL, Toelle BG, Ng K, Marks GB. Effects of gas and other fume emitting heaters on the development of asthma during childhood. Thorax. 2004 Sep;59(9):741-5. PMID: 15333848.

16 WHO recommended classification of pesticides by hazard and guidelines to classification, 2019 edition. Geneva: World Health Organization; 2020. Licence: CC BY-NC-SA 3.0 IGO.

17 Barr DB, Bravo R, Weerasekera G, Caltabiano LM, Whitehead RD Jr, Olsson AO, Caudill SP, Schober SE, Pirkle JL, Sampson EJ, Jackson RJ, Needham LL. Concentrations of dialkyl phosphate metabolites of organophosphorus pesticides in the U.S. population. Environ Health Perspect. 2004 Feb;112(2):186-200. PMID: 14754573.

18 Li M, Wang R, Su C, Li J, Wu Z. Temporal Trends of Exposure to Organochlorine Pesticides in the United States: A Population Study from 2005 to 2016. Int J Environ Res Pub Health 2022 Mar 24;19(7):3862. PMID: 354509545.

19 Cirillo PM, La Merrill MA, Krigbaum NY, Cohn BA. Grandmaternal Perinatal Serum DDT in Relation to Granddaughter Early Menarche and Adult Obesity: Three Generations in the Child Health and Development Studies Cohort. Cancer Epidemiol Biomarkers Prev. 2021 Aug;30(8):1480-1488.

20 Meissner T, Schweinsberg F. Pentachlorophenol in the indoor environment: evidence for a correlation between pentachlorophenol in passively deposited suspended particulate and in urine of exposed persons. Toxicol Lett. 1996 Nov;88(1-3):237-42. PMID: 8920743.

21 Whitemore RW, Immerman FW, Camann DE, Bond AE, Lewis RG, Schaum JL. Non-occupational exposures to pesticides for residents of two U.S. cities. Arch Environ Contam Toxicol. 1994 Jan;26(1):47-59. PMID: 8110023.

22 Patel CJ, Bhattacharya J, Butte AJ. An Environment-Wide Association Study (EWAS) on type 2 diabetes mellitus. PLoS One. 2010 May 20;5(5):e10746. PMID: 20505766.

23 Engelhart S, Loock A, Skutlarek D, Sagunski H, Lommel A, Färber H, Exner M. Occurrence of toxigenic Aspergillus versicolor isolates and sterigmatocystin in carpet dust from damp indoor environments. Appl Environ Microbiol. 2002 Aug;68(8):3886-90. PMID: 12147486]

24 https://www.epa.gov/ingredients-used-pesticide-products/triclosan

25 Savage JH, Matsui EC, Wood RA, Keet CA. Urinary levels of triclosan and parabens are associated with aeroallergen and food sensitization. J Allergy Clin Immunol. 2012 Aug;130(2):453-60.e7 PMID: 22704536.

26 Chrustek A, Hołyńska-Iwan I, Dziembowska I, Bogusiewicz J, Wróblewski M, Cwynar A, Olszewska-Słonina D. Current Research on the Safety of Pyrethroids Used as Insecticides. Medicina (Kaunas). 2018 Aug 28;54(4):61. PMID: 30344292.

27 Wolansky MJ, Harrill JA. Neurobehavioral toxicology of pyrethroid insecticides in adult animals: a critical review. Neurotoxicol Teratol. 2008 Mar-Apr;30(2):55-78. PMID: 18206347.

28 Vanden Driessche KS, Sow A, Van Gompel A, Vandeurzen K. Anaphylaxis in an airplane after insecticide spraying. J Travel Med. 2010 Nov-Dec;17(6):427-9. Erratum in: J Travel Med. 2011 May-Jun;18(3):216. PMID: 21050327.

29 Rossbach B, Niemietz A, Kegel P, Letzel S. Uptake and elimination of permethrin related to the use of permethrin treated clothing for forestry workers. Toxicol Lett. 2014 Dec 1;231(2):147-53. doi: 10.1016/j.toxlet.2014.10.017. Epub 2014 Oct 18. PMID: 25455447.]

30 Duramad P, Harley K, Lipsett M, Bradman A, Eskenazi B, Holland NT, Tager IB. Early environmental exposures and intracellular Th1/Th2 cytokine profiles in 24-month-old children living in an agricultural area. Environ Health Perspect. 2006 Dec;114(12):1916-22. PMID: 17185285.

31 Rodgers K, Xiong S. Effect of administration of malathion for 90 days on macrophage function and mast cell degranulation. Toxicol Lett. 1997 Sep 19;93(1):73-82. PMID: 9381485.

32 Banks CN, Lein PJ. A review of experimental evidence linking neurotoxic organophosphorus compounds and inflammation. Neurotoxicology. 2012 Jun;33(3): 575-84. PMID: 22342984.

33 Abou-Donia MB. Organophosphorus ester-induced chronic neurotoxicity. Arch Environ Health. 2003 Aug;58(8):484-97. PMID: 15259428.

34 Rea WJ, Patel K. *Reversibility of Chronic Degenerative Disease and Hypersensitivity Vol.4* Boca Raton FL, CRC Press; 2010. pg. 650.

35 Miller CS, Mitzel HC. Chemical sensitivity attributed to pesticide exposure versus remodeling. Arch Environ Health. 1995 Mar-Apr;50(2):119-29. PMID: 7786048.

36 Rea WJ, Patel K. *Reversibility of Chronic Degenerative Disease and Hypersensitivity Vol.4* Boca Raton FL, CRC Press; 2010. pg. 697.

37 Mills PJ, Caussy C, Loomba R. Glyphosate Excretion is Associated With Steatohepatitis and Advanced Liver Fibrosis in Patients With Fatty Liver Disease. Clin Gastroenterol Hepatol. 2020 Mar;18(3):741-743. PMID: 30954713.

38 Del Castilo I, Neumann AS, Lemos FS, De Bastiani MA, Oliveira FL, Zimmer ER, Rêgo AM, Hardoim CCP, Antunes LCM, Lara FA, Figueiredo CP, Clarke JR. Lifelong Exposure to a Low-Dose of the Glyphosate-Based Herbicide RoundUp® Causes Intestinal Damage, Gut Dysbiosis, and Behavioral Changes in Mice. Int J Mol Sci. 2022 May 17;23(10):5583. PMID: 35628394.

39 Costas-Ferreira C, Durán R, Faro LRF. Toxic Effects of Glyphosate on the Nervous System: A Systematic Review. Int J Mol Sci. 2022 Apr 21;23(9):4605. PMID: 35562999.

40 Center for Disease Control https://wwwn.cdc.gov/Nchs/Nhanes/2013-2014/SSGLYP_H.htm

41 U.S. EPA. IRIS Toxicological Review of Formaldehyde-Inhalation (External Review Draft, 2022). U.S. Environmental Protection Agency, Washington, DC, EPA/635/R-22/039, 2022.

42 Vardoulakis S, Giagloglou E, Steinle S, Davis A, Sleeuwenhoek A, Galea KS, Dixon K, Crawford JO. Indoor Exposure to Selected Air Pollutants in the Home Environment: A Systematic Review. Int J Environ Res Public Health. 2020 Dec 2;17(23):8972. PMID: 33276576.

43 Abelmann A, McEwen AR, Lotter JT, Maskrey JR. Survey of 24-h personal formaldehyde exposures in geographically distributed urban office workers in the USA. Environ Sci Pollut Res Int. 2020 May;27(14):17250-17257. PMID: 32152860.

44 Rea WJ, Patel K. Reversibility of Chronic Degenerative Disease and Hypersensitivity Vol.4 Boca Raton, FL, CRC Press; 2018 pg. 616.

45 Fujimaki H, Kawagoe A, Bissonnette E, Befus D. Mast cell response to formaldehyde. 1. Modulation of mediator release. Int Arch Allergy Immunol. 1992;98(4):324-31. PMID: 1384864.

46 Garrett MH, Hooper MA, Hooper BM, Rayment PR, Abramson MJ. Increased risk of allergy in children due to formaldehyde exposure in homes. Allergy. 1999 Apr;54(4):330-7. Erratum in: Allergy 1999 Dec;54(12):1327. PMID: 10371091.

47 Tulpule K, Hohnholt MC, Dringen R. Formaldehyde metabolism and formaldehyde-induced stimulation of lactate production and glutathione export in cultured neurons. J Neurochem. 2013 Apr;125(2):260-72. PMID: 23356791.

48 Salthammer T. Data on formaldehyde sources, formaldehyde concentrations and air exchange rates in European housing. Data Brief. 2018 Nov 24;22:400-435. doi: 10.1016/j.dib.2018.11.096. PMID: 30596137.

49 Kelly TJ, Satola JR, Smith DL. Emission rates of formaldehyde and other carbonyls from consumer and industrial products found in California homes. In Measurement of Toxic and Related Air Pollutants, Proceedings of International Specialty Conference on Air and Waste Management Association. 1996. Pg 521-526. Pittsburgh, PA.

50 Namikoshi T, Yoshima TT, Suga K, Fujii H, Yasuda K (1990) The prevalence of sensitivity to constituents of dental alloys. J Oral Rehabil 17(4):337–381.

51 Forte G, Petrucci F, Bocca B. Metal allergens of growing significance: epidemiology, immunotoxicology, strategies for testing and prevention. Inflamm Allergy Drug Targets.2008Sep;7(3):145-62. PMID: 18782021.

52 Loyo E, Jara LJ, López PD, Puig AC. Autoimmunity in connection with a metal implant: a case of autoimmune/autoinflammatory syndrome induced by adjuvants. Auto Immun Highlights. 2012 Dec 15;4(1):33-8. doi: 10.1007/s13317-012-0044-1. PMID: 26000140.

53 Perales RB, Palmer RF, Rincon R, Viramontes JN, Walker T, Jaén CR, Miller CS. Does improving indoor air quality lessen symptoms associated with chemical intolerance? Prim Health Care Res Dev. 2022 Jan 12;23:e3. Pg. 9. PMID: 35019839.

54 Baker BP, Benbrook CM, Groth E 3rd, Lutz Benbrook K. Pesticide residues in conventional, integrated pest management (IPM)-grown and organic foods: insights from three US data sets. Food Addit Contam. 2002 May;19(5):427-46. doi: 10.1080/02652030110113799. PMID: 12028642.

55 Bernhoft A, Clasen PE, Kristoffersen AB, Torp M. Less Fusarium infestation and mycotoxin contamination in organic than in conventional cereals. Food Addit Contam Part A Chem Anal Control Expo Risk Assess. 2010 Jun;27(6):842-52. PMID: 20425661.

56 Edwards SG. Fusarium mycotoxin content of UK organic and conventional oats. Food Addit Contam Part A Chem Anal Control Expo Risk Assess. 2009 Jul;26(7):1063-9. PMID: 19680981.

Publications

Fine AM, Patrick L. Environmental Medicine: Exploring the Pollutome for Solutions to Chronic Diseases. Phys Med Rehabil Clin N Am. 2022 Aug;33(3):719-732. doi:10.1016/j.pmr.2022.04.010. Epub 2022 Jun 23. PMID: 35989060.

Patrick L. Diabetes and Toxicant Exposure. Integr Med (Encinitas). 2020 Feb;19(1):16-23. PMID: 32549860; PMCID: PMC7238916.

Patrick L. Hexavalent Chromium In: Crinnion W, Pizzorno JE. Clinical Environmental Medicine: Identification and Natural Treatment of Diseases Caused by Common Pollutants. 1st Ed. Elsevier 2019:144-149.

Patrick L. Gastroesophageal reflux disease (GERD): a review of conventional and alternative treatments. Altern Med Rev. 2011 Jun;16(2):116-33. PMID: 21649454.

Patrick L. Thyroid disruption: mechanism and clinical implications in human health.

Altern Med Rev. 2009 Dec;14(4):326-46. Erratum in: Altern Med Rev. 2010 Apr;15(1):58. PMID: 20030460.

Dufault R, LeBlanc B, Schnoll R, Cornett C, Schweitzer L, Wallinga D, Hightower J, Patrick L, Lukiw WJ. Mercury from chlor-alkali plants: measured concentrations in food product sugar. Environ Health. 2009 Jan 26;8:2. doi: 10.1186/1476-069X-8-2.

PMID: 19171026.

Dufault R, Schnoll R, Lukiw WJ, Leblanc B, Cornett C, Patrick L, Wallinga D, Gilbert SG, Crider R. Mercury exposure, nutritional deficiencies and metabolic disruptions may affect learning in children. Behav Brain Funct. 2009 Oct 27;5:44. doi: 10.1186/1744-9081-5-44. Erratum in: Behav Brain Funct. 2018 Feb 7;14 (1):3. PMID: 19860886; PMCID: PMC2773803.

Patrick L. Iodine: deficiency and therapeutic considerations. Altern Med Rev. 2008 Jun;13(2):116-27. PMID: 18590348.

Patrick L. Restless legs syndrome: pathophysiology and the role of iron and folate. Altern Med Rev. 2007 Jun;12(2):101-12. PMID: 17604457.

Patrick L. Lead toxicity, a review of the literature. Part 1: Exposure, evaluation, and treatment. Altern Med Rev. 2006 Mar;11(1):2-22. PMID: 16597190.

Patrick L. Lead toxicity part II: the role of free radical damage and the use of antioxidants in the pathology and treatment of lead toxicity. Altern Med Rev. 2006 Jun;11(2):114-27. PMID: 16813461.

Patrick L. Selenium biochemistry and cancer: a review of the literature. Altern Med Rev. 2004 Sep;9(3):239-58. PMID: 15387717.

Patrick L. Toxic metals and antioxidants: Part II. The role of antioxidants in arsenic and cadmium toxicity. Altern Med Rev. 2003 May;8(2):106-28. PMID: 12777158.

Patrick L. Nonalcoholic fatty liver disease: relationship to insulin sensitivity and oxidative stress. Treatment approaches using vitamin E, magnesium, and betaine. Altern Med Rev. 2002 Aug;7(4):276-91. PMID: 12197781.

Patrick L. Mercury toxicity and antioxidants: Part 1: role of glutathione and alpha-lipoic acid in the treatment of mercury toxicity. Altern Med Rev. 2002 Dec;7(6):456-71. PMID: 12495372

Patrick L, Uzick M. Cardiovascular disease: C-reactive protein and the inflammatory disease paradigm: HMG-CoA reductase inhibitors, alpha-tocopherol, red yeast rice, and olive oil polyphenols. A review of the literature. Altern Med Rev. 2001 Jun;6(3):248-71. PMID: 11410071.

Patrick L. Nutrients and HIV: part two—vitamins A and E, zinc, B-vitamins, and magnesium. Altern Med Rev. 2000 Feb;5(1):39-51. PMID: 10696118.

Patrick L. Beta-carotene: the controversy continues. Altern Med Rev. 2000. Dec;5(6):530-45. PMID: 11134976.

Patrick L. Nutrients and HIV: part three - N-acetylcysteine, alpha-lipoic acid, L-glutamine, and L-carnitine. Altern Med Rev. 2000 Aug;5(4):290-305. PMID: 10956377.

Patrick L. Hepatitis C: epidemiology and review of complementary/alternative medicine treatments. Altern Med Rev. 1999 Aug;4(4):220-38. PMID: 10468647.

Patrick L. Nutrients and HIV: part one - beta carotene and selenium. Altern Med Rev. 1999 Dec;4(6):403-13. PMID: 10608913.

Patrick L. Nutrients and HIV: part one - beta carotene and selenium. Altern Med Rev. 1999 Dec;4(6):403-13. PMID: 10608913.

Patrick L. Comparative absorption of calcium sources and calcium citrate malate for the prevention of osteoporosis. Altern Med Rev. 1999 Apr;4(2):74-85. PMID: 10231607.

Patrick L. The treatment of hepatitis C: emerging evidence of the need for change. Altern Med Rev. 1999 Aug;4(4):219. PMID: 10468646.

Part III

Other Triggers and Conditions for the Development of Sensitivity

We've now looked at the underpinnings of sensitization, from the perspective of the all-important limbic/vagal/mast-cell activation systems. Then we studied the most important specific triggers for those systems: Mold toxicity, Lyme disease with its coinfections, other environmental toxins, and EMFs. The more you study any subject, the more complicated it becomes, so while the issues we've examined are extremely important, we've learned that there are other components of sensitization to explore. Some of these are biochemical, specifically difficulties with oxalates, sulfates, and salicylates.

In chapter 12, Emily Givler discusses the role of oxalates in sensitivity, and how to evaluate and treat this condition.

In chapter 13, Greg Nigh discusses the role of sulfur metabolism in sensitivity, and how to evaluate and treat this condition.

In chapter 14, Beth O'Hara discusses the role of salicylates in sensitivity, and how to evaluate and treat this condition. Some important components of a predisposition to sensitivity are structural, including jaw dysfunction and the overall structure of the body, especially involving the cranial bones and their relationship to the rest of the body.

In chapter 15, Tasha Turzo explains the importance of jaw structure, the alignment of our teeth, and how this can profoundly affect sensitization. She then details the evaluation and treatment of these issues. This may seem like rarified air, but I've found that jaw dysfunction creates a uniquely sensitizing process for the body, and if not looked for and addressed, it can prevent any of our other treatments from working.

In chapter 16, Dr. Carmine Van Deven discusses structural issues of the whole body, especially the cranium, from an osteopathic perspective, and shows us how osteopathic perceptions and treatment can be central to healing for many of our patients.

We find that patients who've been prescribed any of several families of medications, such as benzodiazepines (e.g., Valium, Xanax, or Ativan) or SSRIs (selective serotonin reuptake inhibitors) such as Prozac, Lexapro, Celexa, or Zoloft, often have severe difficulties in getting off of those medications. These difficulties aren't always recognized or acknowledged by the medical profession, but the withdrawal symptoms experienced by patients who struggle with this issue has significantly worsened their problems, and need to be understood and treated slowly, carefully, and with compassion. Adding to these issues is the fact that many patients have been prescribed these medications for the purpose of treating anxiety and depression that are actually caused by toxins or infections.

In chapter 17, James Greenblatt discusses these addiction and withdrawal issues in detail, and helps us understand the use and misuse of medications in healing, while addressing the underlying biochemical deficiencies often missed by conventional medical care.

While many of our patients exhibit an array of nutrient deficiencies, we've found that thiamine deficiency (vitamin B-1) is of particular importance in our understanding and treatment. In chapter 18, Chandler Marrs and I discuss the importance of thiamine in healing our chronically ill and sensitive patients, with a clear discussion of the evaluation and treatment of thiamine deficiency.

Biochemically and genetically, we are all unique, and we've learned a great deal about the genetics of sensitivity and chronic illness over the past decade. In chapter 19, Bob Miller offers an epigenetic perspective that helps us understand some of the genetic and biochemical components of sensitization, and which SNPs to measure that can aid in our work with patients.

The various triggers of sensitization, such as mold toxicity, Lyme disease, and other environmental toxins, are known to affect the pituitary gland and the HPA axis in their ability to regulate our hormones. In chapter 20, I review how hormonal dysfunction, with special reference to the adrenal, thyroid, and sex hormones, is affected by many of our triggers. This includes a discussion of how to evaluate and treat these hormonal deficiencies to lessen their impact on sensitive patients.

I've found that when patients are making little progress despite working diligently to reboot their limbic and vagal systems and relieve mast-cell dysfunction, we have to dig deeper into their emotional, spiritual, or energetic issues to help them understand why they're not responding to our usual approaches. In chapter 21, I go into these blocks to help patients who appear to be stuck in their healing program get past their issues and move forward in healing.

Regarding a few other medication conditions that are less common than those already discussed, but still present in some of our patients who are unable to heal, it might be necessary to look at carbon monoxide poisoning and secondary porphyrias. In chapter 22, I review carbon monoxide poisoning as a unique sensitizer, and how to evaluate and treat it.

In chapter 23, I explore the possibility of secondary porphyrias as another contributing factor to sensitization.

The COVID pandemic has made far-reaching changes in our world. The global panic that it engendered still reverberates through our lives, profoundly affecting our limbic and vagal systems to an extent not yet well appreciated. We've observed that the effects of both the viral infections and the vaccines used to treat them, which can trigger prolonged bouts of inflammation, have significantly impacted our patients' sensitivity issues.

In chapter 24, Greg Nigh helps us understand how COVID, either acute or chronic (Long Haul COVID), and the vaccines used to prevent it, have affected our patients who suffer from a chronic, complex inflammatory illness by initiating or worsening their sensitivities.

Chapter 12: Oxalates and Their Role in Triggering Sensitivity

Emily Givler, DSC

Dr. Nathan's Introduction

While not as common as mold toxicity and Lyme disease in setting off the process of sensitization, the accumulation of oxalates in the body's tissues remains an important issue for many of our patients. This is in part because molds make oxalates and partly due to some genetic predisposition, as Emily explains. Of particular importance in this chapter and those that follow is that missing this piece of the puzzle can prevent our patients from making any progress until they are addressed.

✿ ✿ ✿

Fatigue. Weakness. Muscle aches. Cramps. Joint pain. Morning stiffness. Headaches. Eye pressure. Vision changes. Focus/concentration issues, poor word recall, memory issues. Skin sensitivity, light sensitivity. Shortness of breath, dizziness. Lyme disease is often referred to as "the Great Imitator" because its myriad symptoms are commonly mistaken for other conditions. In recent years, mold illness has taken on a similar mantle; many people diagnosed with chronic Lyme discover only much later that they'd been dealing with mold-related illness as well. There is a third condition that mimics both Lyme and mold, presenting with many of the same symptoms and often found either in conjunction with or as a result of the former two: high oxalates. The more sensitive a patient is the more likely high oxalates will be a contributing factor to their illness and sensitivity.

Elevated oxalic acid and the accompanying oxalate precipitates that it produces in the body are often under-recognized, overlooked, or downplayed in terms of significance in hypersensitive individuals, particularly those presenting with pain and fatigue. In this chapter we will examine what oxalates are, how they may present in the body, effective tools for assessment, and treatment options. We'll refer to oxalates and oxalate precipitates interchangeably. These precipitates form when oxalic acid attaches to a mineral.

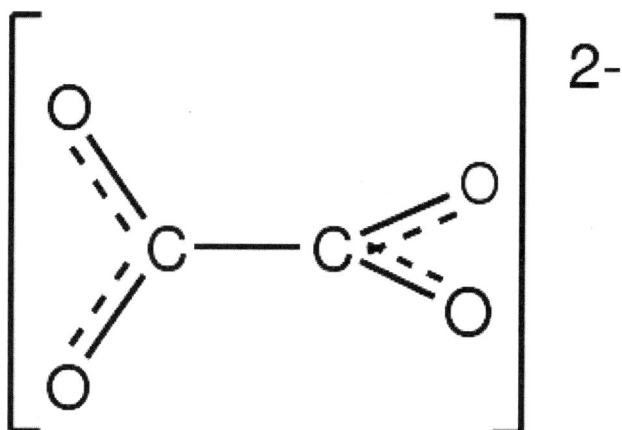

The chemical structure of oxalates.

What is oxalic acid? Oxalic acid is a poison. It chelates, or grabs and binds, minerals. It has a particularly strong affinity for calcium, but can also bind with other metals such as magnesium, potassium, zinc, and iron. Once oxalic acid is bound with these minerals, an insoluble precipitate is formed. These precipitates, or oxalate crystals, are nanoparticles that are essentially like tiny shards of glass in the tissue where they are formed or deposited. Oxalates make up about 80% of all kidney stones, and much like kidney stones, they shred and inflame surrounding tissue. Our cells cannot break them down. Once that precipitate is formed, it can be bound in tissue to sulfate receptors, it circulates in the bloodstream, or it gets excreted. The kidneys are one of our primary oxalate filtration and elimination pathways, but bowels, tear ducts, and perspiration can also be excretion pathways.

When these precipitates clump together in larger masses in the kidneys, they become kidney stones. This is the most easily recognizable presentation of high oxalates. An individual might present with severe flank pain. Often a mass is visible on imaging. When their urine is collected and filtered we commonly find a kidney stone in the urine. The flank pain, often described as among the most intense imaginable, passes as the stone or stones are passed. We can put the stones on a microscope slide and pat ourselves on the back for correctly diagnosing calcium oxalate kidney stones.

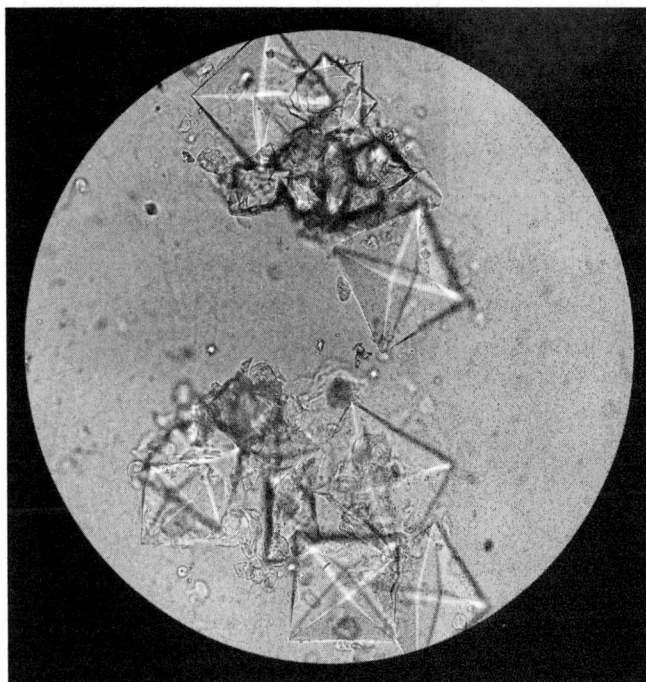

Microscopic image showing Calcium oxalate (monohydrate and dihydrate) crystals from urine sediment.

Fortunately, only 0.5% of people with elevated levels of oxalic acid present with kidney stones. The other 99.5% of high-oxalate individuals deal with oxalate precipitates impacting the body in other, less obvious, ways. Unfortunately for these individuals, retained oxalates are much more challenging to diagnose correctly. Most oxalate precipitates are very tiny and not easily imaged, but their small size doesn't prevent their causing significant damage to the body. The crystalline precipitates can infiltrate cell membranes using sulfate transporters and are then able to shred cellular organelles including but not limited to the mitochondria. This harm to mitochondria can significantly limit the ability to produce adequate ATP, a critical energy-carrying molecule. Is it any wonder that fatigue is associated with hyperoxaluria (the technical name for an excess of oxalates) when the engines of the cells are being destroyed? This is also part of the mechanism by which high levels of oxalates can progressively tip the scales toward hypersensitivity.

One potential symptom of high oxalates in the body is calcinosis, or calcium buildup in soft tissues of the body; the mineral gathers in skin, muscles, tendons, and/or connective tissues. While often benign, calcium deposits in breast tissue can sometimes be an early sign of breast cancer. If there is any calcinosis present, oxalates should be considered as part of the equation.

The presence of oxalate precipitates in tissue is a large component of their relationship to hypersensitivity. Oxalate precipitates can be deposited along nerve sheaths, in the thyroid, in the brain, in connective tissue, in muscle fiber (including the heart), and in the liver, lungs, and kidneys. When it is embedded, oxalate mechanically shreds the surrounding tissue. This can compromise the function of the organ or tissue. It also sets off a biochemical inflammatory cascade as the body tries and fails to resolve the injury. One of these mechanisms is the activation of the NLRP3 inflammasome. If we fail to get rid of the precipitate, we stay stuck in an inflammatory cycle.

When this inflammatory cycle is associated with near-constant or progressively worsening pain, the nervous system becomes more easily dysregulated. Several of my colleagues in this volume address the relationship between the limbic system and hypersensitivity in great detail. I will simply add that oxalates can contribute significantly to chronic pain, potentially contributing to that additional layer of dysregulation.

I find it helpful to remember that pain isn't the problem. As someone who lived with chronic pain for far too long, I know that pain is a problem, but it's not *the* problem. It's the messenger telling us that something is wrong and needs to change. Much of my job as a practitioner is to help people listen to the message their body is trying to send. I never cease to be amazed at how often at least part of that message in the hypersensitive, chronic pain community is *oxalates.*

How do we end up with high oxalate levels? There are many different causes. For most people, high oxalates come primarily from the gut. The simplest source is from our diet, and generally from foods that we would consider very healthy, such as spinach, beets, nuts, soy, and whole grains. This is because oxalic acid is a plant poison—well, poison to us, protection for the plants, which produce it as part of a complex defense mechanism to deter other organisms (like insects, rodents, and us) from eating said plant. Because of this, there's a high degree of variability in oxalate content even among plants of the same species. Measuring the levels of oxalates in certain foods can help provide a guidepost, but we should use care not to overemphasize counting the oxalate content of food.

High levels of oxalic acid are found in tubers (sweet potato, turmeric, ginger), nuts (almonds, cashews), leaves (spinach, chard, beet greens), and whole grains (brown rice, wheat bran). These foods are generally considered healthy, and when a patient makes a shift toward a more whole food-based diet, they may inadvertently open the door for overconsumption of oxalates.

Here is a partial list of the most common foods known to have a high oxalate content:

HIGH OXALATE FOODS

- Spinach
- Beets
- Rhubarb
- Chard
- Chocolate
- Blackberries
- Buckwheat
- Quinoa
- All bran cereal
- Beans
- Almonds
- Sweet potatoes
- Star fruit
- Teff
- Plantains

My Story: Overconsumption to the Max

It's worth taking a moment to note that many people hit a point of frustration, anger, or despair when they first consider that oxalates may be contributing to their health challenges. The high-oxalate foods that find their way into our diets in large quantities often show up as a result of our earnest desire to make healthier choices. We trade white rice for brown rice and the oxalates go up. We swap spinach and kale for lettuce and the oxalates go up. We swap almond milk and flour for dairy and gluten and the oxalates go up. We snack on nuts. We drink green smoothies. We juice celery. Oxalates. Oxalates. Oxalates. It can feel like everything we try to do to support our bodies is actually hurting us. It's so important to forgive ourselves for what we didn't know. As Maya Angelou said, "Do the best you can until you know better. Then, when you know better, do better."

One of the biggest challenges in dealing with high oxalates is realizing that oxalates are the problem in the first place—and now that you know better, you can make better choices for your body.

I've been there. I've made every single one of those mistakes. I started having chronic pain at age fourteen. I didn't realize the connection at the time, but this was shortly after I stopped drinking milk as part of my school lunch and dinner at home daily. I wanted to be healthier, so I switched to water. Shortly after that, I became a vegetarian and loaded up on soy-based fake meat. Much to my surprise, my pain continued to worsen and was then accompanied by significant fatigue. By age nineteen I had a diagnosis of fibromyalgia and my rheumatologist's assurance that it would get progressively worse for the rest of my life. I was told to plan to be disabled by age thirty.

I thought that was a terrible plan. I needed a new plan, so I doubled down on my vegetarian diet. I went away to a college with a vegetarian/vegan cafe on campus as part of the meal plan. I was in early 2000s health-food heaven! Brown rice, organic tofu, spinach, and beets with every meal—and worsening pain with every passing day! There was nothing in my reading about nutrition or in conversations with my doctor that ever led me to believe there was a connection between the foods I was eating and the way I was feeling. My digestion was great. I didn't experience any acute symptoms after eating. I had no idea that I was poisoning myself at every meal.

It took me well over a decade to realize that high oxalate was driving the inflammation in my body. Until that point I continued to overload my system with thousands of milligrams of oxalates every day. This is the good news part of the story. Even after years of missteps, I was able to safely reduce my body burden of oxalates. As they were eliminated, my pain and fatigue started to fade. I passed forty without a thought of disability and had more energy than I'd had as a teenager. I can laugh at how wrong I was about the foods that my body needed to heal, and forgive myself for doing the wrong thing because I genuinely believed it was right at the time. Now I know better, and I can do better. So can you.

The healthy body can handle these "healthy options" in moderate quantities. Humans have been eating plants for a long time, and have multiple mechanisms by which we can bind, degrade, or eliminate oxalic acid. First, we have the protective barrier of the intestinal lumen. This provides a physical barrier against the oxalic acid precipitates that form when dietary minerals like calcium and magnesium bind with oxalic acid from food in the gastrointestinal tract. In a healthy body, these precipitates are either broken down by beneficial organisms in the intestinal tract or excreted harmlessly in the stool.

For some people, adding more calcium-rich foods into the diet when higher-oxalate foods are consumed may be an appropriate strategy to mitigate high dietary intake. Increasing quality organic, grass-fed dairy, provided there is no dairy allergy or sensitivity, is one way to do this. The key is to eat the high-calcium food in tandem with the high-oxalate food. This allows the calcium to bind with the oxalic acid at roughly a 1:1 ratio. Many highly sensitive people are hesitant to add dairy back into their diet because of high incidences of food reactivity. Goat or sheep dairy may be an easier (less reactive) introduction. If camel's milk is available, it can be a wonderful choice for highly sensitive, high-oxalate individuals. The availability of camels milk is limited, however, and the cost is very high: a pint of fresh-frozen camel's milk costs $240; most people would also find the several powdered versions prohibitively pricy.

If dairy allergy or sensitivity is present, calcium or magnesium supplements may be added alongside high-oxalate foods. It's important to note that when supplementing with calcium or magnesium in an attempt to bind oxalates, these dietary minerals will not be absorbed and used in the way we typically think of them. We are using them instead as an oxalate binder. If we've done our job and bound the oxalic acid to the mineral in the GI tract, those minerals and the accompanying oxalate will be excreted harmlessly in stool, meaning that the minerals also end up in your toilet bowl. When working with highly sensitive individuals, magnesium may initially be better tolerated than calcium.

Individuals with leaky gut are more vulnerable to higher rates of oxalate absorption than individuals with healthy GI tracts. When there is increased mucosal-barrier permeability, there is a higher rate of passive diffusion of oxalic acid through the intestinal lumen into the bloodstream. This allows for oxalate precipitates to be deposited in various tissues throughout the body. When leaky gut is the primary factor driving high oxalates, it makes sense to address gut health first. This is a good time to consider temporarily reducing dietary oxalates as opposed to focusing on binding them with calcium. Once the mucosal barrier is healthier, passive diffusion of dietary oxalate should decrease, and some increase in dietary oxalates may be tolerated.

Plants make oxalic acid in response to stress, creating variability in oxalic acid levels among individual plants. For this reason it's important to emphasize again that we can get a ballpark idea of how many oxalates we are eating by looking at tables that lay out that information, but it can be exceedingly difficult to know the exact amount with certainty. In most cases, however, a ballpark idea of oxalic acid content is sufficient. Including a roughly equivalent amount of calcium relative to the amount of oxalate on your plate is a good way to ensure that it is safely bound and eliminated.

Getting a ballpark idea of how much oxalate we eat each day can also help us make smart choices with regard to safe dietary reduction. Too rapid a reduction in dietary oxalate, or for that matter going too rapidly with any intervention that shifts oxalate metabolism, storage, or excretion, has the potential to create problems. It's important to reduce the body burden of oxalic acid slowly, especially in the hypersensitive individual. We need to think about the oxalate reduction process as a marathon rather than a sprint.

Taking things slowly will decrease the likelihood of adverse reactions, including *oxalate dumping;* more on that shortly. Regarding diet, some individuals can tolerate moving more quickly, but hypersensitive individuals are rarely these folks. A dietary oxalate reduction of 5%–10% weekly is often a well-tolerated approach, unlikely to provoke oxalate dumping. This slow progression also allows for healthy substitutions to be made. If we pull something out of the diet, we should put something else in so we don't inadvertently create additional nutritional deficiencies. Well-intended dietary changes are often what get people into trouble in the first place.

What do these substitutions look like? To a degree, that depends on the diet. This is where a general evaluation should be performed. Get a sense of how much oxalate is present in the diet and what the biggest offenders are. If nuts are an omnipresent part of the diet in the form of nut milks, butters, flours, and snacks, consider switching to seed-based options. Usually, these still have a lot of oxalates, but fewer than their nut-based counterparts. If spinach, chard, and kale find their way onto your plate or into your smoothie, consider lower-oxalate vegetables such as arugula, bok choy, tatsoi, or various cabbages. Switch from brown rice to organic white rice. Consider sustainably raised animal protein in place of soy products. Drink water instead of tea. Choose winter squash instead of sweet potatoes. If these high-oxalate foods are making up a high percentage of your diet, never go cold turkey on them; taper slowly, keeping that 5%–10% per week reduction in mind.

As you reduce your oxalate intake, you might start to experience excretion symptoms. For some individuals this could include cloudy urine, sandy stool, or an increase in eye precipitates ("sleepies" as my kids call them). These are healthy signs of oxalate mobilization. Keep up the great work! If these symptoms shift into kidney or bladder irritation or pain, vulvar pain in women, burning bowel movements, pain, or stye formation, the scales have tipped into oxalate-dumping territory.

Oxalate Dumping

Oxalate dumping is the rapid release and excretion of oxalate precipitates from where they have been stored in tissue. If too much of the precipitate is released too quickly, those particulates can aggregate or clump together to form progressively larger crystals and, potentially, kidney stones. The oxalate-dumping process is often incredibly uncomfortable. Symptoms can include headache, nausea, fatigue, brain fog, musculoskeletal pain, flank pain, rectal pain, eye pain and pressure, rash, vulvar pain, and kidney stones.

Anything that shifts oxalate pathways can potentially result in oxalate dumping. The short list of interventions includes: reduce dietary oxalates, add sulfated supplements, introduce Epsom salt soaks, increase dietary minerals as binders, introduce vitamins B6 or B1, and introduce molybdenum (see chapter 13 for more information on this subject). Because this delicate balance can shift quickly, in sensitive individuals it is particularly important to introduce these interventions one at a time. We also need to be prepared with the knowledge of how to properly respond to an oxalate-dumping episode.

If we believe that we are experiencing oxalate dumping because we display one or more of the abovementioned symptoms, we should first hydrate as much as possible. We want to flush out our system and keep the kidneys happy, which is critical. Adding baking soda, potassium citrate, or potassium bicarbonate can be a helpful support as well. Studies show that potassium citrate or potassium bicarbonate are well tolerated and highly effective treatments to dissolve non-obstructing renal stones. Still other studies show that both sodium bicarbonate (baking soda) and potassium citrate can reduce calcium-oxalate supersaturation significantly vs. baseline.

In addition to hydration and renal support with baking soda and potassium citrate or bicarbonate, we should also consider eating something high in oxalate if we suspect we are dumping oxalates. This may seem counterintuitive, as the ingestion of oxalate food is generally considered to shift what the body is doing with oxalate away from excretion and back toward storage. This should therefore be viewed as a short-term strategy to slow down painful symptoms. Ultimately, we want oxalates to be eliminated from soft tissue, but we want it to happen at a safe and comfortable pace.

When we think about the volume of oxalate we should be eating to stop a dumping episode, we should keep it small. Think a tablespoon of nut butter, half of a baked sweet potato, a cup of matcha tea or hot cocoa. When you're hypersensitive and living with very few food options, choose one of the highest-oxalate foods that you tolerate. This increase in dietary oxalate should help prevent further dumping of oxalates, but is unlikely to offer immediate relief. This is critical to note—don't expect to keep eating oxalate rich foods until you feel better. You want to use a single serving to put the brakes on the cycle of oxalate dumping in conjunction with the other strategies for excretion support.

Remember that when we reduce dietary oxalates by limiting our consumption of high-oxalate foods and through the use of calcium and magnesium as binders, there is a cumulative reduction of oxalate and we need to continue to move slowly. Increasing dietary calcium through the inclusion of dairy in the diet is often better tolerated than the use of calcium supplementation in terms of reduction of oxalate precipitates in the body. This applies only to people who are able to tolerate dairy digestively, without any allergies to whey or casein and without lactose intolerance. If you go this route, use the best-quality dairy available and tolerable to you. When in doubt in terms of oxalate content and relative dose of calcium, it's generally better to underestimate calcium rather than overestimate. Magnesium and calcium may be combined so as to not overestimate calcium dosage.

When considering supplementation with calcium or magnesium to bind and reduce absorption of oxalic acid, it is advisable to first support healthy bile flow. Bile plays an important role in the digestion of fat. The first step of that process is emulsification of dietary fats by bile so that they can be broken down by the enzyme lipase and used by the body for energy and for making hormones. If those fats are not emulsified and digested, they can bind with the dietary and supplemental minerals, which results in both fat and minerals being lost in stool and dietary oxalate being over-absorbed. Fat maldigestion due to impaired bile flow is a very frequent (and frequently overlooked) cause of over-absorption of oxalates. Supplements like TUDCA, taurine, and phosphatidylcholine can be helpful in improving bile production and viscosity. This biliary support can play a big role in reducing our absorption of dietary oxalates, and can also improve our mineral utilization overall.

Just as a misguided attempt to increase healthy food in our diets can increase oxalates, incorrect supplementation also has the potential to increase oxalates. I'm talking about over-supplementation with vitamin C. To many, vitamin C feels like a safe and helpful part of a healthy lifestyle. We can go to any drugstore and pick up inexpensive boxes of vitamin C that will give us 500 or 1,000 mg per dose. We seek them out when we're sick, but without knowledge, one man's help might become another man's harm, and so it goes with vitamin C. As far back as 1958 it was reported that oxalate is the major urinary excretion product of ascorbic acid (vitamin C). Because vitamin C is a mast-cell stabilizer and provides immune support, it's commonly recommended to very sensitive individuals. It is worth noting the connection between increasing vitamin C and increased oxalate. This does not mean that we shouldn't use vitamin C if oxalates are high. This is a case where the dose makes the poison. Keeping extra vitamin C below 250 mg per dose should prevent oxalates from forming.

Microbial diversity is another factor that can influence how our body stores oxalates. Our success as a species may prove one day to be tied to the cohort of organisms that have co-evolved deep in our guts. Our ability to break down oxalate in the gut is certainly thanks to them. A specialized microbe called *Oxalobacter formigenes* degrades dietary oxalate. This has likely allowed us to eat plants that might otherwise have given us problems. *Oxalobacter* may be the primary oxalate-degrading bacteria in the gut, but it is by no means the only player: *Lactobacillus sp.*, *Bifidobacterium sp.*, *Eubacterium lentum*, and *Enterococcus faecalis* can all play a role in oxalate degradation.

Because of the critical role that these microorganisms play in preventing over-absorption of oxalates, interventions that disrupt our bacterial balance can have unintended consequences in terms of oxalate balance in the body. Here we find one of the reasons that we see so many issues with high oxalate in the Lyme disease community. *Oxalobacter formigenes* is incredibly vulnerable to tetracycline antibiotics, including doxycycline, which most physicians consider the first-line drug of choice for Lyme disease.

This is where we should use caution in evaluating the success or failure of antibiotic Lyme treatment based on symptoms alone. Symptoms like headaches, joint pain, fatigue, brain fog, and exercise intolerance could be from Lyme. They could also be a result of the Lyme treatment disrupting the microbiome and increasing oxalate burden, particularly if there has been extended antibiotic use coupled with a high-oxalate diet. I would always encourage repeat Lyme testing with a reputable lab to determine whether to continue an antibiotic protocol long term. This can help prevent over-treatment with antibiotics. Keep in mind that like so many things in a highly sensitive body, two things can be true at the same time: we can have high oxalates as a result of antibiotic therapies for Lyme, and we can have chronic Lyme requiring more antibiotics or other treatments.

Despite this knowledge that doxycycline can have a negative impact on our microbiome's ability to degrade oxalate, we should not simply eschew using antibiotics for the treatment of diseases like Lyme. When these drugs are necessary, we should use care to pair them with probiotics and prebiotics. *Oxalobacter* itself cannot be used as a probiotic as of the time of this writing, so supporting the body with other probiotics, including organisms that produce short-chain fatty acids (SCFAs), may be a good choice. Spore-based organisms may be a particularly helpful choice. In my own practice I've seen them support healthy levels of *Oxalobacter* as measured on stool analysis. The use of SCFAs (short-chain fatty acids) supplementally, particularly supplementation with butyrate, may in and of itself help reduce the formation of calcium oxalate crystals in the kidneys and lower the amount of urinary excretion.

It is also of note that tetracyclines are not the only class of antibiotics that can have an adverse effect on microbial diversity regarding oxalate degradation. Fluoroquinolone antibiotics are particularly detrimental to *O. formigenes* levels, and other antibiotics may similarly have a negative impact on some of the commensal species that assist in oxalate degradation. If we follow this line of thinking to its logical conclusion, we can see that long-term reduction of body stores of oxalates necessitates balancing the microbiome.

Another microbial factor potentially contributing to elevated oxalic acid and hypersensitivity is mold, specifically colonized mold. It's important to make this distinction because the presence of mycotoxins or an allergic response to mold, while extremely problematic, does not necessarily translate to high oxalate in the body. When mold species (and some other yeast and fungi) are colonized, or growing in the body, they may produce oxalic acid. Aspergillus, especially *Aspergillus niger,* is well known for its ability to produce oxalate as a fermentation byproduct. This is particularly dangerous when there is mold colonization in the lungs. There have been numerous cases of significant pulmonary damage resulting from the oxalates produced from fungal masses in the lungs.

Most cases of high oxalates come from the gut, and we've discussed several mechanisms by which this may occur. It's important to note that these mechanisms are not mutually exclusive. It's not uncommon for one person to have four or more separate factors contributing to a hyperoxaluric presentation. Like so many other parts of our health, our journey with oxalates often feels like peeling back the layers of the onion— as we address each layer, another presents itself.

The Genetics of Oxalates

Occasionally one of those layers is genetic. True genetic hyperoxaluria presentations are relatively rare. There are specific gene mutations that can result in high oxalates because of increased metabolic production. In these cases, the body is actually making too much oxalate because of a faulty enzyme. We categorize the different types of genetic hyperoxalurias as types I, II, and III.

Type I primary hyperoxaluria is caused because of mutation on the alanine glyoxalate transferase, coded by the AGXT gene, often coded AGT on genetic reports. Variants in this gene can cause the body to produce excessive levels of oxalic acid. Whether we are producing this acid ourselves or consuming it in the diet, the same downstream effects occur. Precipitates form and have to be filtered. If this happens too fast, kidney stones form. This is often the case in type I hyperoxaluria, and such individuals are often labeled as primary kidney-stone formers.

Type I primary hyperoxaluria has an autosomal recessive inheritance pattern; i.e., both copies of the responsible gene, in this case AGXT, must have a pathogenic variant in order for the disease to present in a person.

Type II primary hyperoxaluria presents very similarly to type I, but is caused by a different genetic polymorphism. In this case, the increase in metabolic production of oxalic acid results from a faulty GRHPR enzyme. Like its AGXT counterpart, GRHPR has an autosomal recessive inheritance pattern, necessitating a homozygous polymorphism to interfere with enzyme activity.

Type III primary hyperoxaluria is a little different. The way we support the body in a genetic hyperoxaluria looks a little different from the way we support gut-driven hyperoxaluria. In these cases, vitamin B6 is the supplement of choice. It is the primary cofactor for both the AGXT and GRHPR enzymes. Numerous studies have shown that increasing vitamin B6, either as pyridoxine or P-5-P, can significantly increase the enzyme function even in genetically vulnerable individuals. As the enzyme function improves, oxalate production decreases. In all things oxalate related, we want to start slow and increase our B6 dosage slowly, watching for signs of oxalate dumping as we go. Vitamin B6 also happens to be the primary cofactor for most of the enzymes along our transsulfuration pathway. This is the biochemical pathway through which we make compounds like sulfate and glutathione. This potential increase in sulfate can also help to reduce body stores of oxalate.

Genetic variants on AGXT or GRHPR are no guarantee that a patient will make kidney stones, nor are they the only cause of them, but the likelihood of getting a stone goes up significantly with these rare presentations. This also doesn't mean that kidney stones are the only possible problem in people with this gene mutation. Individuals who produce high levels of oxalates are vulnerable to any and all of the oxalate presentations discussed in this chapter. The National Institutes of Health lists anemia and calcinosis (formation of calcium deposits in any soft tissue) as very frequent symptoms of Type I hyperoxaluria as well as nephrolithiasis (kidney stones) and nephrocalcinosis (too much calcium in the kidneys). Thinking through these presentations can give us insight into what's happening anytime there's an excessive amount of oxalic acid in the body.

Anemia has the potential to present when excessive amounts of iron are bound to oxalic acid: remember, oxalate is a chelator; it binds to minerals. We primarily talk about calcium in this regard, but iron can be bound with oxalate as well. If oxalate levels are high enough, we might see this chelating effect on iron and experience anemia as a result of not enough iron being available for production of red blood cells.

Kate's Story – Anemia and Oxalates

Early in my clinical work in functional genomic nutrition, I began to work with Kate, a woman who had significant health concerns that stretched back decades. Her difficulties were many. Chronic anemia was one that continued to challenge her despite inclusion of iron in the diet from foods like grass-fed red meat and liver as well as iron supplementation. Before you scrunch up your nose at the thought of eating liver, if body stores of iron are low, pâté can be a delicious way to use food as medicine. When Kate ran a urine organic acid test, the level of oxalic acid reported was the lowest I had ever seen—4 mmol/mol creatinine. Kate also experienced significant body pain and fatigue, anxiety, brain fog, and severe immune dysregulation, as well as multiple food and chemical sensitivities. Because she was highly sensitive to supplementation, we started slowly with all of our interventions. Two of the first pieces we brought into her mix were Epsom salt soaks and molybdenum.

The sulfate in Epsom salt can mobilize and facilitate the elimination of oxalate and molybdenum and can help our bodies to produce more sulfate to help this process.

When Kate started soaking in a tub with a small amount of Epsom salt added to the water, she noticed that she was excreting what she described as rust-colored sand in her urine. What she was actually excreting was iron oxalate precipitates. This increased as she added a small amount of molybdenum into her protocol. As she progressed with the reduction of her body burden of oxalate, Kate's inflammation, pain, and fatigue all decreased, and her mental clarity and stamina increased. Repeat lab testing showed that her hemoglobin and ferritin levels, which had been the primary lab values indicating iron deficiency and anemia, began to improve for the first time in years.

There is a profound relationship between oxalate and sulfate. It's vital to understand this relationship if we want to effectively reduce body stores of oxalate. Oxalate and sulfate share transporters. Oxalate moves through the body on sulfate transporters and binds with sulfate receptor sites. A gradient is created between these two ions that allows them to influence one another. As oxalic acid builds up on one side of a cell membrane, it pushes sulfate out across the membrane, which ultimately causes it to be excreted unused in the urine in a process referred to as sulfate wasting. Because of this potential for sulfate loss, we should look for secondary symptoms resulting from under-sulfation in high-oxalate individuals, and because it's a two-way street when it comes to oxalate and sulfate, it also means that we can use sulfate as a tool for reducing stored oxalate.

What does that under-sulfated, high-oxalate, hypersensitive person look like? Like so many other things in the oxalate world, presentation can vary from person to person depending on the system that is most stressed. Loss of sulfate has the potential to influence many different biological processes that rely on sulfate as a substrate. The critical role of sulfate in hypersensitivity will be covered in depth elsewhere in this book (see chapter 13), so we'll cover just some basics here.

Hormones like DHEA and estrogen need to be sulfated. Lack of sulfation along these pathways can dysregulate reproductive hormone balance and may be part of why we see correlations between high oxalates and PCOS (polycystic ovary syndrome), endometriosis, and uterine fibroids.

In addition to hormonal dysregulation, lack of sulfate can have a negative impact on connective tissue. Many different components within joints require sulfate to function properly. Glucosamine sulfate stimulates the biosynthesis of glycosaminoglycans and hyaluronic acid. These are critical for the formation of a healthy joint matrix. Chondroitin sulfate provides additional substrates for the formation of healthy cartilage. Without adequate sulfate, these tissues don't form properly and are more vulnerable to osteoarthritic presentations. We also can become more vulnerable to frequent subluxations, or partial dislocations, as a result of this underlying instability. The bioaccumulation of oxalate and the corresponding loss of sulfate may be a key reason why so many hypersensitive individuals, particularly those with Mast Cell Activation Syndrome, must deal with progressive hypermobility as their illness progresses. This can lead to a downward progression in which high oxalates create instability in the cervical spine or soft palate, creating airway issues at night, and strain the vagus nerve, all contributing to the activation of the mast cells. Hypersensitivity coupled with hypermobility can be viewed as the result of high oxalate and low sulfate.

Heparin sulfate loss is another potentially significant result of elevated oxalic acid. This may be of particular concern in hypersensitive individuals dealing with mast-cell degranulation. Heparin sulfate plays an important role in both acute and chronic inflammatory responses.

The relationship between oxalate and sulfate shows us a second set of pathways that we need to consider when we evaluate an individual's genetics for high-oxalate presentations. Moving beyond the standard view to a deeper understanding, these pathways can help direct us to targeted support for people who are highly sensitive to supplementation. Careful evaluation of sulfite and sulfate levels, for instance, can help us determine whether molybdenum supplementation may be helpful in reducing oxalate levels in the body.

Molybdenum helps support an enzyme referred to in genomics as SUOX, which converts our toxic sulfites into helpful sulfates. In hypersensitive individuals, this pathway is often compromised. Using urine dipsticks to measure sulfite is a simple way to determine whether this support is warranted. If urine sulfites exceed 10 units, molybdenum supplementation should be considered. The addition of molybdenum should help reduce urine sulfite concentrations by increasing its conversion into sulfate. Higher sulfate concentrations can in turn help reduce body stores of oxalate.

The elevation of sulfite beyond 10 units is problematic for at least two reasons. It slows the body's production of sulfate, and studies have shown that low sulfate can be a cause of high oxalates. In addition, high sulfite can in and of itself become an indirect trigger of Mast Cell Activation Syndrome. As sulfite levels elevate, they kick off a multi-step biochemical cascade that my colleague Bob Miller has named the *NADPH steal*. As this cascade occurs, NADPH oxidase increases, which in turn increases superoxide concentrations, which in turn cause the activation of mast cells. High levels of oxalate can also trigger the NADPH steal, making weakness along the SUOX pathway a double whammy for hypersensitivity.

In addition to supplementation with molybdenum and vitamin B6, we can use Epsom salt soaks to increase sulfate levels in the body. Epsom salt, aka magnesium sulfate, is inexpensive, easy to find, and highly effective in reducing body stores of oxalates. Soaking in a tub of Epsom salt water is a simple way to increase serum levels of both magnesium and sulfate. Because of the high level of transdermal absorption of sulfate, highly sensitive individuals need to proceed with extreme caution with this intervention. I recommend starting with foot soaks before proceeding to full-body soaks. The sensitive person should start low and slow in terms of both the time spent soaking and the Epsom salt concentration in the water. It may be necessary to start by soaking for thirty seconds in as little as 1 teaspoon of Epsom salt in a foot basin with several gallons of warm water. Repeat three to five times per week, increasing in five-second intervals up to one minute. After that, increase Epsom salt concentration to 2 teaspoons. Increase both the time spent soaking and the concentration of Epsom salt as tolerated, watching for signs of oxalate dumping.

Glucosamine sulfate and chondroitin sulfate are two more potentially helpful interventions for the low-sulfate/high-oxalate individual who presents with frequent subluxations (slight misalignment of the vertebrae), overt hypermobility (unusually or abnormally great range of movement in a joint or joints), or joint pain. From a genomic standpoint, individuals with variants on the carbohydrate sulfotransferases, the CHSTs, will be most likely to benefit from these interventions. Supplementation with these compounds may help improve the joint matrix. Because they are in their sulfated forms, people with polymorphisms on the CHSTs can use them more readily. Because they are sulfated, however, we should be on the lookout for oxalate dumping. These compounds often have to be used in fairly high doses to be efficacious. In our highly sensitive cohort, we want to be sure to work slowly and progressively up to therapeutic doses.

Evaluation and Testing for Oxalates

How can we measure our body stores of oxalates? We can't, really. We have to be content to measure the amount we're excreting in urine or the amount circulating in plasma. We don't have good tools to assess what may be stuck in the tissue. Recognizing that our tools are imperfect doesn't mean we shouldn't use them. Instead, that knowledge can allow us to read the available tests with a more critical clinical eye. When it comes to measuring urinary excretion of oxalates, there are two main routes to consider. The first is urine organic acids testing (OAT). Through the use of OAT, it's possible to get a measure of glyceric, glycolic, and oxalic acids. Glyceric and glycolic acids, when elevated, can give us an indicator for a genetic predisposition for oxalate toxicity expression. When either of these markers is elevated, we can be certain that excessive oxalate is being produced metabolically.

The third marker we find on this testing is the oxalic acid itself. If this indicator is elevated in isolation, we're looking at a secondary hyperoxaluria: the high oxalates are coming from a gut-related source such as over-consumption, leaky gut, dysbiosis (an imbalance in bacterial composition, changes in bacterial metabolic activities, or changes in bacterial distribution within the gut), colonized mold, or biliary dysfunction. If this marker is elevated in conjunction with glyceric and/or glycolic acid, we know that there's a genetic component, but it doesn't exclude any of the gut-related reasons. This can be an all-of-the-above scenario. In hypersensitive individuals, we often see a pattern of high glyceric or glycolic acid with oxalic acid low or in range. This is one of the more significant patterns, as it indicates that oxalate is being made in high quantities *but not excreted efficiently* (as we saw in my patient, Karen). We should keep this idea of oxalate retention vs. excretion in mind with gut-driven high oxalates as well. Finding an oxalate marker in the normal range can lull us into a false sense of security.

Cross-referencing these markers with OAT biomarkers for mold colonization can give us additional clues as to whether we should look for oxalates as part of the clinical picture. Aspergillus species in particular are oxalate-forming organisms. Their presence in the body should have us on high alert for oxalates. Not seeing elevated oxalic acid when we expect it tells us that there's a high likelihood that it's being retained in the body and not being excreted properly.

If we see signs and symptoms of oxalates—a history that leads us to believe that oxalates are playing a role in a patient's clinical presentation—or one of the patterns discussed previously, but no urine oxalate is found, we could consider plasma-oxalate testing. This blood test is used to assess the body-pool size of oxalate in patients with primary or secondary hyperoxaluria when urinary oxalate is not available or accurate. It's an excellent tool to help avoid oxalate supersaturation (levels above 25 mcmol/L), particularly in individuals with renal failure. As the body-pool size increases, oxalate may precipitate in tissues and cause toxicity. Assessing oxalate levels in this way is a particularly helpful tool for sensitive individuals who may not be efficiently excreting oxalates in urine.

Sensible Sensitive Oxalate-Reduction Strategies

Low and slow is the name of the game with all things oxalate related, particularly if renal function is poor. We should establish the expectation that reduction of the body pool of oxalates can take years for some people, depending on how many of the factors previously discussed are coming into play. Because of the complexity of safe and effective oxalate reduction, it's best done under the guidance of an experienced clinician.

Clearly there are many different aspects to consider when working to reduce the body burden of oxalates. We should remember that we don't need to address all of them at once, especially in sensitive people. Careful investigation of the multiple factors that can contribute to high oxalates can give us targeted tools for reducing their levels and the accompanying symptoms. The progressive layering of interventions specific to the individual oxalate presentation can allow us to reduce your body's store of oxalates and restore health and function safely and effectively, even when, like me, you did everything wrong before you knew better.

EMILY GIVLER is the co-founder of Beyond Protocols, a Functional/Genomic Nutrition Consultant, researcher, and lecturer with a thriving practice alongside her mentor, Bob Miller, at Tree of Life in Ephrata, Pennsylvania. She holds advanced certifications in Nutrition, Herbalism, and Nutrigenomics from the Holt Institute of Medicine, Pan-American University of Natural Health, and Functional Genomic Analysis where she now serves as a researcher and supplement formulator. In her practice, Ms. Givler uses personalized dietary and nutritional protocols based on genetic predispositions, environmental and epigenetic influences, and functional lab testing to help her clients optimize or recover their health.

In addition to her clinical work, Ms. Givler leads the mentorship team at Beyond Protocols, teaching practitioners advanced integration of functional genomics. She also offers one-on-one practitioner mentoring, helping colleagues navigate the complex web of genetic polymorphisms to develop more effective protocols for their chronically ill or complex cases. She sits on the advisory board for the Nutrigenomic Research Institute as well as lending her services as an independent researcher.

www.BeyondProtocols.org

www.TOLhealth.com

Chapter 13: Sulfur Metabolism and Sensitization

Greg Nigh, ND, Lac.

Dr. Nathan's Introduction

In the previous chapter, Emily Givler did a superb job of introducing us to the connection between sulfur metabolism and oxalates, and now Dr. Nigh will expand on this important subject so we can add his information to our understanding of sensitivity and make sure not to miss this piece of the puzzle when our patients aren't responding as we expect them to. For even greater depth, I would encourage readers to read Greg's book, *The Devil in the Garlic,* as well.

✿ ✿ ✿

When, about a decade ago, I became interested in the physiology of sulfur, I had no idea how relevant sulfur metabolism was to a wide range of diseases and symptoms I was seeing in the clinic. I initially believed that aberrant sulfur metabolism was contributing to a relatively small and well-defined set of complaints some patients were experiencing. Over time, though, in collaboration with nutrition therapist Maria Palmer, I developed a treatment protocol to help "fix" impaired sulfur metabolism. As we implemented this protocol with an increasingly broad range of patients, we were shocked to discover how many symptoms and even long-standing diseases were apparently rooted in this underlying sulfur issue.

I will give you a general overview of the protocol we're implementing in the clinic to address these problems with sulfur metabolism. First, though, it's important to understand the basics of how dietary sulfur flows through its various metabolic pathways, what happens when that flow becomes impaired, and the type of symptoms that can result from that impairment. I believe that disrupted sulfur metabolism may be playing a central role in the rising tide of extreme dietary and environmental sensitivity and reactivity I've observed over the past five years.

Sulfur Metabolism: An Overview

Sulfur is one of the most abundant elements of the body, yet it's surprising how little awareness there is about its many critical roles. For perspective, an averaged-sized adult has a total of about four grams of iron in their body, and yet those four grams command a great deal of attention: iron-deficient anemia; iron supplementation and food fortification; and iron storage disease are examples. In comparison, the body of an average adult contains about 140 grams of sulfur. Sulfur is absolutely essential for detoxification and excretion of a wide range of toxins and toxicants, immune function, the production and integrity of connective tissue, and much else.

There are many important sulfur-containing molecules in the body. I'll focus on three: hydrogen sulfide (H_2S), sulfite (SO_3^-), and sulfate (SO_4^{-2}). We take in dietary sulfur contained in various foods and beverages, and a significant portion of that sulfur must ultimately be converted into sulfate. The body needs a constant supply of sulfate to maintain balance and health. In the process of converting dietary sulfur to sulfate, both hydrogen sulfide and sulfite are generated as well.

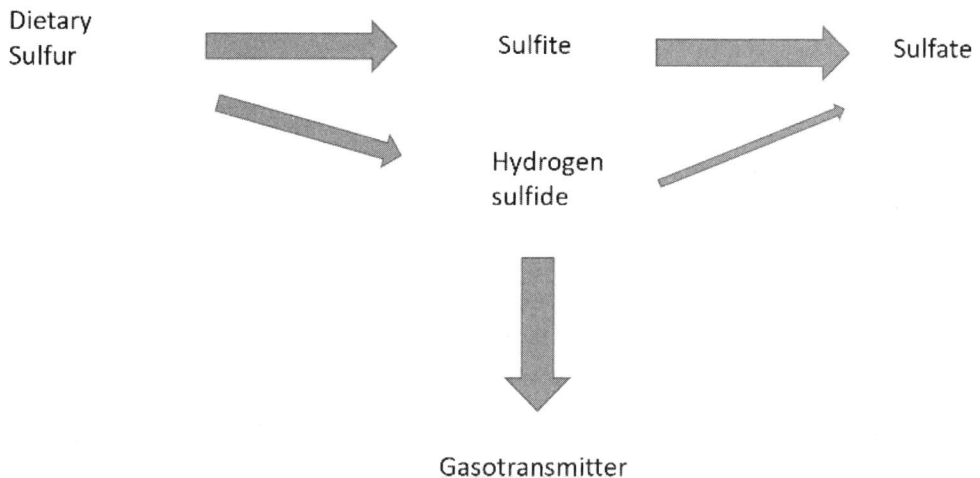

Dietary Sulfur → Sulfite → Sulfate

Hydrogen sulfide

Gasotransmitter

Among many other important sulfur compounds our body needs, the two most relevant for causing symptoms and ultimately driving the hypersensitivity reactions so many are now struggling with are sulfite and hydrogen sulfide. As you can see, these are generated along the pathway from dietary sulfur to the sulfate our bodies need. As you might imagine, anything that impairs the conversion of sulfite to sulfate will lead to a buildup of both sulfite and hydrogen sulfide. That buildup causes problems, but it also triggers solutions. Let me explain.

Bodies are intelligent in what they do and how they do it. There are very few metabolic processes our cells undertake, even those we associate with symptoms and disease, that cannot be viewed as an *attempt* on the part of the cell to correct a problem. Those corrections might cause symptoms we don't like, and if sustained for too long might become classified as a chronic disease, but if we can understand why the correction was needed in the first place, what the correction was trying to accomplish, and ultimately help make this correction, the associated symptoms can simply resolve on their own.

> Sulfite is a sulfur compound that many already know all too well. For those sensitive to sulfites they can cause headaches and other problems. Sulfites are notoriously contained in many wines and are used on dried fruit as a preservative. These dietary sulfites, though, must be processed in the same way as sulfite generated internally. Those sensitive to dietary sulfites are probably sensitive to the sulfites being made in their cells.

In this scenario, the cellular and systemic need is access to sulfate. The problem arises when the normal pathways to sulfate become impaired. This can lead to symptoms that range from mild and occasional to the severe daily symptoms that I believe now encompass the extreme sensitivities and reactivity I increasingly encounter among patients in the clinic.

The correction to this problem revolves around the generation of sulfite and, even more important, hydrogen sulfide, which causes myriad symptoms. To help correct the problem means restoring the normal pathways to sulfate production. This allows sulfite and hydrogen sulfide levels to drop and the associated symptoms to fade away. To offer the right kind of help, it's important to have an understanding of the most common causes of disrupted sulfur metabolism and thus impaired sulfate production.

Sulfate Disruption: The Likely Culprits

My clinical observation is that impairment in the flow from dietary sulfur to sulfate falls under three general causes: nutrient deficiencies; environmental exposures and toxicities; and genetics. I'll run through each of these briefly, because this establishes the foundation for the kinds of therapies that can help correct the problem.

The Nutrients

Every metabolic pathway in our cells is incredibly complex. Each involves at least two and most commonly dozens of proteins interacting in very precise ways. Many of these interactions require enzymes that facilitate the reaction and without which the reaction wouldn't happen. Most enzymes require one or more specific vitamin and/or mineral cofactors, nutrients that must be present for each enzyme to do its work. A list of the most relevant nutrients that are essential to sulfur metabolism will be helpful for us to refer to later on.

Minerals

Molybdenum (Mo)

This is the nutrient most widely recognized as playing a central role in sulfur metabolism and sulfate production. It's an essential cofactor of an essential enzyme—sulfite oxidase (abbreviated SUOX), and the activity of that enzyme is the *only way* for sulfite, SO_3, to be converted to sulfate, SO_4. Not only can this cofactor be lacking in the diet but it can also be drawn away from its sulfur duties because it's needed for other important enzymes as well. One of them is aldehyde oxidase. As the name suggests, this enzyme detoxifies chemical compounds called aldehydes. And what are two important sources of aldehydes that would require Mo to detoxify them? Alcohol intake and yeast, specifically Candida, will both generate aldehydes. For this reason, it's common for people with dietary sulfur sensitivities to also have sensitivity to alcohol intake and/or to struggle with digestive or systemic Candida infections.

Iron (Fe)

Iron plays many roles in sulfur metabolism, but the most essential is that it's required in order to build the SUOX enzyme. Fe is needed to produce molecules called *heme,* which is most familiar to us because it lends its name to hemoglobin, the oxygen-carrying molecule in red blood cells. Heme is present in many other molecules as well, including SUOX. Heme is in fact *essential* to the function of that enzyme. If there's too little iron available, it can compromise SUOX production, which thus compromises conversion of sulfite to sulfate.

Cobalt (Co)

This mineral is most familiar to us in its role as a central atom in cobalamin, which is itself the core molecule of vitamin B12. One antidote used in the event of hydrogen-sulfide poisoning is to give one or a series of high-dose injections of a form of vitamin B12 called hydroxocobalamin. This will oxidize H_2S in the blood, converting it to sulfur dioxide, which can itself go on to be oxidized to sulfite and sulfate if all is working correctly. Cobalt is one of the most common nutrients found to be deficient in those I test, and its deficiency has profound implications not just for sulfur metabolism but for a wide range of neurological issues.

Magnesium (Mg)

This mineral is a cofactor for several of the enzymes involved in the sulfur pathways. Beyond its direct role as a cofactor, Mg plays an essential role in the use of energy in cells, and specifically in the mitochondria. Hydrogen sulfide is oxidized within mitochondria as part of the healthy lifecycle of some portion of that gas. In the process, other important sulfur compounds get produced, in addition to sulfur dioxide, and, as we've already noted, sulfur dioxide oxidizes to sulfite, which is again oxidized to sulfate by SUOX, an enzyme with a large presence right there in the mitochondria. This is a direct link between energy production and sulfate production, a very important link to keep in mind.

Copper (Cu)

One of the most underrated and misunderstood of the minerals, Cu is essential for cellular energy production and for the proper movement of iron into and out of cells. Its central role in cellular energy production is what makes it critical for H_2S regulation and thus sulfate production. If Cu levels are low, iron accumulates in the cell, where it sits and oxidizes, i.e., it rusts. This growing burden of oxidation results in increased production of H_2S, which acts as an antioxidant. It's a vicious cycle that can drive high H_2S levels and resulting symptoms, especially when an inefficient SUOX enzyme can't get it all converted to usable sulfate.

Vitamins/Nutrients

Vitamin D

This vitamin gets a lot of attention for its many important roles in calcium regulation and immunity, but lesser known is its role in promoting intracellular H_2S production, specifically within adipocytes, i.e., fat cells. The H_2S

> It is now widely understood that vitamin D is actually more appropriately categorized as a sterol hormone. This puts it into the same category of hormones as cortisol, progesterone, estrogen, testosterone, and others. Just as taking other sterol hormones should not be considered benign, so too ongoing ultra-high dosing of vitamin D could have unintended consequences. This *could* include overproduction of hydrogen sulfide in cells, and the symptoms that can arise as a result.

acts as an anti-inflammatory in those cells, so this is one important way that vitamin D reduces inflammation. The promotion of this vitamin's health benefits has led many to take very high daily doses. I believe there are several reasons to be cautious about this level of supplementation, reasons that go beyond the potential to drive hydrogen-sulfide production, but a full discussion of that goes beyond the scope of this chapter.

B-Complex Vitamins

I'm going to lump these together rather than discuss each one individually. Essentially, all the B vitamins have some close link to sulfur metabolism; some, like vitamin B6, are linked more strongly than others, like biotin. That said, even biotin has a role to play in scavenging sulfur-containing proteins out of the blood. Either an excess or a deficiency of these vitamins can impact the normal balance of hydrogen sulfide and sulfite within and among cells.

Coenzyme Q10

It was far into my research into sulfur metabolism, and hydrogen-sulfide processing in particular, that I learned about the important role of CoQ10. Its more familiar role is in the mitochondria, buried within the electron transport chain, a necessary stepping-stone as the electrons move toward their final destination: tossed onto oxygen for the production of water. In another role for CoQ10, though, hydrogen sulfide gets transformed into another vital sulfur-containing antioxidant called thiosulfate. Thiosulfate, after doing its antioxidant work, is then transformed into sulfite, which again must go through SUOX to become sulfate.

Environmental Toxins and Toxicants

Mycotoxins

These toxic byproducts of mold are known to play a role in creating intestinal inflammation and general dysbiosis (an imbalance between the types of organisms present in a person's natural microflora—especially those of the gut—thought to contribute to a range of conditions of ill health). It is interesting to note, though, that hydrogen sulfide suppresses the growth of both Candida and Aspergillus, two organisms commonly found overgrowing in the dysbiotic gut. This brings up the interesting possibility that perhaps the overgrowth of bacteria that produce hydrogen sulfide—the sulfur-fixing bacteria—is an adaptive response, an attempt to control the growth of those yeasts.

Toxic Metals

Like the B-complex vitamins, I group these together because a whole chapter could be written about each one and its possible impacts on sulfur metabolism. There are two primary pathways where metals throw a wrench into the sulfur pathways: they impair mitochondrial energy production, which reduces normal H2S cycling in all the ways previous mentioned; or they can displace the mineral cofactors needed for proper enzyme function. In addition to mitochondrial damage, metals such as mercury and arsenic can displace molybdenum within the active center of the SUOX enzyme, severely impairing the oxidation of SO_3 to SO_4, sulfite to sulfate.

Glyphosate

The primary active ingredient in the herbicide Roundup, glyphosate-based herbicides are the most commonly used agricultural chemical worldwide. Glyphosate is now so widely distributed in the planet's food and water systems that most people tested—even those eating a predominantly organic diet—have detectable levels in their urine. Glyphosate possesses a unique ability to

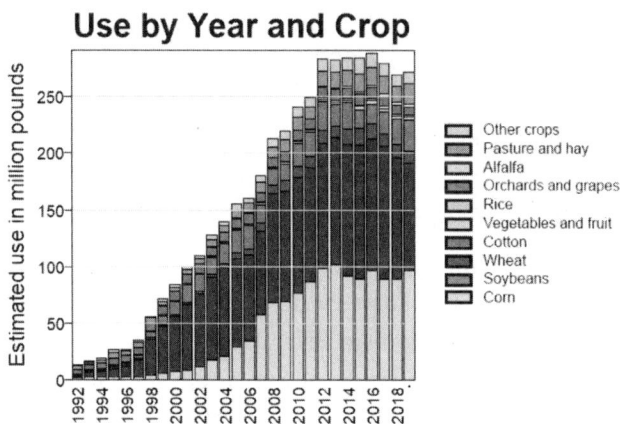

Use by Year and Crop

Source: USGS: https://tinyurl.com/yajcu4s2

disrupt sulfur metabolism because it has such a broad range of impacts on physiology. It strongly binds to molybdenum, copper, zinc, cobalt, iron, and other minerals that are necessary for sulfur metabolism. Beyond this, glyphosate is a modified version of the amino acid glycine and can substitute itself for glycine in the body. Glycine has a calming effect on the brain. It's also an essential component of glutathione, the master antioxidant and detoxifier in the body, and glycine makes up about one third of collagen, the most abundant protein in the body and the fabric of our connective tissue. Whenever glyphosate substitutes for glycine in the body, these and many other aspects of normal physiology could be severely impaired. I believe the astronomical increase in the use of glyphosate-based herbicides that has occurred over the past thirty years might be a very significant contributor to the increase in sulfur dysregulation and related symptoms and diseases that I see in the clinic.

Genetics Impacting Sulfur Processing

There are a handful of genes that have a direct impact on how sulfur gets processed in the body, and a plethora of genes that have an indirect impact. An assessment of patient genetic polymorphisms does not form the basis of any treatment plan I formulate. That said, I believe there are a few genes that appear to me to have a major impact on sulfur processing if they are impacted by polymorphisms (see chapter 19 for more on relevant polymorphisms).

SUOX

This is the gene that encodes the enzyme I mentioned previously. Several polymorphisms in this gene have been documented, and a fraction of them have been studied for their impact on health. For example, a dozen different polymorphisms in *SUOX* result in a deficiency of the sulfide oxidase enzyme. Given what we know about the role of the SUOX enzyme in converting sulfite to sulfate, low levels of this gene should be expected to have a symptomatic impact.

Consequences of Disrupted Sulfate

What does impaired sulfate metabolism have to do with hypersensitivity? I think it's central, and I think the evidence supports that. Impaired sulfate production will ricochet through the body in several detrimental ways, ultimately leading to excess hydrogen sulfide and dysregulation of the autonomic nervous system (ANS). Hypersensitivity is only one of many ways this can manifest symptomatically.

Clinically, the most common manifestations of impaired sulfur metabolism can include one or more of the following:

- Gas, bloating, IBS, and inflammatory bowel disease
- Dermatitis, itching, acne, or other skin manifestations
- Brain fog and/or anxiety
- Temperature-regulation issues, including hot flashes and night sweats
- Headaches, including migraine
- Sensitivity to wine and/or sulfa drugs

I would add to this list hyperreactivity to foods, environmental exposures, and even stress and mental exertion. How does this wide range of symptoms result from impaired sulfur metabolism, and what can be done about it? Let's start with the first question, then move on to treatment strategies.

Suppose for a moment that nutritional issues, exposure to toxins, and/or genetics have conspired to impair normal production of sulfate from dietary sulfur. What should we expect the body to do as a consequence? It can't do without sulfate; we know that isn't an option.

I believe we should expect the body to find another way to produce sulfate, implementing a workaround, so to speak. Bodies do this all the time; it's part and parcel of maintaining health and homeostasis.

Impair blood flow in an artery, and the body creates collateral vessels that literally bypass the blockage.

If instability arises in the spine, the body will create "bridges" between the vertebrae to enhance stability.

If blood pressure around the lungs builds up due to scarring or chronic fluid around the lungs, the heart muscle gets bigger to be able to push more effectively against that resistance.

These are just a few examples of ways that our bodies figure out how to work around obstacles to normal functioning. The bridges created in the spine and the enlargement of the heart are commonly viewed as pathological conditions in need of treatment. Another way to think of them, though, is *brilliant!* They are very sensible solutions to a problem.

What if the problem is impaired access to sulfate? What's a good solution? One readily available solution would be to *facilitate* the growth of sulfur-fixing bacteria in the intestinal tract. These bacteria will generate hydrogen sulfide and sulfite from dietary sulfur compounds. That causes symptoms, sure, potentially lots of them, and no one wants to deal with symptoms, but those bacterial byproducts can be converted into sulfate, restoring cells' access to it and working around the serious problem of impaired sulfate production through the usual routes. Excess levels of hydrogen sulfide are well-documented as causing gastrointestinal inflammation, hypotension, bradycardia (abnormally slow heart rate), concentration and memory issues, and other symptoms. Very important and relevant recent research has shown that high levels of the gas in the intestinal tract leads to visceral hyperalgesia, i.e., a magnified experience of pain in the abdominal organs. This brings us back to what I believe is the fundamental driver of the extreme sensitivities and reactivity I increasingly see in my patients: autonomic dysregulation.

Autonomic Nervous System (ANS): An Overview

The ANS is that aspect of the nervous system that you don't have to think about for it to function: Adjusting your blood pressure and heart rate, salivation, pupil constriction and dilation, the production of digestive juices, bowel motility, and much else. The ANS is divided into two major branches, labeled the sympathetic and parasympathetic branches. These branches typically have opposite effects on physiology, and there should always be a dynamic balance between the two. Sometimes sympathetic signals should dominate, which suppresses parasympathetic signals, and sometimes just the opposite should happen. Both signal types are necessary for healthy functioning. We can imagine a healthy set point to be that easy, fluid, and appropriate transition between these two poles of ANS signaling to the viscera.

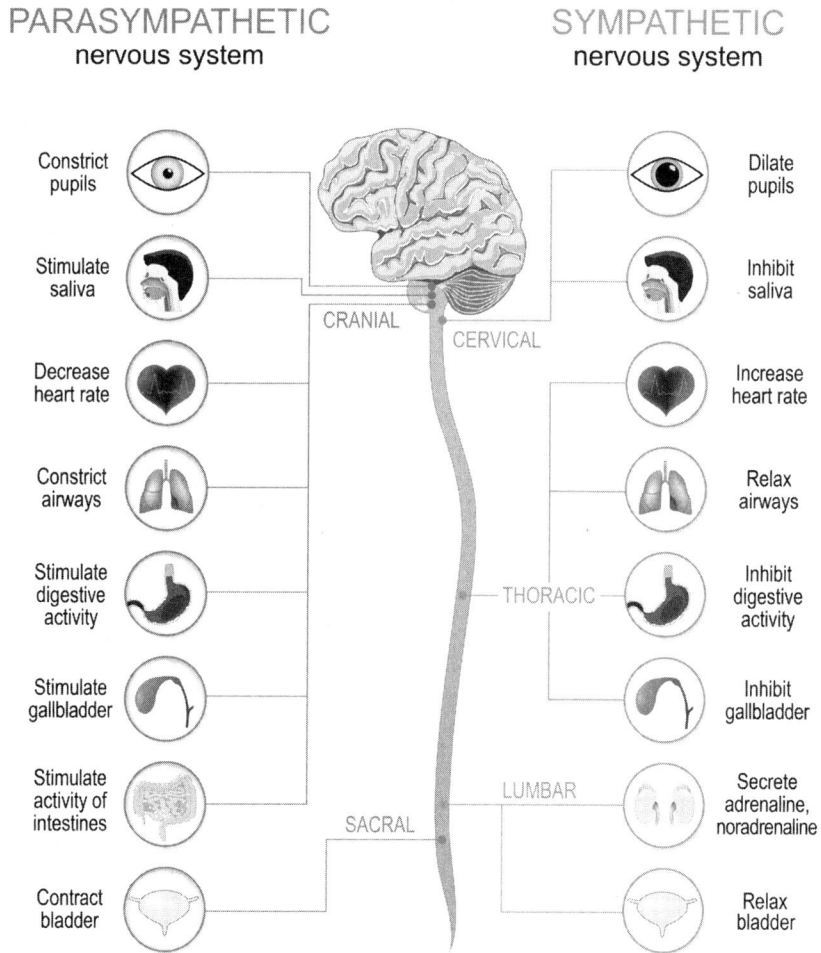

PARASYMPATHETIC
nervous system

SYMPATHETIC
nervous system

Parasympathetic		Sympathetic
Constrict pupils		Dilate pupils
Stimulate saliva		Inhibit saliva
Decrease heart rate		Increase heart rate
Constrict airways		Relax airways
Stimulate digestive activity		Inhibit digestive activity
Stimulate gallbladder		Inhibit gallbladder
Stimulate activity of intestines		Secrete adrenaline, noradrenaline
Contract bladder		Relax bladder

CRANIAL — CERVICAL — THORACIC — LUMBAR — SACRAL

What we know to be true is that virtually all disease states can be characterized by an underlying ANS imbalance. This imbalance is usually, though not always, one in which there is a dominance of sympathetic ANS signaling. See sidebar on page 256 for some of the expected physical manifestations of that activation: reduced saliva, increased sweating, decreased bowel motility, increased heart rate, and much else. These changes, which are supposed to be happening only when under acute stress, can become essentially continuous for those who have an underlying impairment in sulfate production and a resultant excess production of hydrogen sulfide and sulfite. When the nervous system has a strong lean toward ongoing sympathetic activation, for many patients the parasympathetic system maintains a very precarious dampening influence on the sympathetic system. For an increasing number of my patients, those sympathetic signals, already overly active, are on a hair trigger, such that even the slightest perturbance can launch a full crisis-type sympathetic activation.

In this hyperactivated scenario, the whole is greater than the sum of its parts. The nutrient issues, environmental exposures, genetics, sulfur/sulfate issues, and the resulting ANS dysregulation—combine to produce a perfect storm of illness, while none of them separately explains the reactivity completely. I also believe a treatment program that focuses on any one or even a few of these factors can provide short-term symptom reduction but is unlikely to bring about long-lasting resolution of the problem. Compounding this issue is the oft-observed fact that the ANS sympathetic activation has often been a dominant aspect of a patient's constitution for decades. These are deep neurological patterns that can manifest overtly as feeling stressed or irritable or uncomfortably amped up. It's common for patients to acknowledge these or related personal characteristics spanning back to childhood.

This ANS sympathetic patterning presents a unique challenge in the landscape of treatment for this hypersensitivity. It is not enough to address only the underlying sulfur dysregulation; when these two treatment objectives are brought together, in combination with other therapeutic goals as appropriate, the potential to achieve long-lasting relief is very realistic. While individual treatment plans are inherently unique, several components of the plans are common to all.

Building the Plan to Address Hypersensitivity

I always start with sulfur. It's extremely rare that someone with hypersensitivity and seeming pan-reactivity doesn't exhibit at least *some* signs and symptoms of sulfur-metabolism issues. Most commonly there are many indications. I am always clear with patients that it's unlikely all their symptoms will resolve by addressing the underlying sulfur issue, but it's very unlikely their symptoms will fully resolve without addressing a sulfur issue that is present. I start by referring patients to Maria for orientation to the low-sulfur diet she has put together and that she customizes according to individual needs or variances. There are, however, generic low-sulfur diet guidelines available, including one created by Maria. Even general guidelines can bring dramatic benefits for many people. The total plan brings in all the elements I described previously as contributing to sulfur dysregulation, plus additional therapies to directly address autonomic dysregulation and sympathetic excess.

Diet

The strict low-sulfur diet is implemented for two weeks, at which point systematic reintroductions are typically started. The diet is a method for differentiating specific reactive sulfur foods from a general accumulation of sulfur metabolites that eventually spill over into symptoms. These can be overlapping but unique types of sulfur reactivity (see sidebar). While the full set of foods to eliminate is too extensive to list here, the foods we've found to be most reactive are on this short list:

- Garlic
- Onion
- Eggs
- Kale
- Cabbage
- Broccoli
- Cauliflower
- Asparagus
- Brussels sprouts
- Wine

Two weeks of complete avoidance of these nine foods plus wine is a generic application of the diet protocol. At the end, each of these is reintroduced one at a time on an every-other-day basis. Reactive foods are typically very easy to identify. Of course, no one has to introduce foods they simply don't eat or don't like and would not eat or drink otherwise.

Sulfur reactions generally fall into two types: short-term reactivity that might technically be classified as sensitivities, allergies, or intolerances; these are reactions that can happen within minutes of reintroducing a food, or might not manifest for up to twenty-four hours. Once identified, removal of these reactive foods can often allow other therapies to be much more effective.

The second type of reaction is one that develops over time with ongoing sulfur intake. Patients commonly find they have no symptoms eating broccoli once a week, but three times weekly brings symptoms back; or that a bit of garlic powder as a seasoning on occasion causes no problems, but use of too much at once, or adding a whole clove to a dish, overwhelms their capacity to clear out those metabolites quickly enough, and symptoms return.

Supplements

Several nutrients might come into any given treatment program. Here are some details about the few I've already mentioned.

Molybdenum

There are many products with this either as a single nutrient or as part of a combination. My experience is that one particular product called Mo Zyme Forte by Biotics works better than any other. For some patients, simply bringing this product in has lifted years of brain fog or fatigue. It can also raise the threshold of reactivity for those who tolerate some, but not too much, sulfur in their diet. I typically start people out with one tablet twice daily, and have them titrate up to two and even three tablets twice daily to see whether symptoms improve at a higher dose. If so, that tells us that the SUOX enzyme is significantly compromised and can use lots of support. If tolerable, I always recommend these tablets be chewed up prior to swallowing—it just works better and faster that way. If that's not tolerable, swallowing them whole is fine.

Butyrate

Butyrate is not only a great anti-inflammatory for the digestive tract and the primary fuel for cells of the large intestine but also stimulates activity within the vagus nerve, enhancing bowel tone and motility. Studies have also found that oral butyrate has both anti-depressive and anti-anxiety effects. I commonly recommend oral supplementation as well as butyrate added to the coffee solution used in a coffee enema when that detoxification therapy is indicated.

Coenzyme Q10

This is a common recommendation, particularly in those who have fatigue or brain fog as a primary symptom. I dose it in either the ubiquinone form (800mg daily with food), or as ubiquinol (400mg daily with food). It is important to read the label and use a form that does not contain soy lecithin.

Vitamin B12

I recommend the hydroxocobalamin form to optimize hydrogen-sulfide clearance from the bloodstream. This can be a difficult form to find. Clinically, I recommend a product called B12-2000 by Biotics. I have no affiliation with Biotics, but I like many of their products and so suggest them. Usually, I have people chew up one wafer once daily with food.

There are any number of other supplements that might be used in addition to or even instead of these, but in the large majority of patients, I believe these will be quite supportive of the overall therapeutic goal.

Detoxification

This one is harder to generalize because individuals present with such unique exposure histories. There are therapies I commonly advocate. I mentioned coffee enemas. These can be extremely valuable if done correctly. I always suggest the enema be "spiked" with butyrate and a probiotic. It does not need to be more than one half liter each time. Ideally it's retained for ten to fifteen minutes, but this is often an amount of time to work up to. While the enema is retained, I commonly suggest abdominal self-massage, even somewhat vigorously as there often has been long-standing constipation and likely impacted stool that needs to be loosened and expelled. I recommend these enemas as often as daily, depending on the situation. I have heard reservations about their leading to dependency on them, but that has not been my observation. Though it may take a day or two after stopping for normal bowel pattern to resume, so long as appropriate probiotics and butyrate are supplemented, I don't find that they create dependency.

Another very important therapy to do concurrent with the low-sulfur diet and supportive nutrients is Epsom salt baths. Baths are a hassle to many, but for anyone who is able to do them, I think they're an essential component of the therapy. Epsom salt is magnesium sulfate. Soaking in the bath allows both magnesium and, perhaps more important, sulfate, to get into the blood *without needing to go through the digestive tract.* This supplies cells with biologically usable sulfate. It has been amazing to me how many people report dramatic improvement in their digestive symptoms with no change other than starting the bath protocol: The first night use 1 cup salt in a bath as hot as tolerable, soak for at least twenty minutes, then rinse in a shower. The second night use 2 cups, the third night 3 cups. Starting the fourth night and continuing nightly for 7 nights, add 4 cups of Epsom salt to the hot bath and soak. The perk is that the magnesium can help people get into a deep sleep more quickly.

> I had a patient with all the symptoms associated with sulfur dysregulation. She had been taking a high dose of lipoic acid and NAC for three years. She reported to me that through all those years she had been going through "detox." Her detox symptoms, though, had an uncanny resemblance to sulfur symptoms. I had her stop the sulfur-containing supplements and start the protocol. Within just a few days all her "detox" symptoms resolved. She had been reacting to the sulfur in the lipoic acid and NAC.

Other detox therapies might include binders if there are known mycotoxins, or gentle chelators if metals are an issue. Others in this volume will cover detox therapies in detail so I won't go into them here. The only caveat is that when someone is going through the low-sulfur protocol, I remove sulfur-containing supplements, many of which key detoxification nutrients such as lipoic acid, NAC, glutathione, methionine, MSM, DMSA, DMPS, and others.

In the clinic I often have patients use ozone and/or near-infrared saunas, ionic foot baths, pulsed electromagnetic field therapy (PEMF), IV nutrient therapy, or others as indicated.

Autonomic Regulation

Many therapies to help increase parasympathetic tone are widely known and used. They are the therapies we associate with relaxation, including meditation, yoga, exercise, and tai chi. Others, perhaps less widely known but thoroughly studied in this regard, include grounding (also called *earthing*), controlled breathing exercises, and stretching. Another that I recommend to all patients going through the low-sulfur protocol involves finishing each daily shower with tepid or even cold water. Research has shown that contrast temperature involving short-term cold exposure causes an initial sympathetic increase, then a reflex and long-lasting parasympathetic response. Most patients dread the thought of doing this therapy, yet most report feeling completely refreshed and vitalized by it.

A few other common recommendations for ANS regulation are probably also familiar to many. Dynamic Neural Retraining System (DNRS) is a self-guided system framed in the language of limbic retraining and rewiring. It's a therapy that requires both daily physical engagement and a commitment to at least six months of daily practice. It's not a panacea, and it doesn't appeal to everyone. That said, I have witnessed a dramatic improvement in symptoms and response to other therapies including the low-sulfur protocol in several individuals who implemented DNRS as a daily practice.

Another widely known self-guided therapy is Emotional Freedom Technique, or EFT. There are many online training resources. Few therapies are more readily available, and the cost to implement it is as good as it gets. When it's used skillfully, I have witnessed this bring about a dramatic shift in sympathetic/parasympathetic balance as evidenced by a dramatic change in the patient's demeanor and disposition upon presentation in the office.

The final therapy I want to mention is newer in my toolbox, but is one of the most beneficial. It's called Safe & Sound Protocol (SSP), an offshoot of polyvagal theory. SSP involves listening to some relaxing music through a series of days. The audio files, though, have been filtered of specific frequencies. This therapy takes advantage of the close relationship between the auditory nerve and the vagus nerve in order to "adjust" vagal tone. Patients need to work with someone who has been thoroughly trained with the system in order to get orientation to the process and access to the files. I refer to Maria Palmer, the nutrition therapist I work with; she has been through that training, which is closely integrated with the low-sulfur protocol. There are others around the country who can also administer SSP.

Several times each week I get feedback from patients describing their positive experience upon implementing SSP. It's common that reactivity declines overall, sometimes in a short time. People also report more emotional stability, improved digestion and associated symptoms, and a greater general sense of being grounded. I think SSP is one of the most important tools added to the ANS-regulation toolkit, especially for patients who have the clear ANS dysregulation that manifests as hypersensitivity to their world.

Conclusion

Sulfur-metabolism issues are a sign of the times. Our modern world has filled our environment with chemicals that interfere with sulfate production, while the foods we eat are grown on soils depleted of the vitamins and minerals we need. On top of that, the general stress level I'm seeing in my patients—meaning a shift into a general sympathetic activation—has increased dramatically over the past five years, and in the time of COVID-19 the general stress level is truly unprecedented. The confluence of these factors has set the stage for hypersensitivities to become increasingly common. These patients are the canary in the coalmine, likely showing the first manifestations of a rising tide of similar patients to come. With the proper tools at our disposal, which includes addressing both sulfur dysregulation and ANS imbalances, this reactivity can be calmed and life can get back to normal.

DR. GREG NIGH is a naturopathic physician and licensed acupuncturist who has been in practice since 2001. After completing his undergraduate studies at the University of Notre Dame and a master's in Humanities at Arizona State University, he attended the National University of Natural Medicine. There he received his doctorate in naturopathic medicine and a concurrent master's degree in Chinese Medicine. In addition to several peer-reviewed publications, he has spoken internationally on the topic of sulfur and its relationship to health and disease. His practice is at Immersion Health in Portland, Oregon, and can be found online at immersionhealthPDX.com. Dr. Nigh has a clinical focus on naturopathic oncology, Lyme disease, mold-related illness, SIBO, autoimmune illnesses, and, of course, the wide range of symptoms and conditions associated with impaired sulfur metabolism. He is a prolific writer, and his book, *The Devil in the Garlic*, is of particular relevance to this chapter.

Chapter 14: The Role of Salicylates in the Sensitive Patient

Beth O'Hara, FN

Dr. Nathan's Introduction

We are constantly searching for the "missing puzzle pieces." While most sensitive patients respond beautifully to the basics, in the treatment of limbic/vagal and mast-cell issues, a few do not. When we started this work, it was confusing to have a patient embrace our treatment options yet not improve as we expected them to. The question uppermost in our minds as we tried to help these patients was: "What are we missing?" Learning about oxalates and sulfur metabolism added to our ability to help those patients, and here, Beth explains another missing piece—salicylates. For me, one major tip-off that salicylates are problematic for certain patients is when they have flushing and hives that don't respond at all to mast-cell treatments. As Beth explains, however, this is just a small bit of information that will lead us into a larger subject.

☼ ☼ ☼

Introduction

Salicylate intolerance is one of the most challenging of the food intolerances to diagnose and navigate, especially since, at least in my practice, it rarely occurs in isolation from other food intolerances. I'll start by sharing a situation that you might see yourself (or a patient) in.

Maya was in tears when I first met with her. She'd failed protocols with six practitioners before we started. One of her biggest symptoms was hives along with intense redness and flushing after eating. She also had ear ringing that would wax and wane, tightness in her chest, and frequent diarrhea.

What had been so perplexing for the practitioners who were working hard to help her was that a low-histamine diet hadn't improved the hives, redness, flushing, or diarrhea as it does for many people. She was struggling to tolerate a number of supplements as well, but here's where her case became even more confusing: she was taking about 1500mg of quercetin (a high-salicylate supplement) a day and felt it really helped her. This was why I also didn't suspect salicylate intolerance in the beginning. Let's look at what salicylates are; later, I'll tell you more of Maya's story and how we got to the bottom of her health mystery.

What are Salicylates?

Salicylates are compounds found in plants. They're part of the defense mechanisms plants use to protect themselves from invasion by fungi, insects, and bacteria (similar to oxalates as a defense mechanism). Salicylates can be found in:

- medications, particularly aspirin and Pepto Bismol (bismuth subsalicylate)
- a number of plants, especially many colorful fruits, vegetables, and herbs (especially high in mints), as well as some nuts, seeds, and oils
- cosmetics and personal-care products that contain variations of salicylic acid, essential oils, wintergreen, or mint

Certain food additives and colorings—BHA, BHT, and tartrazine—are chemically similar to salicylates. Salicylates aren't a bad thing, just like histamines aren't a bad thing in themselves. Salicylates have a number of anti-inflammatory properties, which is why we're often advised to eat lots of colorful fruits and vegetables. Herbs such as rosemary, basil, and oregano are among the most nutrient-dense foods you can find.

For most people, salicylates have a significant number of powerful health benefits, which is why they're no problem at all if you don't have salicylate intolerance. The problem only arises when you're unable to keep up with the salicylate load.

What is Salicylate Intolerance?

Unlike IgE food allergies or IgG food sensitivities, salicylate intolerance is not an immune-mediated allergy or sensitivity; rather, salicylate intolerance occurs when you take in more salicylates than your body can break down (similar to histamine intolerance).

This means we have to look both at salicylate intake and salicylate breakdown. Consuming more high-salicylate foods, medications, and supplements than can be broken down can be a contributor to salicylate intolerance. For most people, this only happens for those who take high doses of aspirin (salicylic acid) or other salicylate-containing medications like Pepto Bismol (bismuth subsalicylate); however, for others who don't take salicylate medications, this issue can be more due to a difficulty in breaking down salicylates.

There are a few biochemical processes your body can utilize to break down salicylates; these include glucuronidation, sulfation, and glycine conjugation. These primary detox pathways for salicylates are also used extensively in processing mold toxins, which is why salicylate intolerance is much more common in those dealing with mold toxins. Glucuronidation is also the primary phase II detox pathway in the liver for most fat-soluble chemicals and other compounds. When these pathways are compromised by too much toxicity from multiple sources, the load can be too high to process salicylates or even other compounds that use this pathway (such as melatonin, progesterone, estrogen, vitamin D, vitamin E, etc.).

In addition to liver biotransformation (the process by which substances that enter the body are changed from hydrophobic to hydrophilic molecules to facilitate elimination from the body), salicylates are excreted by the kidneys, and kidney issues can lead to challenges with salicylate excretion. There is also a role with the GI tract. Many phenolic compounds (a subcategory of salicylates) are broken down in your gut by certain members of your microbiome, such as *Akkermansia* and *Bacteroides* species. Certain bacteria, such as *Pseudomonas,* are able to produce salicylates, and while more research is needed in humans, it's possible that an excess of these species, with GI dysbiosis such as SIBO (small intestinal bacterial overgrowth), may be another contributor to an excess-salicylate load. Further, intestinal permeability, often called leaky gut, can allow more salicylates to enter the bloodstream from the GI tract than usual, adding to the overall salicylate load in the body.

Symptoms of Salicylate Intolerance

The symptoms are varied and may differ from person to person. Some of the most common tell-tale signs:

- ear ringing (tinnitus)
- difficulty breathing (with or without asthma)
- nasal and sinus inflammation
- hives

- flushing
- itching
- diarrhea
- gas
- GI tract inflammation
- aspirin allergy

Other symptoms that researchers have associated with salicylate intolerance:

- nasal polyps
- tissue swelling
- coughing
- fatigue
- muscle pain
- skin conditions like psoriasis, eczema, and dermatitis
- abdominal pain
- brain fog
- tics
- insomnia
- bedwetting
- ADD/ADHD
- mood swings, depression, anxiety

Of course, not everyone with these symptoms has salicylate intolerance, and most people with salicylate intolerance don't have all of these symptoms. I encourage you to work with a health-care provider who is very knowledgeable and experienced with salicylate intolerance if you suspect you may have it, because you want to check what else may be going on. For example, Mast Cell Activation Syndrome, histamine intolerance, mold toxicity, and some tick-borne infections can manifest the same symptoms.

How Salicylate Intolerance Can Contribute to Sensitivities

Those with salicylate intolerance often feel like they're reacting to most foods and supplements; it can be very confusing. When people start to clean up their diets from gluten, sugar, dairy, and other inflammatory foods, they usually increase their consumption of high-salicylate foods such as broccoli, berries, coconut oil, olive oil, and herbs. Many people switch cane sugar for honey, which is also high in salicylates. It may be tempting to blame the increase in food reactions on the "healthy diet." Those in this situation may feel bewildered about why they develop asthma, rashes, itching, and worsening of tinnitus when they eat healthfully.

A client whom I'll call Aubrey was deeply embarrassed about her diet. When I first met with her, she had realized she was only able to eat foods like iceberg lettuce, wheat, soy, dairy, and meat without reacting. She kept trying to add "healthier" foods like broccoli, raspberries, rosemary, basil, and oregano, but every time she did, she felt sick for days afterward. Her ear ringing became so loud she could barely understand conversations. She would end up using a rescue inhaler multiple times a day, and she'd be covered in hives.

Something similar can happen with some supplements. I've met with many people who thought they were hypersensitive to all supplements, but a few clues helped solve the problem: they were reacting to salicylates, not to everything. Let's look at another example.

Milo didn't have the classic symptoms of salicylate intolerance—hives, itching, or breathing difficulty—but instead complained of muscle pain, weakness, brain fog, facial flushing, and tinnitus. He didn't see a connection between consuming high-salicylate foods and his symptoms, though, so at first it was confusing. He tried a low-histamine diet with no improvements, but the major tip-off came when he kept a journal of his symptoms along with foods, beverages, and supplements. We saw that his symptoms worsened with high-phenolic herbal supplements, particularly quercetin, resveratrol, CBD, and curcumin. Milo didn't have severe salicylate intolerance, and could handle salicylates in foods in moderation. The problem was that the concentrated salicylates in these supplements kept tipping him over the edge.

How do salicylates cause these symptoms? There are many mechanisms, and to cover them all is beyond the scope of this chapter, but I want to touch specifically on the role of salicylate intolerance in MCAS. While salicylates, such as phenolic supplements like quercetin and even aspirin, can often stabilize mast cells for those without salicylate intolerance, for those *with* salicylate intolerance, excess salicylates can trigger release of inflammatory mediators. An excess of salicylates has been shown in some people to trigger mast cells to release inflammatory mediators called leukotrienes along with histamine. Salicylates can also trigger two other immune cells, eosinophils and basophils, to release histamine as well. The release of these mediators can trigger many mast-cell and histamine-related symptoms such as hives, flushing, itching, asthma, etc. Excess salicylates have also been shown to block vitamin K production, reduce magnesium levels, inhibit glutathione production, and increase adrenaline levels. You can see at this point how mold and chemical toxicity can contribute to salicylate intolerance, which can then feed into a number of other problems downstream such as increased mast-cell activation.

How to Determine Whether You Have Salicylate Intolerance

The best way to determine salicylate intolerance is by an elimination trial, but if you search online, you'll find some testing available. There is, however, no simple diagnostic testing available. A common form of testing involves a challenge of consuming salicylates (such as aspirin) and monitoring for symptoms. For someone with salicylate intolerance this can be very dangerous; it can trigger life-threatening anaphylaxis and should never be undertaken without medical supervision. I don't think this form of testing is a good idea for most people. Another form of indirect testing is assessing immune cells, such as an increase in basophils, through blood testing in response to salicylates. Again, a number of other agents could also trigger these immune cells, and these tests aren't readily available, and neither are they considered highly reliable.

Working directly with salicylate intolerance is generally the safest and most reliable way to determine whether someone has salicylate intolerance, though it's still not simple. This involves reducing salicylate intake from foods, beverages, supplements, and, if possible, medications. It's not necessary to eliminate all salicylates, which is nearly impossible anyway. Instead, salicylate levels are lowered through a careful evaluation of, and reduction of, food, supplements, and, if needed, medications that might contain excess amounts of salicylates. Ideally, low-salicylate foods are eaten freely, moderate-salicylate foods are eaten in moderation, and high-salicylate foods are completely avoided. This needs to be done for a few weeks to allow the load of accumulated salicylates to gradually clear. For those with better detoxification pathways, lower chemical and mold-toxin loads, and better gastrointestinal function, clearing can occur within one to two weeks. For those with poor detoxification, high chemical and mold toxin loads, and challenged GI tracts, it can take a few weeks to clear the excess salicylate load. If, after a period of time, symptoms are improving, this is a fairly good indication of salicylate intolerance.

I want to emphasize that not everyone with Mold Toxicity or Mast Cell Activation Syndrome has salicylate intolerance. In my practice of extremely sensitive clients with mast-cell dysregulation and Mold Toxicity, only about 20% have salicylate intolerance. If you aren't sure, and are eating a standard Western diet of high levels of simple carbohydrates, inflammatory fats, gluten, corn, sugar, and dairy, you'll want to explore shifting to a healthier diet first to see how much your symptoms improve. If your symptoms worsen, though, it's important to work with a practitioner who is well educated in these areas. One of the food intolerances that many people with sensitivities explore next is histamine intolerance. For 70%–80% of sensitive people, this can make a big difference. I say this because if you don't have salicylate intolerance, you don't want to eliminate healthy foods unnecessarily. If, however, you've tried the things above, you might want to look into salicylates and read chapter 12 on oxalate issues, which often co-occur with salicylate intolerance.

I caution that if you suspect salicylate intolerance, be sure to only use a well-researched list of foods that could contain large amounts of salicylates; don't rely on most lists you can find online (even on generally reputable sites). For example, cauliflower has been listed as high in salicylate on numerous websites, yet testing data generally agrees that white cauliflower is low to moderate in salicylates, depending on growing conditions, variety, and how it's cooked. I've also seen high-salicylate foods listed as low salicylate. These errors occur due to misinterpretation of the research data, or errors in copying and pasting from one website to another, which is unfortunately rampant on health sites. I've found this issue even on medical websites with a high trust level on Google. If you're trying to determine whether you have salicylate intolerance, these mistakes can at best lead to the needless—and perhaps dangerous—elimination of foods. At worst, it can mean you think you've reduced salicylate foods when in fact you haven't.

You'll find some online groups dedicated to salicylate intolerance, which can be a wonderful community resource, but it's essential you do your own research on what you can tolerate and what you can't. Just because someone else does or doesn't tolerate a food is not a reliable way of knowing whether it's high or low in salicylate. People can react to foods for numerous reasons unrelated to salicylates, which can become quite confusing. If you suspect salicylate intolerance, it's much better to start with clearly studied lower-salicylate foods and then slowly introduce foods you're unsure about to build your own individual tolerance list over time.

Sources of Salicylates

While there is a body of research on salicylate levels in foods and supplements, this research is still in its infancy. Further, the existing research can be contradictory based on a number of factors. These include whether the tested food or herb was raw or cooked, whether it had been frozen, and which cooking methods were used. The growing season and growing conditions can also affect salicylate levels, including how long the plant had grown before it was harvested. All of this means there is no perfect salicylate foods list.

I've listed a selection of foods that are generally considered high in salicylate for you to explore. In the next section, I'll discuss high-salicylate herbs and supplements. These lists are by no means complete; for more detailed information on salicylate levels in food, I refer you to the excellent work of Sharla Race (see the resources section at the end of this chapter). You can also find a cross-referenced list of low-histamine, low-salicylate foods on my website, mastcell360.com, under the Foods Lists menu.

High Salicylate Foods

High-salicylate seasonings include: basil, rosemary, sage, turmeric, paprika, dill, mint, oregano, thyme, cumin, black pepper, ginger, allspice, cloves, cinnamon, nutmeg, apple cider vinegar, balsamic vinegar, and yeast extracts.

High-salicylate fruits include: most apples, grapes, raspberries, blackberries, apricots, blueberries, cranberries, oranges, pineapple, plums, strawberries, loganberries, avocado, cantaloupe, cherries, grapefruit, mandarins, mulberries, nectarines, and watermelon.

High-salicylate vegetables include: sweet potato, canned tomatoes, tomato puree, watercress, alfalfa sprouts, broccoli, cucumbers, eggplant (with peel on), peppers (hot and sweet), radishes, water chestnuts, and green olives.

High-salicylate fats include: almond oil, coconut oil, peanut oil, sesame oil, walnut oil, corn oil, and olive oil.

High-salicylate nuts and seeds include: macadamias, almonds, peanuts with skins, Brazil nuts, pine nuts, pistachios, and sesame seeds.

High-salicylate sweeteners: honey.

High-salicylate beverages include: peppermint tea and most herbal teas, fruit and vegetable juices, and caffeinated coffee.

If you have salicylate intolerance, it doesn't mean you can't consume even a bit of these foods; it just means you'll likely have to watch your overall salicylate load until your salicylate pathways are much improved. Also, keep in mind that artificial flavorings and colors, and preservatives such as BHT and sodium benzoate, often put additional load on the same pathways that clear salicylates, and may also trigger reactions.

Low- and Medium-Salicylate Foods

While a number of foods are high in salicylate, fortunately, there's a great variety of foods that are low in salicylate. For those who have salicylate intolerance, it can take an adjustment and some creativity to shift salicylate consumption, but it's possible to remain nutrient-balanced while eating a lower-salicylate diet. Here's a selection of negligible-, low-, and medium-level-salicylate foods. While some foods such as wheat, sugar, and soy oil, are low in salicylate, they aren't necessarily best for those with chronic health issues, but I've included these types of foods here for reference. Please note also that many people with salicylate intolerance are also affected by oxalates and sometimes by histamines, and might need a cross-referenced list for all of these food intolerances.

Low-to-medium-salicylate seasonings and flavorings include: salt, saffron, soy sauce, poppy seeds, cilantro, carob, cocoa, parsley, and garlic.

Low-to-medium-salicylate fruits include: banana, lime, lemon, pears, peeled Red or Yellow Delicious apples, passion fruit, mango, pawpaw, fresh figs, rhubarb, custard apple, kiwi, loquat, lychee, and tamarillo.

Low-to-medium-salicylate vegetables include: bamboo shoots, cabbage, celery, rutabagas, brussels sprouts, peeled eggplant, carrots, lettuces, mushrooms, beets, asparagus, black olives, fennel, turnip, spinach cauliflower, green beans, onions, potatoes, pumpkin, tomatoes, summer squash (zucchini and yellow), chayote squash, leeks, mung-bean sprouts, and shallots.

Low-to-medium-salicylate fats include: sunflower oil, soy oil, butter, ghee, and canola oil.

Low-to-medium-salicylate nuts and seeds include: poppy seeds, cashews, pecans, sunflower seeds, hazelnuts, fresh or dried coconut, walnuts, and peeled peanuts.

Low-to-medium-salicylate grains include: corn, millet, oats, rice, wheat, rye, buckwheat, and barley.

Low-to-medium salicylate sweeteners include: maple syrup, white sugar, light treacle, and molasses.

Low-to-medium-salicylate beverages include: water, decaf coffee, milk, soymilk, rice milk, dandelion coffee, rose hip tea, and fennel tea.

Low-to-medium-salicylate miscellany: beans, lentils, split peas, dairy (milk, cheese, plain yogurt), unprocessed meat, fish, shellfish, eggs, and tofu.

Supplements, Medications, and Topicals

Another place where salicylates are commonly found is in medications and supplements. Not many supplements have been tested at this point, but I've observed that most herbal supplements, such as CBD, perilla, astragalus, milk thistle, St. John's wort, valerian, Chinese skullcap, sulforaphane (broccoli-sprout extract), quercetin, aloe, resveratrol, propolis, DGL, holy basil, ginkgo biloba, pycnogenol, ginger, black cumin seed (*Nigella sativa*), and mangosteen tend to be problematic for those with salicylate intolerance. Often, oral and topical medications that contain salicylates are also challenging. These include aspirin, Pepto Bismol (bismuth subsalicylate), magnesium salicylate, diflunisal, salsalate, Alka Seltzer (original and extra-strength, which contain aspirin), and choline salicylate.

Fortunately, there are many low-salicylate supplements and medications. Vitamins and minerals, such as B vitamins, magnesium, calcium, chromium, etc., don't contain salicylates by themselves. Further, fish oils and their active form, SPMs, are low in salicylate—just watch for other ingredients like lemon flavor, which could add some salicylate load depending on how concentrated it is.

Salicylates can also be absorbed through the skin in topical products, whether medicated products or personal products, such as deodorants, sunscreen, shampoo, soap, lotion, toothpaste, mouthwash, etc. Many topical medications contain salicylic acid, menthol, mint, birch, and a variety of other high-salicylate herbals. Look for variations of the word "salicylate" on the ingredients label; look for *sal-ethyl carbonate* and *stroncylate* too.

Other sources can include cleaners and significant contact with plants that are high in salicylates, if one is crushing the leaves or releasing the oils in some way.

Addressing Salicylate Intolerance

Fortunately, salicylate intolerance is reversible for most people. The first step is to determine whether you have it. Then, as you learned at the start of this chapter, identifying the root triggers that affect salicylate degradation and lowering the load are key to recovery. To recap, here are the major contributors to salicylate intolerance:

- Overconsumption of salicylate compounds (particularly an overuse of medications like aspirin and Pepto Bismol)
- Mold toxicity and chemical toxicity
- Oxalate issues (due to oxalate load on the sulfation pathways also needed to break down salicylates)
- Depletion of nutrients needed for the various detox pathways due to food restrictions, absorption issues, or toxicity depleting nutrient levels
- Lack of sulfurous veggies in diet (for sulfation pathway support)
- Lack of d-glucaric acid-containing plants in diet (for glucuronidation pathway support)

Here are the major steps that I've seen help many people with salicylate intolerance:

- Temporarily reducing salicylate load in foods, beverages, medications, supplements, and topical products
- Reducing mast-cell activation
- Introducing some key supports that help with salicylate breakdown and mast cells
- Reducing chemical toxin and mold toxin load on the liver and kidney pathways
- Reducing pathogenic bacteria in the gut
- Improving healthy gut microbiome and gut lining

Regarding the abovementioned key supports, I'll briefly mention a few. For those who are very sensitive, these should be introduced in the correct order at the right time, and you can review the mast-cell chapter (chapter 4) for more details on this approach and the mast-cell supports I mention next. These are a few of the low-salicylate, low-histamine mast-cell supplemental supports that can be very helpful: SPMs, DAO, bicarbonates, D3, magnesium, vitamin B1, low-salicylate vitamin C, and dye-free H1 and H2 blockers. Charcoal can bind to excess salicylates. Epsom salt baths support the sulfur pathways that help with both salicylates and oxalates, but for those with a high oxalate load, Epsom salt may need to be started as low as 1–2 tablespoons in an entire bath, or just a sprinkle for the most sensitive. Further, calcium-d-glucarate and astaxanthin are low-salicylate options to support the glucuronidation pathway. While the implementation of these is outside the scope of this chapter, you now have an idea of how salicylate intolerance can be approached.

Conclusion: Ending with Hope

This chapter is meant as a starting point, but it's not comprehensive enough to guide you fully in addressing salicylates. Salicylate intolerance (along with oxalate issues) is one of the most challenging food intolerances to navigate, and if you're concerned about salicylate intolerance, I strongly recommend you work with a healthcare provider who is experienced in this area.

I can't emphasize enough that you don't want to whittle down your foods list unnecessarily. This can lead to serious nutrient depletion, which can worsen issues like salicylate intolerance, oxalate issues, histamine intolerance, mast-cell activation, and detoxification, to name just a few. I made this mistake many years ago. I was reacting every time I ate, and thought that if I kept a food diary and eliminated the foods I'd eaten when I reacted, I'd be able to unlock what was causing my issues. In a matter of just a few months with this approach, I was down to only ten foods plus some seasoning I tolerated. My reactions reduced for a few months, which brought me some short-lived relief, but then I spiraled into severe sensitivities and mast-cell activation with anaphylaxis. At the time, I couldn't find anyone who understood these issues and could help me, and I learned many lessons the hard way. Fortunately, practitioner knowledge and experience has grown exponentially since then. Be sure to think about swapping and replacing foods rather than eliminating unnecessarily, and please seek professional help if you're dealing with these types of issues. It's not something that's easily done properly on one's own.

That said, it does get better! Working with the underlying root causes of salicylate intolerance can help you improve your detoxification pathways and GI tract and allow you to safely return to adding salicylate foods and possibly herbs back into your life. I now enjoy a widely varied diet and can eat salicylate foods again with no issues. My histamine, oxalate, and lectin issues have greatly improved as well. I'll end, however, with telling you about Maya, whom you read about earlier. Maya greatly reduced her salicylate load, and we worked on switching her to a variety of low-to-medium-oxalate foods to maintain variety and enjoyment. About three months into lowering her salicylate load, the flushing, hives, tightness in her chest, and diarrhea completely resolved. Six months later, Maya's ear ringing was down by half. She'd failed numerous protocols previously, so we took a different tactic: Over time, she introduced most of the supports I mentioned above, and did a gentle, low-salicylate mold detox. Her tinnitus stopped completely after one year into the detox protocol. Her mycotoxin levels gradually came down over two years, and she's now reintroduced many high-salicylate foods, such as raspberries, all herbs, cinnamon, nutmeg, olive oil, and coconut oil. She's able to eat in restaurants and with friends without any problems. She can take some herbal supplements now as well, including a lower-dose quercetin called isoquercetin, perilla seed extract, and milk thistle extract. Maya worked hard over the past two years, and it's really paid off.

Reversing salicylate intolerance takes time. It's not an overnight experience, nor is it simple to navigate. It takes several weeks to several months for a person's salicylate load to reduce, but if you keep your mind focused on the fact that healing is possible and keep taking small steps each day, you'll eventually get there. Know that you aren't in this alone, and there are excellent resources out there to support you. Many others have reversed their salicylate intolerance, and you can too!

Resources

Books

The Salicylate Handbook by Sharla Race
Beyond the Salicylate Handbook by Sharla Race

Blogs

www.mastcell360.com/salicylates

Find low-salicylate recipes (that are also low histamine, low lectin, and low oxalate) at www.mastcell360.com.
Visit www.foodcanmakeyouill.co.uk/salicylate-in-food.html

BETH O'HARA is a Functional Naturopathic Consultant who specializes in complex, chronic cases of Mast Cell Activation Syndrome (MCAS), histamine intolerance, salicylate intolerance, and Mold Toxicity. She is the founder and clinical director of Mast Cell 360, which she designed to be the kind of practice she wished had existed when she was severely ill with Mast Cell Activation Syndrome, histamine intolerance, mold toxicity, neural inflammation, Lyme, *Bartonella,* Babesiosis, fibromyalgia, and chronic fatigue.

Her mission today is to be a guiding light for others with MCAS, histamine intolerance, and related conditions in their healing journeys. She holds a doctorate in Functional Naturopathy, a master's degree in Marriage and Family Therapy, and a bachelor's degree in Physiological Psychology. You can find a number of resources at mastcell360.com including blogposts, courses, and information about the Mast Cell 360 practice. You can also join the Mast Cell 360 community and get access to a number of free educational videos by liking the Mast Cell 360 page on Facebook. We look forward to having you join us!

Chapter 15: Dental and Facial Components of Sensitivity

Tasha Turzo, DO

Dr. Nathan's Introduction

At first glance, a reader might think *Maybe I can skip this chapter; after all, what in the world do the face and jaw have to do with sensitivity?* From personal experience that I shared with Dr. Turzo, including the story of the patient featured at the end of this chapter, when patients are unable to tolerate *any* of our treatments (including limbic/vagal/mast cell and supplements), I have to consider the possibility that the difficulty in healing comes from a compromised structure of the face and jaw. This was alluded to in chapter 5, on the Spiky-Leaky Syndrome, but here Dr. Turzo provides you a full understanding of the critical role of these structures in the development of sensitivities. These issues are far more common than is usually appreciated, so consider this chapter a guide for delving more deeply into factors that might be setting off your sensitivities.

✿ ✿ ✿

This chapter is about the often-missed—and vital-to-survival—craniofacial and jaw function, and the serious health consequences associated with head, face, neck, and dental-occlusion compromises. My hope is that it will lay the foundation for a broadened perspective and treatment plans for our sensitive patients, some of whom will be unable to respond to the usual treatments until these craniofacial issues are properly addressed.

People who have chronic inflammation such as mold toxicity and other biochemical imbalances and also have craniofacial dysfunctions can have a much more complicated healing process.

Optimal craniofacial structural development begins in utero. If the mother's facial structures are compromised with an underdeveloped upper and lower jaw that creates a suboptimal airway (the space behind the tongue), the baby's growing face is formed in this oxygen-deprived state, resulting in an underdeveloped upper and lower jaw. This situation demonstrates one of the basic principles of osteopathy: the dysfunction of a system (suboptimal oxygenation) creates a dysfunctional structure (underdeveloped facial structures).

A mother with a compromised facial breathing structure will create a child with an underdeveloped facial airway. Our health begins with our capacity to breathe and to oxygenate our tissues for growth and repair. If we don't have optimal oxygenation, our biological system will be dysregulated and will function in survival mode, which can dictate our experiences in life as fright, flight, fight, or paralysis. Unfortunately, over the generations since the industrial revolution, processed foods, poor soil nutrition, and a softer diet have stunted our facial growth and have created an underdeveloped upper and lower jaw structure. Thus most of our patients these days have some degree of a suboptimal airway, leading to a heightened survival-mode-wired nervous system with less ability to meet other life challenges.

The birth process is the second experience that can compromise craniofacial growth and development. As the baby's head molds and compensates to deal with the forces of birthing as it comes through the birth canal, cranial-nerve injuries and entrapments can occur in an attempt to prevent injury to the head and neck. Some of our sensitive patients were compromised at birth with vagal nerve-entrapment syndrome, creating a whole-body compromise with suboptimal vagal tone. A compromised vagus nerve decreases the body's ability to detoxify biotoxins, including mycotoxins, which could explain why some patients' detoxification process is slower, tolerating smaller amounts of binders or none at all.

Other cranial nerves can also be entrapped during a traumatic birth, such as the hypoglossal nerve, which controls the muscle contraction and coordination of the tongue. Compromise to this nerve will create a narrow palate with an underdeveloped face, a compromised airway, potential jaw-joint problems, and chronic neck pain. Who knew that our birth could create such significant health issues? Actually, throughout life, any injury to the head and neck can have effects similar to those of a cranial birth trauma, and affect the entire functioning of the central and peripheral nervous system, leading to a dysregulated nervous and immune system. This concept is central to understanding how these imbalances may contribute to the development of sensitivity in patients who are at risk, especially through their effects on the limbic system and vagus nerve, which are paramount in this discussion.

For a person with craniofacial dysfunction, the function, motion, and structures of the cranium and face are compromised, creating increased sensory input to the brain. Because the face and head houses our functions of survival (airway, swallowing, and chewing), this area of our body sends exponentially more neural signals to the brain than other parts of our body do. The increase in sensory input to the brain optimizes adaptability toward survival. We grow toward maximizing our airway just as plants grow toward sunlight. The sensory input from our craniofacial complex drives our facial growth, body posture, and even our dental occlusion. When there's a compromise to the function and structure of the craniofacial complex, the excessive sensory input to the brain can create a neuronal crisis, leading to a cell-danger response with overwhelming sensations. Increased pain in the craniofacial complex can increase pain in the rest of the body. The limbic system can be repeatedly activated with a craniofacial dysfunction as the neural input informs the brain that survival conditions are being threatened. This situation can also be stimulated by an injured tooth or a subacute infection associated with a bad root canal. The neural input through the trigeminal nerve, which contains the largest sensory nerve input to the brain, can create an overstimulation of the brain. As the sensory input from the trigeminal nerve is received in the reticular formation in the brain, the overloading input creates disintegrated neural output responses that can leave the nervous system in a state of heightened sensitivity, panic, and sensations which are chaotic. There is a biological reason for the trigeminal nerve to take up so much space in the brain: it's the sensory input from the face that holds our vital survival functions of breathing, chewing, and swallowing. This information is essential for the body to make adaptive compensations to optimize health. If there is craniofacial dysfunction, the overstimulation of input to the brain creates a condition that compromises the healing process. Relieving craniofacial dental dysfunction can give the system immense mental, emotional, and physical relief, allowing the body to heal itself with greater ease and peace.

Causes of craniofacial dysfunction include:

- Birth trauma to the craniofacial area
- Plagiocephaly (asymmetrical head at birth)
- Torticollis (spasm of the neck muscles at birth that causes the neck to twist to one side)
- History of head/face/neck injury
- Temporomandibular joint dysfunction
- Tongue-tie
- Abnormal swallowing pattern
- Misalignment of the teeth

Symptoms of craniofacial dysfunction include:

- Vagal nerve compromise and dysautonomia (disorder of the autonomic nervous system)
- GI dysregulation
- Brain fog
- Head and neck pain
- Trigeminal neuralgia (sudden, severe facial pain)
- Bell's palsy
- Difficulty with mycotoxin detoxification
- Difficulty nursing
- Torticollis
- Allergies
- Open-mouth posturing with narrow palate and dental crowding
- Dysfunction of the temporomandibular joint (the hinge joint between the temporal bone and the lower jaw)
- Abnormal swallowing pattern
- Misalignment of the teeth
- History of being a colicky baby
- Facial asymmetry
- Visual disturbances
- Chronic sinus and ear infections
- Sleep apnea
- Facial tics

Craniofacial structure and function are important to overall health, but how does trauma specifically affect the functioning of the head, face, and neck? Basically, trauma affects the motion and function of these structures, and it's essential for health that the body has sufficient motion to optimize function. Motion is the basis of life and is the essential component in a biotensegrity system such as our bodies. (Biotensegrity: Our bones are held in position by tension from our muscles and fascia. The shape of our body is maintained by the balance of this tension across our entire structure.) The capacity for expansion and contraction or compression of the body is vital for the pumping action needed to drive vital nutrients (blood, venous, and lymphatic) into and out of our cells. Flexibility and stability are also essential to the capacity for movement of the body as a whole. The body is one functioning unit. The cranium and face have a subtle physiological motion that is crucial to optimal health, and trauma can affect the motion and function of the system.

The biotensegrity model explains the complexities of movement and stability of an interdependent, integrated, complex system in living organisms. This principle is based on the ability of all parts of the system to be in motion. If one area is restricted by an injury or compromise to the tissues, the entire system is constantly compensating for that restriction, which creates a disintegrative biological system.

Our fascial matrix is an interconnected tensional network. Our bones are not in direct contact with each other; rather they float in the tension structure created by our fascial network. Bones and tissues make up a dynamic balance of compression (pushing forces) and tension (pulling forces). Through this fascial network, any force can influence and adapt to any part of the whole, from cells to the entire body. In other words, our structure functions to create stability and a homeostatic neural input to the brain. (For more on this subject, see chapter 16 on osteopathic manipulation and its role in the sensitive patient).

Twenty-nine bones, including the three inner ear bones and the hyoid bone, participate in the integrity of the craniofacial complex. These bones interdigitate with one another in a unique pattern, creating a specific motion for each bone. The subtle movement of each bone is essential not only for providing a cushion for compression to protect the brain from injury but also to provide a flexible container for the breathing (movement) of the central nervous system, which is paramount for the brain-drainage detoxification process, called *glymphatic drainage.* This process keeps the brain healthy by pumping out toxic products of cellular respiration along with other toxins that can damage neighboring healthy brain cells. This subtle inherent physiological motion of the face and cranium is our protection against neurodegenerative diseases, which are now understood to result from an inflammatory process that the body is unable to regulate properly. The motion and compressible nature of the craniofacial bones are vital to the optimal functioning of the brain and cranial nerves. A compromise to the motion or position of any of the twenty-nine bones can have a profound effect on the health of the individual by affecting the brain-detoxification process and/or impinging on key cranial nerves.

Let's circle back to how our birth process can affect our healing capacities. The birth process is one of the most formative processes most of us will encounter. The compressive forces that shape the cranium affect the craniofacial structure and functions. It's never too late in one's life to receive cranial osteopathic treatment to address craniofacial birth compressions. We continue to heal and remodel until we are no longer breathing.

During birth, the baby's head compresses the mother's cervix to stimulate dilation and open the tissues. Any compromise to the opening of the cervix (secondary to malposition of the baby's head and other causes) that creates less stimulation to the tissues or lack of softening of the cervix can lead to an increase in compression into the baby's head, creating cranial injuries. A birth in which Pitocin, vacuum extraction, or forceps are used, or that exceeds the "pushing stage" of two hours, is considered a traumatic birth from the baby's perspective. The area of the baby's skull that is most vulnerable to compression and displacement is the back of the head. The cranial bone in the back of the head is called the occiput, and it articulates with the first cervical vertebra. This is the most resistant area to molding and compensation of the birth forces. The first joint that the compressive forces encounter is between the occiput and the first cervical vertebrae. The four very important cranial nerves which exit the skull at the base of the cranium, between the occipital, temporal, and first cervical vertebrae are the glossopharyngeal (IX), vagus (X), accessory (XI), and hypoglossal nerves (XII).

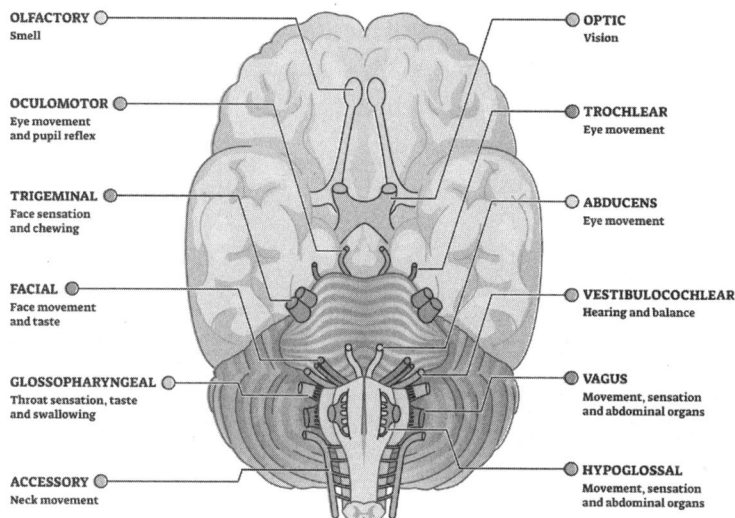

OLFACTORY
Smell

OCULOMOTOR
Eye movement
and pupil reflex

TRIGEMINAL
Face sensation
and chewing

FACIAL
Face movement
and taste

GLOSSOPHARYNGEAL
Throat sensation, taste
and swallowing

ACCESSORY
Neck movement

OPTIC
Vision

TROCHLEAR
Eye movement

ABDUCENS
Eye movement

VESTIBULOCOCHLEAR
Hearing and balance

VAGUS
Movement, sensation
and abdominal organs

HYPOGLOSSAL
Movement, sensation
and abdominal organs

Cranial Nerves

The glossopharyngeal aids in the swallowing process. The vagus nerve has the widest effects in the body, ranging from gastrointestinal health to emotional well-being and cardiac function. Any compromise to this nerve can have vast health effects. The accessory nerve innervates the trapezius and sternocleidomastoid muscle (SCM) and is responsible for turning the head and neck. Compromise to this nerve creates torticollis (wry neck). The hypoglossal nerve is the motor nerve to the tongue. When this nerve is entrapped, the baby is unable to nurse and swallow properly. The atypical swallowing pattern will affect normal facial growth and thus compromise the development of an optimal airway, which is a growing, undiagnosed compromise to one's health.

The consequences of compression of these nerves include issues with swallowing, sucking, digestion, range of motion of the neck, torticollis, spitting up after feedings, gas, bloating, and constipation. A functional swallow is a primary driving force for facial growth and development which creates space for all thirty-two teeth. If the hypoglossal nerve has been compromised by a head injury or birth trauma, there will be suboptimal formation of the palate and airway, leading to crowding of the teeth and misalignment of the dental occlusion. The position of our teeth is a consequence of our breathing, swallowing, and chewing pattern, tongue-resting position, and the position of the craniofacial bones. The teeth will erupt and move to form an occlusion, in which the teeth in the upper jaw touch the teeth in the lower jaw, forming the largest "joint" in our bodies in order to support an upright physiological position and neurological neutrality. If the teeth are not in a supportive occlusion, the neural sensory input to the brain through the trigeminal nerve can create an overwhelming constant feedback that "something's not right."

This constant feeling of dis-ease provides ongoing, relentless stimulation of the sympathetic nervous system that continually signals the limbic system and vagal nerves to be alert to the possibility of danger or threat, and can be an important stimulus to the creation of a hypervigilant, sensitive patient.

Common symptoms of compression at the base of the head (occipital condylar compression) include:

- Nursing problems
- Poor milk supply
- Painful nipples with nursing
- Baby falling asleep on the breast
- Difficulty sucking and latching
- Reflux and vomiting
- Spitting up after nursing
- Colic
- Opisthotonus (arching of the head)
- Constipation/gas and bloating
- Airway issues/snoring
- Crowding and misaligned teeth

Craniofacial Dysfunction and the Vagus Nerve

The vagus nerve has been named the King of the Nerves because of its myriad effects and influences. It's the longest cranial nerve, traveling between the head and the gut, and is thus at greater risk for compressive forces and injury compared to the other eleven cranial nerves, which travel shorter distances. The most common areas of structural compromise to the vagus nerve are as it exits the base of the cranium between the occiput and temporal bone and as it travels in front of the upper cervical vertebrae. Head and neck traumas can injure the nerve and create "vagal compression syndrome." Many studies cite the relationship between the vagus and the brain-gut connection. There is also evidence of the onset of "leaky gut" within two weeks of a head injury, which will affect the capacity to detoxify biotoxins, including mycotoxins. Birth trauma, cervical whiplash injuries, head injuries, and temporomandibular dysfunction (TMD), including all its etiologies, are the most common causes of the compressive dysregulation of the vagus nerve that creates vagal compression syndrome.

As the vagus exits the cranium between the occiput and temporal bones, the motion of the temporomandibular joint and the temporal bone can affect vagal tone. Restriction of the joint and temporal bone can compress the fascial-filled space called the jugular foramen, which is a space between the occipital and temporal bones. This provides the exit for the vagus, glossopharyngeal, and accessory nerves out of the cranium to their endgame innervations. If the temporal bone has been slightly displaced and/or compromised in its motion, the jugular foramen will have less space, creating an entrapment of these cranial nerves and lymphatic and venous drainage.

Most of the lymphatic and venous drainage from the brain also exits the skull through this space. Our lymphatic and venous system is completely dependent on motion for drainage. This is why the lymphatic and venous vessels are located between muscles and bones. They need the pumping action of those structures to create a negative pressure that is the driving force for fluid drainage. So, yes, our brains drain toxins through the space between the occiput and temporal bone, and the health of our brains is dependent on our cranial motion and most specifically our temporal bones.

Temporomandibular Dysfunction

The temporomandibular joint (TMJ) is crucial in balancing the cranio-cervical mandibular dental complex. We still have much to learn, however, about its contribution to craniofacial dysfunction, vagal dysfunctions, neurodegenerative diseases, glymphatics, airway dysfunction, and movement disorders, as well as diffuse and localized chronic pain syndromes.

Traumatic injuries are an important cause of TMD disorders affecting the vagal tone. Individuals who sustained whiplash injuries in automobile accidents have an increased risk of developing TMD. Many people have experienced pain, popping, crepitus, and/or a change in the opening width of the mouth after a car accident. The TMJ is the accommodator for the changes in the cranium, cervical vertebrae, vision, dental occlusion, tongue function, and neuromuscular integration, as well as vagus-nerve function. It connects the face with the cranial bones, hyoid, and cervical vertebrae. What is commonly missed about this joint is that it stabilizes the functioning and volume (space) of our airway (the space behind the tongue and in front of the neck), as well as swallowing, chewing, speech, and cervical stability. We need our jaw joints to have peak functioning for optimal capacity for airway, chewing, swallowing, and brain drain for neurological function and capacity to maintain an upright position. Craniofacial dysfunction and vagal compression syndrome play a large but often unappreciated role in our patients who have developed POTS (postural tachycardia syndrome), many of whom have lost the ability to stand upright without getting unusually dizzy or light-headed.

There is clear evidence that patients who have experienced a traumatic brain injury (TBI) are more prone to neurodegenerative diseases. The osteopathic perspective in understanding these illnesses is that the central nervous system, the dural membranes, and the cranial bones have had their inherent motion restricted through the compressive forces of an injury, and thus brain drain or glymphatic flow has been compromised. When there are obstacles to brain drain, products of normal cellular respiration become toxic waste products and build up within the brain, damaging the surrounding healthy brain cells and leading to neurodegenerative diseases, almost all of which are associated with the accumulation of these cellular waste products in the brain and the inflammatory reaction this creates. Having an open outflow, which includes soft mobile cervical tissue, helps keep the brain draining and healthy. There also needs to be freedom of movement in the front of the neck—scalene and sternocleidomastoid (SCM) muscles—for optimal lymphatic draining out of the head and into the neck. Brain fog is a common experience when there is suboptimal craniofacial motion, as the cells in the brain are compromised with toxic cellular debris. Suboptimal sleep also relates to suboptimal glymphatic drainage. Most of the brain drain happens while we sleep, as the brain cells contract and allow the toxins to exit into the fluid between cells and out of the brain through the glymphatics. Thus the less sleep we have the less brain drain we get. An increase in sensitivity and fragility of health could be a consequence of a functional/structural injury to the head, face, and/or neck area, which can compromise optimal brain drain and lead to vast health challenges.

The Current Epidemic of Airway Compromises

Today, with our upper and lower jaws underdeveloped, our faces have more of a "bulldog" look than they did thousands of years ago. This shorter face from front to back leaves a smaller space behind the tongue for air to travel to our lungs, leading to airway deficiency. This is another cause of craniofacial dysfunction for the sensitive patient. Many factors contribute to this development. The human diet has been softening ever since the use of fire for cooking, and it softened further in the transition from hunting to farming, but it was not until the rapid spread of industrialization in the nineteenth and twentieth centuries that food became so soft that it deprived the jaw system of the exercise needed by the jaw muscles to develop properly and stimulate facial growth. The resulting loss of healthy chewing exercise and the consequential changes in the form and function of the jaw system have significantly altered the pattern of modern human facial growth. This produces a number of significant health issues, including sleep apnea, diabetes, cardiovascular disease, hypertension, stroke, depression, dementia, dysbiosis, CFS, poor vagal tone, and attention deficit disorder (ADD/ADHD). These are all consequences of airway compromises. (See chapter 5 for the connections of these interweaving issues in the creation of the Spiky-Leaky Syndrome).

There is also a significant rise in the incidence of tongue-ties. Presently, one in three children is tongue-tied. A limited and dysregulated tongue function will create distortion and dysfunction to the craniofacial complex. Why is there a decrease in facial development over time, an increase in sleep apnea, crowding of the teeth in children, and tongue-tie? They are all related and have to do with the interplay of our modern diet, environmental toxins, nutrient-poor soil, invasive birth interventions, and loss of the functions that create the face.

The nutrient-poor condition of our lands and foods has also created softer, weaker bone structure. We are now born with a degree of osteopenia (weak bones). We see this in children as changes in the arch structures of the body, all the way from a narrow high palate to collapsing foot arches (pronation). A collapse in structure is occurring. The cranial bones are also softer and less dense, which can lead to less protection during the birthing process as well as predisposition to traumatic brain injury. The combination of increased forces used at birth (vacuum extractions and Pitocin) and a less protective cranium creates a setup for increased cranial nerve injuries.

The consequence of the above conditions is that our faces are compromised for airway patency; thus we have less adaptive capacity to optimize full function. Sometimes just one too many required compromises leads to a collapse of the system.

Treatments for Craniofacial Dysfunction

Osteopathic treatments engage areas of the body that have tissue restrictions and are compressed, usually secondary to injury or repetitive-use injuries. Through engaging the restricted tissues as a fluid state, these treatments can resolve the restricted tissue and restore physiological motion. The separated hard and compressed tissue is then able to integrate with the whole of the system back into its physiologically fluid state, thus restoring inherent motion and optimal health.

The osteopathic perspective is to first remove the obstacles to health by restoring normal physiological motion, and then see how the body can heal itself. When motion has been restored, the need for specific interventions becomes clearer and less invasive.

I like the image of a stormy sea as the complicated, sensitive patients. By engaging tissues to create a "neutral" in the tissues of the storm, the areas that are the fulcrum of the problem become clear, and the sea and tissue can tell us where we need to intervene. It helps to differentiate what the primary dysfunctions and compensations are, clarifying and potentially simplifying the treatment process.

Other modalities besides osteopathic treatments that I've found extremely helpful in treating patients with craniofacial dysfunctions are functional medicine, mycotoxin binders, homeopathic constitutional remedies, prolotherapy/PRP (platelet-rich plasma) injections, cold laser therapy, and Fotona 1064 laser treatments.

Osteopathic treatments can increase motion and improve tissue flexibility, but if the ligaments are hypermobile secondary to injury, inflammation (triggered by MCAS), EDS (Ehlers-Danlos syndrome), or poor nutrition, the implementation of prolotherapy and PRP has been extremely helpful. This modality in the hands of an osteopathic physician is very potent, as we can feel which tissues need the support, and that can guide the injections to be very specific to address the instability. Some patients are finding relief from craniocervical instability (CCI) with PRP. From a holistic perspective, it's important to address all the cervical instability, not just the first cervical vertebra. Laser therapy is one of the cutting-edge treatment modalities. There is so much potential to heal with photobiomodulation, which helps regenerate tissue. I use this method daily with most of my patients. I have also been providing constitutional homeopathic remedies for nearly thirty years in my practice. It's been a miracle turnaround for many of my patients.

The osteopathic, myofunctional, and orthodontic ALF (advanced lightwire functionals) appliance has also been extremely helpful for patients with airway, tongue, and temporomandibular dysfunctions and/or malocclusions. This is a light wire that is placed behind the teeth and is adjusted monthly by an ALF-trained dentist while an osteopath trained in the ALF approach also treats the patient. More about this can be found in my book *The ALF Approach*. As an osteopathic physician, I am committed to finding the Health first and then using "do no harm" interventions as much as possible to help patients heal themselves.

Signs to look for to diagnose craniofacial dysfunctions:

- Facial and cranial asymmetry
- Inability to stick tongue out beyond lower lip (one can definitely still be tongue-tied even if a patient can stick their tongue out farther than the lower lip, but this is the first obvious sign). More information is in *The ALF Approach*.
- Hold cheeks apart and swallow. If you're unable to swallow with lips apart, you may have an abnormal swallowing pattern and should see a myofunctional therapist.

- Popping or clicking (or pain) when you open and close your jaw
- The lower center of your teeth not lining up with the center of your upper teeth. This could indicate that your lower jaw is shifted to one side.
- Any of the upper teeth occluding inside of the lower teeth (cross-bites)
- Any openings in your dental occlusion where the teeth do not come together
- Open-mouth breathing during the day or night
- Head is held forward of the neck.
- When opening the mouth you can see the back tissue arches and the airway opening underneath.

Those are just some of the physical expressions that indicate craniofacial dysfunctions. To help you to get a picture of how profoundly these issues can affect a patient's health, driving a sensitivity so intense that it literally takes over their life, I present the following case, some of which is told in the patient's own words.

Barry's Story

Dr. Nathan referred Barry to me because of his craniofacial dysfunction and history of an *inability to tolerate* any *binders or limbic retraining or vagal treatments or mast-cell activation supplements.* He was so compromised that the effort of picking up his kids would induce a HERX reaction. His facial pain was so intense he didn't know how he would survive. He, like so many of our patients, had been to dozens of practitioners and was holding on to a thin thread of hope.

Barry presented to my office with extreme facial and jaw-joint pain. He was restless with pain. He had a history of chronic sinus infections as a kid and grew up in a moldy house. He had a class 3 dental occlusion, in which the upper jaw is smaller than the lower jaw, and the upper teeth are occluded behind the lower teeth.

It's a classic representation of an airway-deficient facial structure with midface deficiency, typically caused by a tongue-tie and/or an open-mouth breathing habit. Given the history of growing up in a moldy house and a strongly positive mycotoxin urine test, the obvious conclusion was that Barry was unable to breathe through his nose secondary to the mold allergies, so he had to breathe through his mouth. The low tongue posturing (the normal resting position of the tongue is in the upper palate) as a result of open-mouth breathing affected the growth and development of his upper palate (the upper jaw bone, or *maxilla*). On initial examination, a tongue-tie was also diagnosed. Barry not only had open-mouth breathing influencing his underdeveloped facial growth but the limited range of motion of his tongue had impeded its resting position to the upper palate in order to grow the face in a forward direction.

Barry had had two surgeries in an attempt to correct his dental occlusion. Both included cutting the upper and lower jawbones and repositioning them to fix together. Barry had metal plates and screws in his face that were left from the surgery to stabilize the jawbones. After the first facial surgery, he began to have severe digestive issues, dizziness, and sleep disturbances. He later learned that this was the beginning of a vagal dysautonomia created by compression into the temporal and occipital bone connection with TMD. He then sought help from a functional-medicine doctor who suggested supplements that crashed Barry's life. Because his vagus severely compromised his neurogastric immunological capacity to react to detoxifying supplements, the detoxifying supplements created a complete shutdown of function. As Barry described the experience:

> Over those months of supplements and dietary restrictions, on a scale of 1–10, my quality of life went from 8 (before treatment) to 0 (after treatment). The only way to describe my life was "torture." I had lost the ability to fall asleep for more than five minutes, as I would be awoken by an electrical jolt throughout my body. My body had developed a constant internal vibratory sensation that felt like a second heartbeat, which was terrifying. I had continuous vertigo and dizziness. I became extremely sensitive to lights and sounds, and had vision impairments. I had tremors and fasciculations throughout my body. My face became numb with a constant tingling sensation. I started to itch all over, as though bugs were crawling through my skin. I had an incredible amount of brain fog and confusion and short-term memory problems. On top of that, my GI issues and pain were now much worse. All I could do was cry.

Barry was also severely impaired with pain which had been aggravated by several osteopaths who didn't understand the dental occlusal dysfunction and how it affects cervical and cranial function. After reading Barry's surgical reports, an MRI of his jaw, and a CBCT scan, it was clear to me that he needed an ALF-trained dentist to help stabilize and restore a physiological dental occlusion. This intervention would support his jaw joints as the osteopathic treatments unwound the craniofacial cervical trauma. It also became clear that Barry would need two more surgeries to remove the metal plates and screws from his face. Over the next three years, Barry would fly coast to coast to receive osteopathic treatments and laser treatments from me, and then see Dr. Bronson, DDS, in Virginia for adjustments to his ALF appliance. Barry also had a frenectomy, which gave his tongue the range of motion to reach his palate. With each functional swallow, the pressure from the palate into the base of the cranium augmented Barry's cranial motion and allowed his body to continue to heal itself. It was a three-year process, but slowly, and with a nonlinear pattern, Barry's health improved. He stated:

As my swallowing function continued to integrate and my craniofacial structures released, my body transitioned itself into detoxification mode. Every day, my doses of binders were increased until I was taking 2 teaspoons of activated charcoal, 4 *Saccharomyces* capsules, and 2 Welchol capsules. In the previous five-plus years, I had barely been able to remove any toxins from my body without exacerbations. Now, in a matter of two weeks, I had removed all the mycotoxins from my body. On January 4, 2022, a lab test confirmed that I was mold-free. With a proper swallow, my TMJ continues to heal and reposition my structure. My metabolism has shifted back to eating more carbohydrates. I can even eat gluten without a reaction now that the toxins are removed and my digestion has improved. I'm exercising every day or two, after not having been able to do any physical exertion for more than five years.

To this day, Barry is the most compromised and complex patient I've ever treated—and the greatest success story. His case demonstrated how treating the craniofacial system restored the cranial nerve functions, opened the airway, and improved the dental occlusion to help stabilize his temporomandibular and facial dysfunction. This treatment in turn simplified the process of detoxifying the mycotoxins. Barry was able to clear all the mold with a minimal amount of binders, and no follow-up antifungal treatment was needed.

The obstacles to his health needed to be identified and removed. Once the motion and health of his systems were integrated, his body was able to heal itself with less need for intervention.

Dr. A. T. Still, DO, founder of osteopathy, stated: "Anyone can find the disease, but who can find the Health?" We heal from our Health, not from our Dis-Ease. By restoring normal physiological motion, Barry was able to heal himself, and his body will continue to function at its optimal capacity. Thank you to Barry and Dr. Nathan for the opportunity to participate in his healing journey.

A take-home message: If your patient is struggling to quiet their nervous system despite heroic efforts to use the methods that can reboot the limbic and vagus-nerve systems or to take mast-cell supplements, consider the possibility of craniofacial dysfunction. Dig a little deeper into the patient's history and ask about possible birth trauma, injuries to the head and neck, and jaw dysfunction. It's possible that you might need to start their healing journey by first restoring craniosacral mobility.

TASHA TURZO, DO, graduated from Western University, Pomona, California, in 1994 where she received a Post Graduate Osteopathic Manual Medicine/Anatomy Fellowship. She completed her internship at the UCSF Family Medicine Residency. Since 1995 she has practiced osteopathy, homeopathy, functional medicine, and prolotherapy/PRP, and has specialized in craniofacial dysfunctions. Dr. Turzo has taught extensively in the field of craniofacial dysfunctions since 1997. Awarded a Fellowship of the Cranial Academy (FCA), she has been recognized as a leader in cranial osteopathy. She began co-treating patients with Dr. Nordstrom (creator of the ALF appliances) in 1995.

A founding member of AEI (ALF Educational Institute), she has taught many weekend courses to osteopaths, dentists, and myofunctional therapists. Dr. Turzo presents a two-day on-demand course, "The ALF Approach," as well as a hands-on course, "Treating Craniofacial Complexities." She is the administrator of The ALF Mentorship Program, which is an interprofessional online discussion group. She is an internationally recognized expert in the application of osteopathy and functional dentistry, with a focus on the use of Advanced Lightwire Functional (ALF) devices and TMD. Dr. Turzo published her book, *The ALF Approach,* in 2020. She is also medical director of two nutritional IV and injectables clinics, BeWell IV. Her website is drtashaturzo.com.

Chapter 16: Structural Components of Sensitization

T. Carmine Van Deven, DO

Dr. Nathan's Introduction

In the previous chapter, Dr. Turzo laid the groundwork for understanding the importance and relevance of looking at a patient's physical structure, especially of the face and jaw, as another component of the development and perpetuation of sensitivity. Here, Dr. Van Deven expands that discussion to include the entire physical structure and how it relates to the health of every patient. For those trained as MDs, the study of structure isn't given much importance, nor is it connected to every aspect of a patient's health. For osteopaths (DOs), however, it's a vital part of their education. Soon after I completed medical school, I was fortunate enough to stumble into osteopathic studies, and am grateful for the osteopathic physicians who trained me to feel the physiological phenomena Dr. Van Deven refers to. At times, he waxes rhapsodic about these perceptions and the sacred gift that allows him to connect deeply to the needs of his patients. I corroborate his perceptions: they're no exaggeration; rather, they are what can be taught, to those who will embrace this journey, as a unique skillset that resonates to the sensitivity of our patients. This allows us, through the sense of touch, to communicate our compassion at a level beyond the spoken word and thereby convey to our patients a sense of safety and trust that facilitates healing. It would be a rare patient who, having acquired a complex illness, didn't have related structural issues that would respond well to structural treatment. In fact, for some patients, this is the "stuck" realm that needs to be addressed for healing to become possible.

✧ ✧ ✧

Introduction

The human body is a functional whole with tremendous ability to overcome challenges, adapt, and thrive. Motion is integral to this dynamic process as an expression of health and is essential to life itself. This includes all aspects of anatomy and physiology, animated by spirit, thus creating the living presence of human form.

When the many structures of the body are in the correct three-dimensional position, movement is fluid and easy. Anti-gravity mechanisms suspend and balance all bones, tissues, and organs. Fluids circulate and physiology is self-regulating. The body is expansive and free, and inherent healing forces are free to act.

Sometimes, however, an acute event or prolonged strain can significantly derail normal functioning and lead to a cascade of health challenges. This is especially so with sensitive and chronically ill patients, who would likely benefit from an osteopathic approach to health.

Osteopathy

The unity of body, mind, and spirit and our innate capacity to heal from within are the founding principles of Osteopathy. Dr. Andrew Taylor Still, originally trained as a traditional allopathic physician, developed Osteopathic Medicine in 1874 to include hands-on diagnosis and treatment, which was ultimately the catalyst for the resolution of a wide range of diseases and conditions. This system of medicine recognizes that the structure and function of the body are inseparable, acting as one event.

William G. Sutherland, DO, a student of Dr. Still's, continued to expand the osteopathic concept as it relates to the cranium. His appreciation of the movement at the sutures and of the tissues within the skull introduced new diagnostic and treatment applications throughout the body. Over time he became increasingly aware of subtle forces that are at the heart of maintaining and restoring health. This was the basis for what is known as cranial osteopathy.

Many people are not aware that the medical training of osteopathic physicians (DOs) parallels that of allopathic physicians (MDs), and both are licensed to prescribe medications, deliver babies, and perform surgery as per their training. The difference is that DOs are additionally trained to sense health and disease with their hands by way of extensive hands-on training, enhancing their ability to feel structural and functional imbalances in their patients and to properly treat them using a variety of approaches.

In the following pages we will explore the osteopathic concept and shine light on underlying mechanisms that predispose and contribute to illness and sensitivities. We will then review the osteopathic exam, common findings, osteopathic treatment, and relate Mary's story to bring it all together. All of this is specific to the sensitive patient, though the principles presented apply to patients of all ages and conditions.

Structure and Function

Continuity exists throughout the body, and is interwoven at every level. The physical body is not simply a physical container but rather the direct extension and expression of underlying function and physiology. From the perspective of wholeness, structure and function are one activity. This is a fundamental principle of all living beings.

On the physical level, changes to our structure will impact function and vice versa. An injury such as a fall may compress and distort the bony frame, muscular, and connective tissue elements, altering motion and function of the joints. It may also affect the position and function of various tissues, organs, and fluids of the body. Conversely, disease and other disruptions of normal physiology will alter the anatomy. A lesser-known example is a viscerosomatic reflex, whereby dysfunction of an internal organ may lead to hypertonicity (muscle overactivity) and tenderness of paravertebral muscles at the corresponding spinal level. This occurs by way of nerve signals to the spinal cord, and may assist in identifying the cause of a patient's symptoms.

It is important to also acknowledge the impact that emotional, mental, and spiritual health have on both function and structure. Sudden and profound emotional stress is known to trigger an acute heart failure in those previously without heart disease, for example. Meanwhile, positive emotions, such as hope and faith, will reduce the risk of heart disease as well as other diseases. Thus patterns of thoughts and feelings may be profoundly influential. The entirety of who we are is manifest in our physical being and its underlying motion.

Motion

The living body is a symphony of motion. We experience this on a macroscopic level as we walk, dance, and play. Joints move smoothly through their range of motion, held in balanced tension by muscles, tendons, ligaments, and a three-dimensional web of fascia that extends from head to toe. Concurrently, the whole, undivided body expresses inherent rhythmic motion. There is a lengthening and shortening, while laterally paired structures internally and externally rotate in cycles. In addition to the mobility of internal organs with gross motion, each moves on a specific axis at its own tempo. For example, the brain gently coils and uncoils, suspended in cerebrospinal fluid, while motion at the cranial sutures allows for the bones to move in relation to one another and the shape of the skull to change accordingly. As we broaden our awareness beyond mechanical motion, we see that the body moves through a three-dimensional process of inhalation and exhalation, expansion and contraction. We are a drop in the ocean being breathed by a unifying source.

Simultaneously, physiology is also in motion. Electrical impulses extend from the brain, heart, and gut and travel through nerves to their target tissues and organs. Endocrine glands produce and release hormones into the bloodstream. Blood and lymphatic fluid glide through vessels and channels, driven by the beat of the heart, pulsation of vessel walls, contraction of skeletal muscle, and the pumping of our diaphragms. Nutrition is delivered to every cell, absorbed and used within, while metabolic waste and toxins are expelled and removed from the immediate environment. Effortless communication takes place across all systems and tissues. Ideally, the living continuum of function and structure is seamless throughout the body at every level, made possible through motion and driven by spirit. From the perspective of the natural world, there is no anatomy, only inherent function.

The principle of motion also applies to mental and spiritual health. One of the most important aspects of the human experience is personal evolution, the ease and speed of which is determined by the individual. This includes accepting and embracing new and sometimes radically different perspectives, ideas, and belief systems that empower health and embody love. The end result of this process is the discovery and pursuit of a life purpose that is in alignment with The True Self. This involves stepping forward into the unknown and even feared spaces as an act of faith. While illness invites these opportunities, patients tend to have trouble moving in this direction, often secondary to traumatic events that have limited their abilities to heal and to trust.

Trauma

Trauma is a common underlying cause of disease, particularly for sensitive patients. It has many forms, all of which can alter both structure and function. Subsequent dysfunction of the hypothalamic pituitary adrenal (HPA) axis, limbic system, and autonomic nervous system can affect every tissue and organ. The resulting physiological hyperreactivity, such as chronically elevated cortisol, prevents the ability to rest and reset, with ensuing disease and over-sensitivity throughout the body. Trauma is often greatly under-recognized, underappreciated, and not appropriately treated.

Physical trauma comes in many forms. When we take a fall, for example, those forces are ideally absorbed and then dissipated by various tissues of the body in an adaptive way. It's not uncommon for the specific force and its direction, known as a force vector, to continue to impact the body and alter its function long after the original insult. Tissue may remain hypertonic and bone may contain the force, affecting joint mechanics, reducing motion, and leading to pain and inflammation. In addition, nerve and organ function, blood flow, and lymphatic drainage may all be affected.

The body is exceedingly intelligent as it adapts to injury and keeps moving. Physical pain and dysfunction and altered physiology are often secondary to compensation from the original and underlying disruption. The initiating cause, however, is frequently not identified or treated, leaving the individual to manage their symptoms completely unaware of the full picture.

Not all physical trauma is easily remembered or even thought to be significant. A physical strain from passing through the birth canal can influence growth and development throughout one's life, and don't forget Mom. Carrying a child is a beautiful process that stresses the anatomy and physiology of the body, especially during delivery. Surgery and most any reason to be in a hospital are common traumas. Also, car or bike accidents that we walked away from with "no injuries," or an ankle sprain that seemed to heal on its own, are examples. These events may continue to impact the way we move and function as a whole, weakening the individual's health over time.

Often overlooked are nonphysical forms of trauma. Environmental exposures and chronic infections can be easily hidden from our awareness. Emotional, mental, and spiritual trauma may be the result of childhood abuse or daily stress and anxiety, for example. The functional response of the body may include organ dysfunction such as irritable bowel syndrome (IBS) or shortness of breath, increased tension and pain, insomnia, and disturbances to the autonomic nervous system, often triggering a vast array of autoimmune diseases, furthering the stress response, and sending the individual in a self-perpetuating cycle. Many of those reacting to trauma have become so accustomed to it that they accept it as normal. For further insight, see chapters 1 and 2 on the limbic system, chapter 3 on vagal dysfunction, and chapter 21 on emotional, energetic, and spiritual considerations.

Shock

When we experience or witness a sudden and overwhelming event that's beyond our ability to handle in the moment, we are in a state of shock. (Please note: This is not the same as the conventional medical definition of shock, which requires emergency care). We neither fight nor flee, but rather experience a level of disassociation to remove ourselves from the situation, and the body is left in a bracing pattern, "frozen." An injury, surgery, illness, or witnessing the sudden death of a loved one are examples of sudden stressors that can trigger this response. This is a natural protective mechanism. Muscles react by becoming unusually tight, especially along the spine. The body feels stiff, and every biological system is affected by the heightened stress response. On a subtle level, the experience may create a void in certain areas of the body where there is a lack of life and potency. After the initial shock, the individual is left to deal with the trauma. Sometimes, however, the paralyzing impact of the shock does not fully dissipate. Many of our most sensitive patients have been impacted in this way.

Being in shock will prevent healing by treatment modalities that would otherwise be very effective. This was brought to light by Robert Fulford, DO. Most sensitive patients have been or are currently in this state of internal tension with resistance to motion. Therefore, identifying and releasing shock is a necessary step to create an opportunity for a complete healing process. This can be complicated, requiring a high level of skill from a physician who can appreciate the complexity of these vector forces and understand the delicate order in which such imbalances need to be addressed.

Osteopathic Exam

Osteopathic physicians use their hands to evaluate the living function and structure of the body. With seasoned hands, each physical layer is appreciated, not by increasing pressure but rather allowing the information to be brought to the perception of the physician. The most gentle contact may provide tremendous insight into every coexisting biologic system while also being aware of subtle activity outside the body.

The specifics of the exam will vary among physicians, but common themes exist. Visually, posture and biomechanics are observed when first greeting the patient, and can be telling of previous trauma. Bones, tissues, and organs are evaluated in a specific manner related to their function. This might include characteristics such as three-dimensional position, tension, density, and motion. The quality of the tissue, fluid, and potency are ideally also taken into account, thus leading the physician to specific areas to work with in order of priority, as directed by The Health of the patient. Combined with medical training and the standard physical exam, this awareness provides tremendous clinical utility to both diagnose and treat even the most complex cases.

Common Findings – Structural and Functional

Structural Findings

Patients display a variety of abnormal physical findings that limit motion, contribute to their condition, and restrict the healing process. Common themes involve the components of the autonomic nervous system (ANS), heart, abdominal diaphragm, digestion, and detoxification. The cause and specific dysfunction of each of these areas is unique to the patient and their history.

Autonomic Nervous System

The ANS normally maintains internal homeostasis by controlling the activity of smooth muscle and internal organs, and is primarily composed of two divisions, the sympathetic and parasympathetic nervous systems. The sympathetic nervous system (SNS) activates a "fight or flight" response to stress, while the parasympathetic nervous system (PNS) has an opposite and complementary function known as "rest and digest." Imbalance of the ANS with the scales tipping in favor of the sympathetics is virtually ubiquitous with this population, with anatomical contributions frequently overlooked. See chapter 3 for a detailed understanding of this dynamic system, which will also help make the following structural implications more meaningful.

Sympathetic Nervous System

Structural dysfunction impacting the SNS tends to stimulate its activity, creating an increased level of stress. The implications are widespread, such as increasing the perception of pain, initiating anxiety and insomnia, and interrupting digestion and immune function. The SNS originates in the thoracic and lumbar regions of the spinal cord, with initial bundles of nerve fibers, called ganglia, located on either side of the spine, extending down to and meeting at the coccyx. The ganglia may be compressed or strained due to pressure from abnormally positioned ribs or trauma to the sacrum or coccyx (tailbone). Injury to the coccyx may also interrupt the fire that ignites the engine of life and lead to chronic fatigue. Structural irritation of the sciatic and median nerves, which have more than 80% sympathetic fibers, may stimulate the SNS, even without symptoms of sciatica or carpal tunnel syndrome.

Parasympathetic Nervous System

When the PNS encounters structural challenges its activity is often inhibited, thereby allowing the SNS to predominate and ultimately contributing to hyperreactive physiology. Its nerves extend from the cranium and sacrum, two areas that are often dysfunctional in chronically ill patients. This is often the case when the cranial bones exhibit little to no motion and the head feels very hard and dense as a result. Within the restricted cranium, the brain, the dura that encases the brain, and the fluids thereof are also not moving normally. Thus the function of the brain and its natural detox mechanisms are affected. This could occur in a patient with no physical trauma to the head, as chronic stress, anxiety, and toxic exposures are common causes. To learn about the implications of dental issues, tongue-tie, and temporomandibular joint (TMJ) disorder, see chapter 15. Parasympathetic function of the vagus nerve is commonly interrupted along its course due to compression as it exits the cranium and as it continues through tight suboccipital muscles, and from limited motion of the abdominal diaphragm that would otherwise stimulate it. Similar dysfunction may occur at any point along the wandering course of the vagus nerve. As seen here, and in the general sense, vagal-nerve dysfunction is not the problem, it's an effect. Meanwhile, often secondary to a fall or other trauma, the sacrum may be internally compressed and malpositioned, often too high in the pelvis. This distorts the function of the parasympathetic nerves that extend from the sacrum, and can also create a compressive force that extends up through the spine and into the base of the cranium, furthering dysfunction of the PNS.

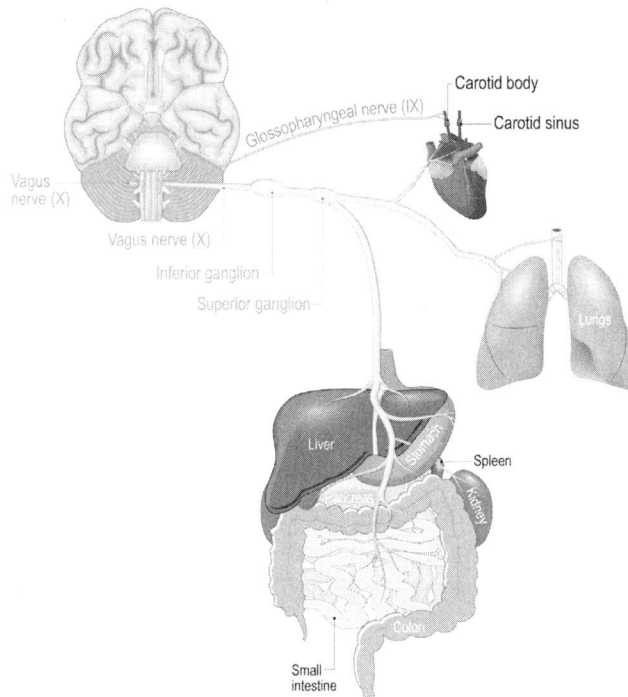

The vagus nerve

Heart

The heart and chest area are home to both physical and emotional strain. Heartbreak may create layers of dense, contracted tissue that act as an anchor, mechanically pulling on tissue continuity that extends into the cranium and with the fascia of the entire body. This pulls the head, neck, and shoulders down and in toward the heart. The increased tension of the pericardium and of the heart itself restricts its power output and dampens the potency that it instills into the blood. On the surface, the sternum is abnormally hard, like protective armor against future emotional intimacy and vulnerability. This creates a physical draw into the area, much like the tension of the heart, distorting posture and biomechanics.

Abdominal Diaphragm

The simple act of breathing may be abnormal. Instead of healthy belly breathing, they tend to take shallow, chest breaths. The abdominal diaphragm is tight and elevated, limiting its descent during inhalation. This is a common response to stress and trauma, with widespread implications. With reduced motion of the diaphragm, the lungs have less space to expand into during inspiration, and the decreased amount of oxygen drawn into the body may lower cellular metabolism and contribute to fatigue. Respiratory-assist muscles overwork in compensation and can lead to chronic headaches, neck, back, and shoulder pain. Venous and lymphatic circulation also suffer, contributing to fluid stasis and impeded immune function.

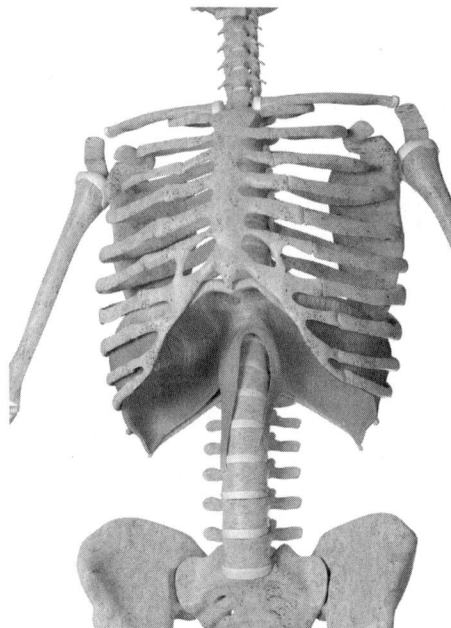

Diaphragm

Digestion

The digestive function of the stomach, gallbladder, pancreas, and intestines is compromised. As a combination of dysregulated ANS function and being pulled upward with the abdominal diaphragm, the stomach produces less acid. The reduction of stomach acid has numerous functional implications, such as nutritional deficiency, indigestion, abdominal bloating, and intestinal dysbiosis. The elevated position of the stomach also creates a susceptibility for stomach acid to reflux up into the esophagus due to distorted function of the lower esophageal sphincter. ANS imbalance from causes previously mentioned may also diminish the digestive function of the gallbladder and pancreas and reduce intestinal peristalsis, contributing to maldigestion, constipation, diarrhea, bloating, and development of irritable bowel syndrome (IBS) and small intestinal bacterial overgrowth (SIBO). Additionally, the origin of the connective tissue from which the small intestines are suspended, called the root of the mesentery, often elicits increased tension. This compresses the blood vessels, lymphatic channels, and nerves that pass through it to the small intestines, potentially compromising nutrient absorption and maintenance of the intestinal epithelial barrier.

Detoxification

Without the normal descent and function of the abdominal diaphragm acting as an internal pump in coordination with the other diaphragms, fluid motion throughout the body suffers. For sensitive patients the greatest impact is impaired detoxification as it relates to circulation of lymphatic fluid and the function of the liver itself. Sluggish or stagnant lymphatic drainage contributes to the buildup of toxins and metabolic waste before arriving to the heart and eventually to the liver and kidneys for clearance. The downward pressure that the abdominal diaphragm places on the liver during inhalation would normally help expel filtered blood and then draw unfiltered blood within during exhalation. This process is greatly reduced if the diaphragm is not moving fully. As a result, the liver often has a palpatory sense of being heavy, congested, and with diminished inherent motion, reflecting its reduced function and the toxic load throughout the body.

It's no coincidence that the head, heart, gut, and sacrum are commonly disrupted in sensitive patients. The head, heart, and gut all possess independent, complex neural networks and are major centers of intelligence, often referred to as the three brains, with the autonomic nervous system connecting them. In addition to regulating our physiology, each possesses a unique perspective and awareness, offering guidance in our daily lives. Simply stated, their functions include the logic of the brain, feeling of the heart, and instinct of the gut. Interestingly, the heart sends more signals to the brain than it receives. Whether we're listening or not is another story. Structural distortion of any of these locations will disrupt their normal function. The more of these areas that are involved, the greater the impact and the more ill the patient becomes.

Functional Findings

In addition to structural findings, there is a vast realm of underlying functional disturbances detected within the body and in the space around it. These are common subtle findings brought into awareness while the physician listens to the whole of the patient with the hands and heart.

Increased Density

The most significant observation is often the sense of increased density. As the body originally develops from embryologic fluid, we retain this underlying transparent and fluid nature. Stress, trauma, and shock disrupt this expression of health. The intention of the physician and the way they palpate the patient can also increase the density and disturb the ANS. The natural transparency solidifies, creating the perception of a solid mass and limiting the ability of The Health to manifest in treatment.

Reduced Motion

With the increase in density comes a lack of motion. What was once free to move in every direction is now stiff and restricted, like water becoming cement. There is a disturbance of the effortless inhalation and exhalation of every cell, tissue, and subtle being of the individual as a whole. Active resistance, often secondary to fear, prevents progress of healing on mental and emotional levels. Ease of motion is replaced with restriction and bracing.

Fragmentation

Shock and trauma may lead to fragmentation of the body and spirit as an adaptive measure to protect the individual from further damage. Wholeness is lost. No longer operating as a unified function, the different parts are not well integrated, and additional dysfunctions arise as compensations. From a musculoskeletal perspective, for example, limbs may be subtly displaced from the central midline. The patient may feel like the troublesome arm or leg is not connected to the rest of their body or its chronic issues are not resolving as expected. Similar disintegration of function may occur with any region or body system. This is the case with autoimmune disease, as the immune system attacks the self as if it were a separate, foreign threat.

Autonomic Dysregulation

Imbalance of the ANS may present in a variety of ways. The sympathetic and parasympathetic nervous systems may be individually overactive or underactive, and both may be dysfunctional at the same time. The two systems may also lose their sense of connection to one another, no longer one coordinated matrix. Initially in the disease process, in most cases, the sympathetics predominate, increasing the rate of the system and creating a heightened sense of electrical activity that is scattered and disorganized. This makes it very difficult for the patient to rest and experience stillness. The ability to maintain the high output declines over time as the PNS assumes the dominant role in the chronically ill patient. With low potency, the system slows and becomes denser with the lack of activity.

Reduced Vitality

Vitality may suffer. As a reference point, young children are the perfect example of high vitality. Health beams through them unimpeded as they light up a room. The chronically ill patient feels depleted of this natural resource. There is a drag on the system, and the spark is lost. Potency might no longer extend from the midline and move through the skin. If it is present, it tapers off quickly. The light is out and even the patient's eyes appear relatively dull.

Biological Signatures

Biochemical, metabolic, and immune activity is palpable. With a refined sense of perception, it is possible to decipher specific toxins and infections, as well as nutrient and hormone levels, within the body. This provides guidance for follow-up laboratory testing to assist in diagnosis and treatment. Anemia, hypothyroidism, autoimmune disease, and terminal cancer can all slow down the system, whereas acute infections, hyperthyroidism, tachycardia, and acute toxicity, to name a few, can cause it to speed up. To the physician, Lyme disease specifically feels like a buzzing. In addition, the evaluation of the effects of medications should not be overlooked, as they can impact the rate of the system in either direction, lock up the potency, and cause fragmentation.

Osteopathic Treatment

Osteopathy in its truest nature is a dynamic, inherent process facilitated by the physician to open doorways to The Health. This can be achieved in a variety of ways, ultimately engaging a healing process with a benevolent, omnipotent consciousness that is as old as the heavens and can never die. As stated by Dr. Sutherland: "Allow physiologic function within to manifest its own unerring potency rather than apply a blind force from without." Treatment is dictated and directed by this innate function that leads to cause with each successive treatment. This is a personal journey for each patient, for which the physician is not to interfere but rather synchronize with and augment. Setting the stage for this process to unfold is an art and science.

For sensitive patients, physical contact might not feel safe. In these cases, extra time and care must be taken to put the patient at ease. With divided attention, the physician may patiently wait until the patient feels safe enough to allow themselves to relax and accept the touch of the osteopathic physician. Once acknowledged, gentle hands-on contact is permitted and welcomed.

For both the physician and patient to reach a neutral state is crucial to experience The Health as it unfolds. The concept of neutral state refers to the moment when a patient has shifted from simply lying down on the treatment table, still stressed, with all of their personal and physical concerns still prominent, to settling down into a state of relaxation and receptiveness. The physician will guide the patient as needed to reach this state of neutral, which may include addressing structural lesions to help put the patient at ease. The importance of the neutral state is to achieve one homogenous density. Once it is achieved spontaneously, the physician waits, only to synchronize with the innate therapeutic forces that enter and begin treatment as directed by The Health. The more the neutral encompasses the whole of the patient, the more potent the treatment.

At times The Health of the patient may place its attention on releasing structural lesions, which the physician may augment with their hands. This includes facilitation of every aspect of the body, from bones and tissues to the brain, viscera, and blood flow, to improve position, motion and function. If force vectors from previous trauma are found, they are released accordingly. A wide variety of techniques are applied, from very gentle to more direct, but all are applied with little force. Regardless of the technique, patients' comfort and sense of well-being are the most important aspect of any treatment.

If the patient is in shock, this must be resolved before the body can fully respond to treatment. This can be accomplished with a gentle approach in cooperation with the patient's health at the first visit, creating the potential for further progress.

The process of reaching neutral and engaging indwelling therapeutic forces is the foundation of osteopathy. The most subtle and profound approach to treatment is Traditional Osteopathy as described here, also known as Biodynamic Osteopathy, a term created by James Jealous, DO. This is an extension of the latter experience and teachings of Dr. Sutherland and osteopaths who followed him. Well-intentioned manual therapists providing craniosacral therapy may be helpful, but lack the breadth and depth of cranial osteopathy and its full potential of treatment. Specialists in Osteopathic Manipulative Medicine (OMM) often complete years of training after medical school and participate in lifelong study of osteopathy. It's best to seek care from a physician trained in Cranial Osteopathy, ideally also Biodynamic Osteopathy. To find them visit www.cranialacademy.org and www.traditonalosteopathyedu.com respectively.

Mary's Story

Mary was a thin sixty-one-year-old with many health challenges. These included chronic pain, a constant headache, and severe bilateral temporomandibular joint disorder, back and neck pain, mold toxicity, anxiety, depression, insomnia, brain fog, adrenal fatigue, immune deficiency, autoimmune disease in the form of Sjogren's and Raynaud's disease, elevated biomarkers to chronic infections, IBS with constipation and bloating, pre-diabetes, scoliosis, and osteoporosis. She was sensitive to light, various supplements and foods, and had severe reactions to medications.

Mary's medical history was significant for trauma of various kinds. She was the subject of childhood abuse, and her father was an alcoholic, which led to her parents' divorce when she was twelve. As an adult, from subconsciously chewing on a soft bite guard overnight for four years, she slowly and completely wore down the discs of her temporomandibular (TMJ) joints and developed a bone spur on the left side. This not only increased TMJ pain but ignited a deeply engraved pattern of muscle spasms at the neck and a non-stop headache at the base of the skull at variable levels of severity. Mary experienced at least nine significant physical traumas, which included motor vehicle accidents, falls, and blows to the head. Excessive stress and air travel left her with significant and permanent vision loss. Surgical history included the removal of her uterus and ovaries in separate procedures due to endometriosis, two low-back surgeries due to ruptured discs, left bunion correction, and twelve dental procedures involving root canals and extractions. In preparation for travel to Taiwan, she received numerous vaccines within a short time. Mary was exposed to weekly pesticide fogging for roaches in a previous home for over five years, and was directly sprayed with pesticide while biking near a cherry orchard. To top it all off she was also exposed to toxic mold on two occasions, each lasting two years, whose effects continued to haunt her.

In search of help, Mary had seen a multitude of other clinicians over the years. When we met, she brought in a suitcase full of her daily supplements and a homeopathic agent that she had to micro-dose due to her sensitivity. All of these were intended to treat symptoms and individual abnormalities seen on lab testing. Despite her efforts, Mary's was a low quality of life.

When Mary presented to our office, she was very apprehensive about any hands-on treatment, especially after a recent major exacerbation of pain from a seemingly mild manipulation of her neck by another clinician. Just prior to her first appointment she prayed that the Lord would heal her or take her.

After slowly reviewing the basics of traditional osteopathy and answering Mary's questions about treatment, we proceeded with a blend of a conventional and osteopathic exam. As she eased onto her back on the treatment table in the quiet room, she immediately asked for the lights to be turned off, stating that her eyes were sensitive.

The excessive tension throughout her tissues held Mary's body very stiff and braced against any further distress. This was the overall theme of her body. Her skull was mildly misshapen, extremely compressed, and had virtually no motion. Her spine was also very rigid, most notably at the neck and upper back, with advanced scoliotic curvature. Both abdominal diaphragms were exceedingly tight and drawn up toward her head, with minuscule descent during inhalation. Mary's abdomen was moderately bloated and there was excessive tension of the mesentery. Her sacrum felt compressed, with no motion, and was stuck too high in the pelvis. Finally, her right leg was pulled up toward the pelvis, which made it appear shorter than her left leg.

Sitting at the head of the table, I paused for a few moments before my hands made gentle contact at the lateral aspect of her shoulders. The most significant sense of Mary at that moment was that of increased sympathetic activity. There was also the overall perception of significant density, heaviness, and contracture, with little motion, and low vitality. Taking the whole picture into account, it was clear that Mary was in a state of shock.

Synchronizing with her health and keeping her wholeness in my awareness, the stage was set for treatment. At that moment, Mary's greatest stillness presented itself, and with divided attention I softly sat in that fulcrum and waited. And waited. Slowly but surely, Mary began to settle. As her body became more and more at ease on the treatment table she reached neutral. Her system was idling and ready to make a shift. The stillness grew and deepened, enveloping the room as her sympathetic activity dissolved. Mary was finally able to rest. She underwent a deep therapeutic process in which transmutative forces restored midline function and resolved compensatory lesions, and a gentle unwinding process was set in motion.

When we reached the endpoint of the treatment, the sensation of Mary's body was vastly different from where we'd started. The generalized rigidity and hyper-alertness was replaced with a soft, diffuse warmth and overall sense of well-being. She reported feeling very relaxed as she slowly rose from the table a few minutes later, pleasantly surprised by the experience. She also felt and appeared taller and more upright as she left the office, a dazed smile on her face.

When I saw Mary in follow-up two weeks later, she happily shared that she felt the greatest relief of pain in twenty-two years of various therapies. Her posture also remained improved, with no extra effort on her part, and her leg-length discrepancy was resolved. She was fascinated and eager to continue.

Since that time we've continued to make progress with osteopathy, and have added functional medicine to Mary's treatment. A tongue-tie release also provided significant relief of anxiety and dramatically improved her sleep. Her pain is now up to 90% better, brain fog and abdominal bloating have greatly decreased, and she has more energy to enjoy activities such as pickleball for the first time.

The reason Mary is doing so well is that she's finally being treated as a whole. Shock was released, she is now able to rest, and inherent healing forces are being engaged. The many previous therapies targeted a variety of dysfunctional parts, with limited improvement of her condition. Now that the underlying cause is being cared for, Mary is well on the way to her greatest state of health.

Summary

Osteopathy is a sacred science and healing art ideally suited for those in need, including the sensitive and chronically ill. This system of medicine, practiced by osteopathic physicians (DOs), recognizes the unity of body, mind, and spirit, and our innate self-regulating, self-healing mechanism. Inherent motion is the matrix upon which this is possible, as an expression of health and essential to life itself.

The structure and function of the body are one event, inseparable in the natural world. The position, tension, and motion of tissues, organs and fluids, when normal, support optimal health and function, and when abnormal, contribute to disease. Altered physiology and distortion of structure are often secondary to trauma of various kinds. The hands-on application of osteopathic principles, known as Osteopathic Manipulative Medicine (OMM), provides unique diagnostic insight into the underlying cause of illness and an opportunity to restore health.

Sensitive patients exhibit common physical and physiologic disruption that contribute to their condition. Structurally this involves the components of the autonomic nervous system, heart, abdominal diaphragm, digestion, and detoxification. Subtle functional disturbances are perceived as increased density, reduced motion, fragmentation, autonomic dysregulation, low vitality, and biological signatures.

Osteopathic physicians who specialize in OMM use their hands to cooperate and communicate with indwelling therapeutic forces. To fully engage this potential, the patient is to reach neutral and shock must be released if present. This is true to my experience (some sense of neutral before releasing shock) and in agreement with the process presented in the "Osteopathic Treatment" section. Addressing specific structural lesions is guided by the intelligence of The Health and augmented by the physician. Successive treatment leads to cause, assisting the patient in their healing journey and creating an opportunity for personal evolution. The service of osteopathy is a gift to humanity.

T. Carmine Van Deven, DO, is an osteopathic physician with expertise in identifying and treating the underlying cause of complex illness from a place of health. He is a graduate of Illinois State University where he earned a B.S. in Computer Science, and of the Arizona College of Osteopathic Medicine where he taught and conducted research as an OMM Scholar.

Dr. Van Deven completed a Family Medicine Residency in Mount Vernon, Washington, and NMM Fellowship in Pittsfield, Massachusetts. Cranial and Biodynamic Osteopathy are a continual focus of study. He is dual board-certified in Family Medicine and Osteopathic Manipulative Treatment (FM/OMT) and Neuromusculoskeletal Medicine/Osteopathic Manipulative Medicine (NMM/OMM).

Dr. Van Deven has a private practice in Scottsdale, AZ, where he provides a synergistic blend of Traditional Osteopathy and Functional Medicine. His heartfelt holistic approach embraces the spiritual nature of each patient as a vital component of the healing process. Evaluation and treatment are applied in cooperation with natural law, to resolve disease and to assist in the embodiment of The True Self. For more information visit www.drvandeven.com.

Chapter 17: Benzodiazepine and SSRI Withdrawal As Contributing Factors to Sensitization

James Greenblatt, MD

Dr. Nathan's Introduction

Our sensitive patients live in fear. This is understandable in that the simple act of walking to their mailbox might bring them into contact with another individual who's walking down the street, doused in perfume or cologne, or who washed their clothes in detergent with a strong scent. For many of our patients, this chance meeting can trigger profound fatigue, brain fog, or even neurological events such as dyskinesias or pseudo-seizures, which can bring our patients quite literally to their knees. Never knowing what they'll encounter, from a stimulus perspective, as they navigate through life, becomes a growing source of anxiety. Given that many of our patients have had, in addition to their sensitivity, considerable anxiety and depression triggered by mold toxicity and Lyme disease, a large percentage have presented to us already having been placed on antidepressant medications such as SSRIs and/or benzodiazepines for anxiety.

Most of my patients are eager to get off of those medications, and unfortunately, either under the direction of their treating physician or of their own volition, they discontinued their medications far too abruptly for their sensitive systems. This has added medication withdrawal to the complex spectrum of what's making them sensitive, and before I've had a chance to wean them very slowly and carefully, they've come to my practice in various stages of withdrawal.

I believe this is far more common than is currently appreciated, and in this important chapter, Dr. Greenblatt helps us to understand the withdrawal process and how to treat it with precision and compassion.

✿ ✿ ✿

Carl Jung was one of the first psychiatrists to describe sensitive patients and how innate sensitivity can affect an individual's life. Highly sensitive patients (HSPs) often struggle more with emotional lability, and it's not unusual for them to have stronger responses to stress and challenging situations. This often puts HSPs at greater risk of developing clinical symptoms of depression and anxiety, and when they seek treatment, a doctor invariably prescribes medication in an attempt to provide relief.

In the United States, rates of depression and anxiety continue to increase. The COVID-19 pandemic produced a near-perfect storm of increased stress over health concerns, financial needs, work, and other factors that put individuals, especially HSPs, at higher risk of developing depression and anxiety.

While many people don't seek treatment for depression and anxiety symptoms, a huge percentage do. Antidepressants, including selective serotonin reuptake inhibitors (SSRIs) and serotonin norepinephrine reuptake inhibitors (SNRIs), are among the most prescribed medications, considered the first-line treatment for depression and anxiety. About 10% of the US population is on antidepressant medications, and numbers have been increasing (Johansen, 2021).

If antidepressants don't relieve anxiety symptoms, doctors often turn to a different class of medications: benzodiazepines. About 13% of adults are on benzodiazepine medications such as Valium and Xanax, typically prescribed for anxiety. Due to the serious side effects and the risk of addiction, benzodiazepines are typically recommended for short-term use only; however, since mainstream psychiatry doesn't have much in the way of additional tools for relieving anxiety symptoms, benzodiazepines regularly get prescribed long-term, which often leads to devastating side effects when these medications are discontinued.

Antidepressants and benzodiazepines blunt or reduce the experience of emotions. While this may feel like a benefit, it can also be a concerning side effect. When emotional blunting is more severe, individuals feel unable to access their emotions, which can dull or flatten life experiences. In sensitive individuals, this can cut both ways: it might feel like a relief or it might feel like a loss of connection with the colorful emotions that our experiences provide.

Unfortunately, antidepressant medications are not as effective as we'd hoped. They're often no better than an active placebo, providing a clinically insignificant level of improvement. Worse, they make sweeping changes to brain chemistry, influencing receptor and neurotransmitter levels throughout the brain. Once established, these changes can be difficult to reverse. If medications are discontinued, even ineffective ones, it can lead to further disruptions in normal brain functioning.

Brain skips, brain zaps, fatigue, dizziness, insomnia, rebound depression, and anxiety are all common symptoms of medication withdrawal. In sensitive patients in particular, these symptoms can be debilitating. They are also often experienced as exacerbations of the anxiety and depression caused by mold toxicity, Lyme disease, and mast-cell activation, which makes it even harder to tease apart the understanding of what's triggering a patient's suffering.

If withdrawal symptoms were short-lived, they would be much easier to deal with. Knowing that relief is days away, a patient could struggle through the acute phase. Unfortunately, it's not unusual for withdrawal symptoms to last for weeks, months, even years in some cases. With brain chemistry unbalanced from medication, the effects for some sensitive individuals can be overwhelming. The patient might feel as though the only viable response is to retreat further from life and from trying to cope with a seemingly never-ending array of side effects due to a sensitive brain dysregulated by medication and withdrawal.

As an example of this, after ten years, one of my patients, John, suddenly stopped his antidepressant medications when he and his wife were trying to get pregnant. John soon developed multiple symptoms including the feeling of "bubble head," (a prickling or tingling sensation in the head), the feeling that he was always underwater, insomnia, and random brain zaps. These symptoms persisted for over a year, even after John restarted his medications.

A Short History of Benzodiazepines and Antidepressant Medications

When benzodiazepines and SSRIs were first introduced, they were touted as breakthrough treatments that were safer than their predecessors. Benzodiazepines replaced barbiturates, the previous option, which had even higher addictive potential and life-threatening side effects. They caused more significant respiratory depression, which was often lethal in overdose. While benzodiazepines still carried risks, they were lower than for barbiturates. As such, these risks were initially minimized or outright ignored as benzodiazepines became one of the most prescribed medications throughout the 1970s. Their popularity was understandable, since, in the short term, benzodiazepines are very good at reducing anxiety, stress, and phobias and helping to treat insomnia. Unfortunately, these initial positive effects can boomerang when the medications are taken long term and tolerance erases their positive effects.

Interestingly, the same general pattern occurred with selective serotonin reuptake inhibitors. Older, first-generation, antidepressants had more severe side effects. They were also significantly more dangerous in overdose, a serious concern for depressed patients who might be suicidal. When Prozac, the first SSRI, was introduced, it was heralded as a game-changing treatment. The drug was safer than the tricyclic antidepressants that had come before. Due to this, physicians felt comfortable prescribing Prozac and it quickly became a blockbuster medication.

In fact, Prozac became so popular that it was thought to help treat more than just clinical symptoms. "Are you lacking motivation at work? Try Prozac." "Are you too sensitive to criticism? Prozac can help." As both doctors and patients initially embraced the medication, prescriptions skyrocketed, and due to their sensitivity, HSPs were often prescribed Prozac or other SSRIs in an attempt to medicate away their troublesome sensitivity.

As such, SSRI medication became first-line therapy for both depression and anxiety. Millions of prescriptions were written as well-meaning prescribers tried to improve their patients' mood or stress levels through a simple prescription.

Over time, it slowly became clear that these medications were not panaceas. Due to the effects on brain chemistry, the changes caused by both benzodiazepines and selective serotonin reuptake inhibitors made the individuals taking them susceptible to tolerance, addiction, and withdrawal.

While tolerance and withdrawal are readily acknowledged with benzos, when these side effects began to come to light with SSRI and SNRI antidepressants, the pharmaceutical industry developed the misleading terminology "discontinuation syndrome." This change in language was meant to downplay the problems, though studies have clearly shown that "withdrawal" is a more accurate description.

As research into the benefits of these medications gained steam, people began to realize they were not as effective as initially believed. This led to a conundrum: millions of patients were taking ineffective medications that were not significantly helping their symptoms; however, stopping the medications led to disabling side effects. Patients were trapped into continuing ineffective meds in order to avoid the severe withdrawal associated with them.

Even more distressing, sensitive patients commonly have it worse. Due to their sensitivity, drug side effects are often worsened, and while side effects may be problematic when taking the drug, the level of discomfort from stopping can be intolerably worse.

Rebecca: A Case in Point

Rebecca, a young patient, had struggled with depression since her teenage years. A family physician prescribed citalopram. For nine months, Rebecca diligently took it, even though it wasn't helpful for her symptoms and she often felt emotionally blunted, unable to connect with others. While she did well in school, she struggled with her emotions and sensitivity to social situations, which led to symptoms of low self-esteem and low mood. After a nonconstructive discussion with her doctor, Rebecca decided to stop the citalopram on her own.

Within days, the side effects were overwhelming: Rebecca felt feverish, anxious, and horribly fatigued. Getting off the couch or out of bed took supreme effort. Worst of all were the brain zaps, an electric shock-like sensation that would start in her brain and extend down into her extremities. When she came for help, even though the medication was providing no benefits, Rebecca swore that she would stay on citalopram for the rest of her life. The alternative—dealing with the severe withdrawal, worsened by her sensitivity—was untenable for her.

How Psychiatry Often Makes Matters Worse

Due to their sensitivity, HSPs often seek professional help, and, not having much in the way of tools to help them, health-care providers invariably turn to antidepressants, benzodiazepines, and other medications in an attempt to medicate away the symptoms associated with being sensitive, including higher highs and lower lows or increased sensitivity to stress and anxiety. Since sensitive patients are, well, sensitive, they often experience stronger side effects. While this alone is of concern, many patients are never even told about the risks for side effects and withdrawal from these medications.

Informed Consent

When any treatment is prescribed, patients are supposed to be informed about alternatives, risks, and benefits. This "informed consent" is considered a mandatory part of medicine, giving patients the appropriate autonomy to make educated decisions. Unfortunately, in practice, informed consent is often seen as an annoyance or a legal formality, with patients forced to hurriedly sign an informed-consent document before the initiation of treatment. Even worse, often due to time constraints, doctors forgo informed consent completely, depriving patients of a proper understanding of a medication's risks.

As such, it's not surprising that research shows that patients are typically poorly informed about psychiatric medications. Surveys often find that patients are unaware of the risks and side effects. For HSPs, this is a serious disservice. If sensitive patients were properly informed about the minimal benefits and the added risks of medication treatment, many would likely choose a different path. One study found that only around 1.8% of clinical sessions with patients prescribed antidepressants included any discussion of side effects (Linden, 2011). This is a shockingly low number, especially considering the high rates of side effects and withdrawal symptoms from these medications. A recent survey of antidepressant users found that 61% of the respondents reported at least ten of twenty adverse effects, most commonly (Read, 2018):

- Feeling emotionally numb, reported by 71%
- Feeling foggy or detached, reported by 70%
- Feeling not like myself, reported by 66%
- Sexual difficulties, reported by 66%
- Drowsiness, reported by 63%
- Reduction in positive feelings, reported by 60%
- Suicidality as a result of the drugs, reported by 50%
- Withdrawal effects, reported by 59%
- Addiction, reported by 40%

Considering these high levels of side effects, it should be of the utmost importance to inform patients of the potential risks. For numerous reasons, however, this often does not occur, which is clearly of concern, and due to this lack of informed consent, many patients are trapped on medication, stuck between the rock of ongoing side effects and the hard place of severe withdrawal.

Many HSPs who do manage to stop medications face increased or worsening sensitivity due to the brain changes induced by medication; and while the data from published research is minimal, it still suggests that many individuals have withdrawal symptoms that can last for years after stopping benzodiazepine and antidepressant medications (Authier, 2009; Davies, 2019).

These long-standing withdrawal effects can be devastating for sensitive individuals.

Overmedicated Anxiety: An Example Case

Mike was a high-functioning business executive. While he recognized that he was sensitive, often internalizing the stress from other people's actions and emotions, Mike's sensitivity also proved valuable for securing business for his company. Due to the pressure and stress from work, his primary-care doctor had started him on Xanax. When Mike's anxiety increased as his business was flourishing, the doctor added Klonopin to the mix.

While the medications seemed helpful initially, over time, Mike started to feel his business edge slipping. As the medication dosages increased, Mike's business acumen began to falter and his memory became poor, often forgetting key information about clients—and still the prescribing physician kept increasing the dose.

Trusting his doctor and caught in a spiraling web of severe anxiety and medication side effects, Mike continued to increase his dose of the medications. This further worsened his memory and started to cause a noticeable slurring of his speech. His business partners and clients thought he was drunk, and overnight the successful company Mike had worked so hard to build began to crumble.

As his business declined, Mike sought a second opinion on his mental health and was horrified when he was confronted with his own dependence on prescription medication. Tapering the medication only exacerbated his mental deficits, which now included serious short-term memory problems. Due to his sensitivity, he was even more keenly aware of his blunted cognitive abilities. Out of sheer desperation, Mike looked into alternative treatment approaches to help with his severe dependence and withdrawal symptoms.

A New Understanding: Sensitivity and Withdrawal

Psychotropic medication typically targets neurotransmitter systems in the brain, including serotonin, GABA, dopamine, and norepinephrine. Changes to these systems can alter how they function, upregulating or downregulating receptor levels and changing receptor sensitivity. These changes can be difficult to reverse. When the drug that induced the changes is removed, dysregulated brain systems are thrown further into disarray.

A Journey of Clinical Discovery

It's interesting to note that some patients have minimal withdrawal symptoms when they stop antidepressant or benzodiazepine medication. When I first began to encounter patients, especially sensitive patients, who were having severe withdrawal, this fact stuck out like a road sign, suggesting that physiological differences must allow for the spectrum of patients' different levels of withdrawal symptoms.

Based on this understanding, I've documented those physiological differences in thousands of patients I've treated over thirty years. By applying a functional medicine model, I began to systematically evaluate my patients for the underlying causes of their severe withdrawal symptoms. Over the years of my practice, patterns emerged, demonstrating the existence of core nutritional deficits that, left untreated, were major players in withdrawal severity. By identifying and treating these core deficits, it was often possible to help even the most sensitive patients restore balance.

Sensitive Patients: Recognizing Individuality

While standard medicine and psychiatry often apply a one-size-fits-all approach, functional medicine recognizes patient individuality. This is especially critical for HSPs.

Considering that about 20% of the population qualifies as sensitive, identifying and treating these individuals *as individuals* is often the key to their health and wellness.

When someone who is sensitive has a disruption in their neurotransmitter systems, it can cause more intense and disconcerting symptoms. Sensitive individuals are more aware of their thoughts, feelings, and sensations. While this acute awareness can be extremely useful, in situations of medication withdrawal it can also be overwhelming.

In many cases, sensitivity may come down to genetic differences, which can also play a part in the variability of a person's nutritional needs. The two often go hand in hand. While the list of underlying factors that cause or contribute to medication withdrawal can include nutritional deficiencies, dysbiosis, genetic factors, toxicity, hormonal dysregulation, occult infections, and others, a large percentage of patients benefit from focusing on three factors: core nutritional deficiencies, gut health, and inflammation.

Core Nutritional Deficiencies

Mainstream medicine ignores or downplays the significance of nutrient deficiencies and overlooks the available evidence suggestive of the beneficial role of nutrition and mental health. While other nutrients can play a part, vitamin B12, vitamin B6, folate, vitamin D, and magnesium are often key for withdrawal. Individual amino acids or broad-spectrum amino-acid support can also provide profound benefits. Evaluating for deficiencies or a higher need for any of these core nutrients can be very helpful in treating withdrawal symptoms, including increased sensitivity.

Vitamin B12

B12 plays a role in the formation of red blood cells. When deficient, anemia can result. The vitamin also plays a critical role in both the central and peripheral nervous systems through helping with the production of myelin, a fatty material used for wrapping neurons in a protective sheath. This sheath needs to be constantly repaired. If B12 is in low supply, the sheath can degrade, causing serious damage to nerves. In severe cases, this can cause neuropathy that, left untreated, can be difficult to reverse.

Vitamin B12, along with folate and vitamin B6, also plays an important role in neurotransmitter production. A deficiency of any of the three can impair serotonin or dopamine production. For sensitive individuals, impaired neurotransmitter function can be a core contributing factor to worsening sensitivity. Problems with neurotransmitter production are also likely a contributing factor to why vitamin B12 deficiencies worsen withdrawal symptoms.

Vitamin B12 is one of the most underutilized treatments in modern medicine due to a number of misconceptions: First, a person can be low in vitamin B12 without having signs or symptoms of anemia; second, blood levels of vitamin B12 can be normal while levels in the central nervous system are low; and third, blood levels are commonly elevated when taking B12; this is not dangerous and does not indicate a need to stop taking the vitamin.

While not an overly reliable indicator, if blood levels of B12 are midrange or lower, individuals may still benefit from supplementation. Functional blood testing for B12, by checking for high homocysteine levels, can also be useful. Generally, supplementing with methylcobalamin or hydroxocobalamin is preferred over cyanocobalamin. A typical dose is 2,000 micrograms of sublingual methyl B12 twice daily. In cases of more severe deficiency, injections can be useful to restore levels more quickly.

Folate

With similarities to B12 for supporting blood-cell formation, neurotransmitter production, and myelination, folate, if deficient, can play a similar role in exacerbating sensitivities, especially during medication withdrawal.

Folate has also been shown to be a key support for mental health, especially when used in the active L-methylfolate form. Maintaining serotonin levels is critically reliant on adequate levels of folate.

When testing for folate levels, blood levels have been shown to be poorly characterized, leading to inaccurate results. High homocysteine blood levels can indicate a need, though generally, genetic testing for methylene-tetrahydrofolate reductase (MTHFR) single nucleotide polymorphisms (SNPs) is the preferred approach. In patients who are heterozygous or homozygous for either of the most problematic SNPs, 677 or 1298, supplementation is recommended.

When indicated, start supplementation with L-methylfolate between 1 and 3 milligrams, and raise levels slowly as needed. Some individuals will benefit from up to 15 mg per day. Proper dosing can significantly improve mood and decrease sensitivity symptoms related to medication withdrawal.

The most common form of folate is folic acid; however, folic acid is an inferior synthetic version that is not effective, and even potentially harmful, in patients with MTHFR SNPs.

Vitamin B6

The final B vitamin that shouldn't be overlooked in patients who struggle with worsened sensitivities after medication withdrawal is vitamin B6. The active form of the vitamin, pyridoxal 5'-phosphate, plays a role in the synthesis of neurotransmitters, the utilization of amino acids and glucose, and gene regulation, among other functions. Its specific effects on supporting serotonin and gamma-aminobutyric acid (GABA) production are key for helping with both antidepressant and benzodiazepine withdrawal.

While testing plasma B6 levels has some utility, confounding factors can affect the results. Another functional approach for assessing the need for vitamin B6 is through so-called "kryptopyrrole testing."

Kryptopyrrole, a misnomer for a similar molecule, 2-hydroxyhemopyrrolene-5-one, or HPL, is a compound excreted in the urine due to disturbed hemoglobin synthesis. When present in higher amounts, HPL is neurotoxic and appears to contribute to a number of different mental health conditions. In individuals with high levels of HPL, vitamin B6 and zinc are typically useful for reducing it. Patients with mold toxicity and Lyme disease have an altered biochemistry that leads to a higher percentage of patients with elevated HPL.

Typically, dosing is 25–50 mg of vitamin B6 combined with 30 mg of zinc, both taken twice daily. Retesting levels in three months can help to determine whether higher doses are needed. Keep in mind, however, that long-term dosing of zinc above 40 mg can cause copper deficiency, which can lead to neuropathy. Higher doses of B6, typically over 200 mg, can also cause neuropathy over time. Patients should be monitored carefully, and if any symptoms of concern arise, dosing should be reduced.

Vitamin D

Our understanding of vitamin D has undergone a profound transformation over the past thirty years. Initially, vitamin D was considered important for bone health and calcium absorption, but little else. With the discovery of vitamin D receptors throughout the body, effects on immune function and mental health, among others, continue to be documented.

In the brain, vitamin D plays a role in maintaining serotonin levels. Evidence suggests that vitamin D plays a role in supporting GABA function as well. These mechanisms are likely key for why adequate vitamin D can aid in withdrawal and reduce symptoms of sensitivity due to neurotransmitter imbalances. By helping support neurotransmitter levels, proper brain function can be maintained, keeping mental-emotional symptoms in oversensitive patients under better control.

For supplementation, vitamin D levels should be tested. In cases where 25-hydroxy vitamin D is less than 40 ng/ml, supplementation should be initiated to a target level of 50–60. For individuals who are very deficient, 5,000–10,000 IU per day is not an unusual dose to restore levels and keep them in the optimal range. Generally, if supplementation is stopped, levels just slowly drop back down to the previous level of deficiency. Unless there is a significant change in daily sun exposure, continuous supplementation is needed to maintain adequate vitamin D in the vast majority of cases.

Magnesium

One of the most common nutritional deficiencies, magnesium is crucial for maintaining health. The mineral plays a role in muscle function, energy metabolism, and the synthesis of protein, deoxyribonucleic acid (DNA) and ribonucleic acid (RNA). It also has a significant impact on brain function, including through the often overlooked neurotransmitter glutamate.

Glutamate is an excitatory neurotransmitter. It's likely that many individuals struggling with sensitivity have overactive glutamate circuitry. The glutamate neurotransmitter system has been implicated in a number of mental health conditions, including depression, anxiety, and schizophrenia.

One of the brain benefits of magnesium is that it acts like a brake on glutamate activity, helping calm things down. This can be incredibly useful for HSPs. When you consider that about 50% or more of people don't consume enough magnesium daily. it makes sense how important magnesium supplementation can be. Magnesium is also important for enhancing serotonergic activity and activating GABA pathways.

Through all these far-reaching effects, magnesium is a critical piece for reducing problematic levels of sensitivity and improving mood. It also commonly helps decrease withdrawal symptoms, especially in deficient patients.

Unfortunately, as with a number of other nutrients, testing for magnesium levels is not overly accurate. Due to the mineral's importance, it's often a good idea to supplement most individuals as a way to help calm overactive and oversensitive brain circuitry. Dosing of 400–600 mg of magnesium as magnesium citrate or glycinate per day with food is typical. Side effects from too much can include diarrhea, which can necessitate switching forms or using a lower dose. In some people, magnesium threonate can also help due to its enhanced ability to cross into the brain and improve gastrointestinal tolerance.

Neurotransmitter Support

Numerous vitamins and minerals can strengthen and support neurotransmitter function throughout the brain; sometimes, however, indirect support isn't enough. Many brain neurotransmitters are formed from amino acid precursors. By taking these direct precursors, you can effectively raise neurotransmitters to restore proper levels when needed. For sensitive individuals, finding the proper balance of neurotransmitter support is often key.

When using amino acids, there are two main approaches: target individual neurotransmitters, or give a broad-spectrum amino acid product. The main amino acids used for supplementing:

- 5-hydroxytryptophan (5-HTP) to raise serotonin
- Tyrosine and phenylalanine to raise dopamine and norepinephrine
- GABA to directly raise GABA levels and function
- Free-form amino acids, to raise essential and some nonessential amino acid levels for broad-spectrum support

5-HTP

5-HTP is the direct precursor of serotonin. While some 5-HTP is lost upon digestion and absorption, whatever makes it into the bloodstream will rapidly raise serotonin levels in the brain. Generally, 5-HTP has been shown to have antidepressant and antianxiety effects and can help treat individuals during antidepressant withdrawal. When selective serotonin reuptake inhibitors, or SNRI medication, is discontinued, lower serotonin levels can result, and 5-HTP can help directly treat lowered serotonin.

Caution is warranted, however; if 5-HTP is combined with antidepressants, it can predispose individuals to too much serotonin, which can cause serotonin syndrome. Severe serotonin syndrome is a life-threatening emergency that can include fever, muscle rigidity, and seizures. Generally, dosing starts at 50 mg of 5-HTP and is slowly increased to avoid gastrointestinal side effects.

Tyrosine

The amino acid phenylalanine is a precursor to tyrosine, which in turn is a precursor to dopamine. Dopamine can further be used to make norepinephrine and epinephrine. Phenylalanine also has some appetite-reducing effects, which can help patients who struggle with overeating.

Tyrosine has been shown to help people function better under stress. For sensitive individuals who function poorly in stressful situations, tyrosine may provide some benefits. It can also be used to shore up dopamine and norepinephrine production in patients who have withdrawn from SNRI antidepressants or Wellbutrin. Dosing of tyrosine is often between 500 mg and 2000 mg per day, based on symptoms and treatment response.

GABA

GABA is the main inhibitory neurotransmitter in the brain. In essence, GABA slows everything down. Benzodiazepines work through the GABA system, and during withdrawal, GABA activity is often reduced. By supporting the GABA system during and after withdrawal, it's possible to help mitigate symptoms, especially in sensitive individuals.

The efficacy of GABA seems somewhat variable. It likely stems from individual differences in how well GABA can get into the central nervous system to affect the brain.

There's also a subset of individuals who have a reverse response to GABA, which can ramp them up and cause anxiety. Still, in those who benefit, GABA can be quite useful. Dosing 500–1000 mg as needed for anxiety up to two or three times per day for withdrawal symptoms can help. In sensitive individuals with significant anxiety, start low until it's clear that GABA is having a positive effect.

Free-Form Amino Acids

One of the simplest yet most profound supports for mental health is free-form amino acids. Individuals with mental health issues, especially sensitive individuals, often have gastrointestinal symptoms or problems. Protein digestion is frequently impaired, often depriving the brain of needed amino acid precursors.

By providing the body the proper amino acids in a predigested form—as individual amino acids—digestive issues are effectively bypassed. This gives the brain and body all the needed amino acid building blocks to function properly and fuel neurotransmitter synthesis.

Dosing of free-form amino acids is typically 4 grams twice daily, best on an empty stomach. Most sensitive patients will benefit from free-form amino acids, even more so in patients with digestive issues.

Dysbiosis and Gut Health

When it comes to helping treat sensitive individuals, one of the most important areas of focus is gastrointestinal health. The gut is one way that we directly experience the world. The outside world (as food and drink) interacts directly with our intestinal tract, and nutrients are taken up by the body, with waste left behind. Due to this interaction, about 70% of the immune system is present to defend us from bacteria and other invaders that we ingest through food and drink.

When the gut is out of balance, our personal interactions with the outside world are often out of balance as well. Research has repeatedly shown how important gastrointestinal health is to mental health, for healthy aging, for immune function, and for keeping inflammation in check. In many cases, problematic sensitivity can have roots in gut health. This often presents as dysbiosis, in which bad bacteria or yeast have taken up residence, with detrimental effects on digestion and the rest of the body.

Dysbiosis can be obvious in patients who suffer from gastrointestinal problems such as constipation, diarrhea, and irritable bowel syndrome, or it can be more occult, causing inflammation but having fewer direct effects on digestion.

For individuals with any form of mental health diagnosis, testing organic acid levels in the urine can often yield important findings about gastrointestinal health. One key analyte, 3-(3-Hydroxyphenyl)-3-hydroxypropanoic acid (HPHPA) can indicate an overgrowth of damaging clostridia bacteria. HPHPA is thought to be a metabolite of a pathological form of tyrosine that can disrupt brain circuitry, potentially contributing to autism, schizophrenia, and other mental health conditions.

In cases of clostridium overgrowth or other types of dysbiosis, high-dose probiotics and a diet low in sugar and rich in whole foods is often helpful. If these changes aren't enough, treating the clostridia directly with antimicrobials may be necessary in some individuals.

Individuality and Inflammation: Polyphenols to the Rescue

In general, excess chronic inflammation worsens everything. In sensitive individuals, doubly so. Chronic inflammation is well known to be a component of almost every chronic disease. Even mental health conditions, including depression, anxiety, schizophrenia, ADHD, obsessive compulsive disorder, and others, have all been shown to correlate with increased inflammation.

If excess inflammation is present, it will exacerbate withdrawal, making the process even more miserable. The solution is to target the inflammation, helping quench the overactive immune system and restore more normal functioning.

While mainstream medicine does not have good side-effect-free options for reducing inflammation, nature has provided numerous plants to safely help. One type of compound found in plants, called polyphenols, is often helpful.

Polyphenols are found in a number of herbs known for their anti-inflammatory effects, including turmeric, pine bark, green tea, and grape-seed extract. For sensitive individuals dealing with excess inflammation, a mixed polyphenol supplement with curcumin can be quite useful. As inflammation begins to be tamed, symptoms of sensitivity and withdrawal are often reduced if not eliminated.

Helping Patients With Withdrawal

When a sensitive patient still needs to taper and eliminate an antidepressant or benzodiazepine, start by identifying and treating these core deficiencies for three to six months. Once levels are replete, begin a slow taper based on the individual's clinical response. Always go slowly, with only small changes in dosing. During the taper, major side effects should be avoided. If serious side effects arise, go back to the last stable dose and reassess for other needed support. Typically, something may have been missed, or other treatments, as detailed throughout the rest of this chapter, can restore stability, and the taper can then continue with reduced side effects.

Throughout any taper, there needs to be a strong doctor-patient relationship built on trust and open communication. The patient should be in charge of when to taper, unless they are trying to proceed too quickly. It's also worth remembering that every individual is unique, especially sensitive individuals, and that their process will require a personalized approach. In patients who struggle with overeating and are also withdrawing from SNRIs or Wellbutrin, phenylalanine may be of assistance. Dosing can be similar to tyrosine, at 500–2000 mg per day. During any withdrawal process, identify and treat core deficiencies for three months while evaluating for other aspects of an individual's health that could be affecting or worsening withdrawal. During the withdrawal process itself, go slowly, with only small changes in dosing. If serious side effects emerge, increase to the last stable medication dose and evaluate further for additional needed support before continuing.

Respecting Individuality and Sensitivity

While the treatments outlined here will help many people who are struggling through withdrawal as a contributing factor to sensitivity, they won't help everyone. The causes of withdrawal and oversensitivity are numerous. It's always possible that there could be other nutritional deficiencies, like iron, niacin, or zinc, that are contributing. There could be hormonal imbalances that need to be addressed with the thyroid or sex hormones. In some cases, toxicity may be a major player, including mold toxins or heavy metals. For every case of withdrawal and sensitivity, it's critical to recognize the individuality and uniqueness of the patient.

Cookie-cutter approaches don't work well. Evaluating an individual's symptoms and doing the proper laboratory evaluations can help identify many of the underlying causes. People are unique, with a unique genetic makeup, unique life experiences, and a unique history. Celebrating and treating this uniqueness is the key to the success of functional medicine.

Considering that estimates suggest that about 20% of the population is considered highly sensitive, patients who become over-sensitized upon withdrawal are not uncommon. Through the use of a functional, individualized approach, the vast majority of these patients can bring their symptoms under control and find relief.

The most common causes of HSPs struggling with increased sensitivity after withdrawal are from nutritional deficiencies that include vitamin B12, folate, vitamin B6, magnesium, and vitamin D. Neurotransmitter systems should be supported with precursor amino acids and GABA, and gut problems addressed. If symptoms remain, adding anti-inflammatory polyphenols will often provide relief. Proper laboratory testing can help guide any treatment approach to identify deficiencies of concern.

Other problems that shouldn't be overlooked but that don't contribute to symptoms as often include thyroid and sex hormone imbalances, which can be measured and addressed. A dietary analysis and workup may also uncover other nutritional deficiencies, including omega-3 fats, zinc, additional B vitamins, and other nutrients. Unfortunately, in this day and age, toxicity concerns must also be considered, including heavy metals, flame retardants, solvents, fluorinated compounds, plastics, plasticizers, pesticides, herbicides, and mold toxicity.

An individual's current life situation and stress levels can also play a part. Family, relationships, work, and other social dynamics can play a huge part in a person's symptoms, depending on the amount of stress that they contribute. When, if possible, these stressful components are changed, it can also often help provide relief.

Summary

HSPs more often seek medical care for symptoms related to different aspects of their health, and are more likely to experience withdrawal when discontinuing medication for depression, anxiety, or other mental health conditions. By understanding the components that can cause or increase withdrawal symptoms, it's possible to mitigate withdrawal-induced sensitivity.

Addressing nutritional deficiencies, supporting neurotransmitter systems, and providing supportive therapies based on an individualized approach makes a difference. By recognizing the unique characteristics of our highly sensitive patients we can more effectively understand and address their medical needs and concerns.

References

Linden M, Westram A. What do psychiatrists talk about with their depressed patients parallel to prescribing an antidepressant? Int J Psychiatry Clin Pract. 2011;15(1):35-41. doi:10.3109/13 651501.2010.527007.

Read J, Williams J. Adverse Effects of Antidepressants Reported by a Large International Cohort: Emotional Blunting, Suicidality, and Withdrawal Effects. Curr Drug Saf. 2018;13(3):176-186. doi:10.2174/1574886313666180605095130.

Davies J, Read J. A systematic review into the incidence, severity and duration of antidepressant withdrawal effects: Are guidelines evidence-based? Addict Behav. 2019;97:111-121. doi:10.1016/j.addbeh.2018.08.027.

Authier N, Balayssac D, Sautereau M, et al. Benzodiazepine dependence: focus on withdrawal syndrome. Ann Pharm Fr. 2009;67(6):408-413. doi:10.1016/j.pharma.2009.07.001.

James M. Greenblatt, MD, a pioneer in the field of functional and integrative medicine, and a dually board-certified child and adult psychiatrist, has treated patients since 1988. After receiving his medical degree and completing his psychiatry residency at George Washington University, Dr. Greenblatt completed a fellowship in child and adolescent psychiatry at Johns Hopkins Medical School. He currently serves as the Chief Medical Officer at Walden Behavioral Care and is the founder of Psychiatry Redefined, an online educational platform dedicated to the transformation of psychiatry, which offers online courses, webinars, and fellowships for professionals.

Dr. Greenblatt has lectured internationally on the scientific evidence for nutritional interventions in psychiatry and mental illness. He is the author of seven books, including *Functional Medicine for Antidepressant Withdrawal* and *Finally Focused: The Breakthrough Natural Treatment Plan for ADHD.* Dr. Greenblatt was inducted into the Orthomolecular Hall of Fame in 2017 by the International Society of Orthomolecular Medicine. Find more information at www.PsychiatryRedefined.org and www.JamesGreenblattMD.com.

Chapter 18: Thiamine Deficiency and the Sensitive Patient

Neil Nathan, MD, and Chandler Marrs, PhD

The importance of thiamine (vitamin B1) first came to my attention when a patient I'd been working with shared his recent research with me. He had improved greatly from long-term struggles with Lyme disease, *Bartonella*, and mold toxicity, but his biggest complaint was that he was unable to exercise as he used to. Prior to getting ill, he was heavily into martial arts and enjoyed long, strenuous workouts and how strong his body felt. While his other symptoms were markedly improved, this one area of dysfunction remained a constant frustration. Ever the researcher, he discovered the book by Derrick Lonsdale and Chandler Marrs called *Thiamine Deficiency Disease, Dysautonomia, and High Calorie Malnutrition*. Within two weeks of starting thiamine replacement, he was able to return to two-hour intense workouts and felt the strength return to his body. This got my attention.

As I studied that book, it became clear to me that thiamine deficiency was an important piece of the puzzle that I had been missing. The connection to my work with mold came from the realization that new research showed that mold toxins made it difficult for the body to absorb and then use this vitamin for the myriad biochemical reactions that depend upon it. With this new information, I began to treat all my mold-toxic patients with thiamine—with great results.

While other vitamins, notably B-12 and B6, are also deficient in many of our patients, the work done by Lonsdale and Marrs is especially relevant to our patients and deserves a special place in our comprehensive discussion of sensitivity.

I had the honor of working with Chandler Marrs to distill information from their book to bring this knowledge to you. I graduated from medical school at the University of Chicago (Pritzker) in 1971. At that time, the few references to nutrition involved how we'd begun to learn about vitamins in terms of their importance to body chemistry.

(Alas, fifty years later, it's a rare medical school that discusses the wonderful advances in nutritional information to any degree at all, but that's another story.)

Thiamine (vitamin B-1), was named that because it was the first B vitamin to be discovered. There was an awareness of some kind of illness in medieval Japan, described as "leg disease," characterized by partial paraplegias and edema of the legs. Of course, there was no understanding of vitamins or nutrition in those times, so no treatment was available. In the 18th and 19th centuries, this became known as beriberi, but it was not until thiamine was identified as the source of this condition that treatment became possible.

The cause of beriberi was eventually discovered to be the consumption of polished rice; i.e., rice whose husks were discarded after milling. It turns out that the B vitamins are in the husk, so those who consumed large amounts of polished rice were set up for thiamine deficiency. Part of the irony of this is that since the milling of rice is expensive, polished rice was associated with affluence and was a goal to be reached as a symbol of wealth and status in Japan and China.

When I traveled to China in 1985 as a part of an international effort to build relationships with the newly opened country, we lived in the Wu Yi mountains of southern China and studied tai chi and calligraphy with Al Huang's group. Our hosts were aghast at our pleas to be served what they called red rice (i.e., brown rice) because it would have been viewed as absolutely unthinkable to treat honored guests without serving them polished white rice.

By 1962, after the vitamin was successfully synthesized, hundreds of papers were published in the medical literature suggesting this vitamin for a wide variety of possible applications. While a great number of symptoms have been noted for beriberi, none of them is considered pathognomonic (specifically characteristic or indicative of a particular disease or condition). The designations for beriberi then included "wet" beriberi, in which edema was a dominant symptom, and "dry" beriberi (non-edematous). Now, however, we see a far more expansive set of symptoms, and we have to look deeper into the biochemistry of the illness to understand its varied manifestations.

If we view the symptoms through organ systems, a brief overview would look like this:

Neurological Symptoms

- Peripheral neuropathy
- Ataxia
- Polyneuritis
- Paralysis
- Horizontal nystagmus (rapid, repetitive, uncontrolled side-to-side eye movement)
- Reduced visual acuity
- Changes in mental status

Cardiovascular Symptoms

- Tachycardia
- Decreased diastolic pressure/normal systolic
- Labile hypertension

Gastrointestinal Symptoms

- "Full sensation"
- Constipation/SIBO
- Heartburn/Esophagitis
- Nausea/Vomiting/Loss of appetite
- Decreased peristalsis (gastroparesis)
- Dysautonomia: Increased sensitivity of the limbic system
    - Decreased tears
    - Decreased sweating
    - Emotional lability
    - POTS
    - Sympathetic/Parasympathetic imbalance
- Edema, particularly in the pretibial area, and to a lesser extent the face

These symptoms are insidious; they develop gradually over months to years. For that reason, they can escape detection in the early stages. Symptoms may also wax and wane relative to thiamine availability in the diet and thiamine demand from life stressors. Modern medicine often misses the gradual decline of health and the waxing and waning of symptoms. We tend to focus on the end stages of the disease process and not the early indicators. Hundreds of years ago, before thiamine was discovered, 7th-century Chinese physicians described what later would become the diseases of thiamine deficiency, now called beriberi and Wernicke's encephalopathy. From a translation of Chinese texts published in *Understanding the Jiaoqi Experience: The Medical Approach to Illness in Seventh-Century China*:

> When they get this illness, many people do not immediately feel it. Some first have no other disorder and then suddenly get [this one]; some contract it after suffering multiple other illnesses. In the beginning, the symptoms are trivial; the patient eats, drinks, and amuses himself the same as ever, and his physical strength is the same as before. At this time one must observe the illness carefully....
>
> Its symptoms: numbness from the knee to the foot, sometimes aching, sometimes a creeping sensation like insects crawling around. In some cases, the area from the toes to the knee and calf is especially sensitive to cold. In some cases, the lower leg is bent and weak and [the patient] cannot walk. In some cases, the lower legs have slight

swelling, extreme sensitivity to cold, or pain. In some cases [the lower legs] are relaxed and do not obey [the patient's intentions], or twitch acutely. There are some whose condition is dire [yet] they can still eat and drink; [but] there are some who cannot eat, or who vomit upon seeing food and drink and can't stand the smell of food. Some [patients] feel a thing like fingers, dispatched from the meaty part of the calf, which travels upward and attacks the qi of the heart system. Some have spasms over the entire body. Some have a serious fever and headache. Some people's brains and hearts rush and throb [as though frightened], and they do not want to see light in the places where they sleep. Some patients have a bitter pain in their bellies and simultaneously have diarrhea; in some, their language is sloppy and error-filled and they easily forget or mistake things. Some have cloudy eyes and a confused aura. All of these are signs of the illness…. When one first contracts this illness, one should treat it quickly. It is different from ordinary illnesses.

This ancient description adeptly characterizes how diversely thiamine deficiency manifests. No two people have the same symptoms, at least early on. As the disease progresses, the final common pathways are primarily the central and peripheral nervous systems and cardiovascular damage.

Of particular interest in our study of patients who have become unusually sensitized, is that the core issue here is the instability and imbalance of the autonomic nervous system, especially noting limbic dysfunction. This should alert us to the possibility that we should consider thiamine deficiency in all of our patients who've become sensitized.

Marrs and Lonsdale remind us (p. 13): "there has been an emerging body of evidence showing that functional dysautonomic syndromes can be initiated by environmental stressors, including dietary constraints, and pharmaceuticals by mitochondrial damage."

The Cell Danger Response described by Dr. Robert Naviaux stresses the important role of mitochondria as cellular monitors for stressors, especially toxins and infections, and the central role of mitochondria as regulators of the Cell Danger Response. The key role of thiamine in energy metabolism, with which the mitochondria are so importantly connected, clearly takes center stage here.

Quite a few medical conditions have been associated with thiamine deficiency, including:

- Alcoholism (notably Wernicke's encephalopathy)
- AIDS
- Alzheimer's disease
- Parkinson's disease

- Cancer
- Hyperemesis Gravidarum (prolonged vomiting in pregnancy)
- Prolonged total parenteral nutrition
- Diabetes (even more likely with the use of metformin)
- Vaccine reactions
- Psychiatric disorders
- Mold toxicity
- Chronic Fatigue Syndrome/Myalgic Encephalitis
- Post-exertional malaise or myalgia
- Mitochondrial disease
- High-calorie malnutrition (a common American dietary concern)

It's notable that a number of medications also induce thiamine deficiency. Among the most common:

Metformin (also blocks B9, B12 and CoQ10; several million Americans are currently on this medication).

Many classes of antibiotics such as Bactrim, Flagyl, and the fluoroquinolones (Cipro, Levaquin, and the others) block thiamine and other B vitamins such as folate.

SSRIs such as Zoloft deplete thiamine. SSRIs in general damage mitochondria by multiple mechanisms, which makes them especially bad for health.

Proton pump inhibitors such as Prilosec, Prevacid, and Nexium block thiamine but also block B12.

Diuretics such as furosemide deplete thiamine, which when used in patients with heart or kidney disease and who may already be at risk for thiamine deficiency, increases the probability of diminished thiamine.

Last but not least, what we consume daily has an enormous impact on thiamine availability. It's well known that continued heavy alcohol use induces thiamine deficiency, but did you know that regular alcohol consumption, below the threshold for alcoholism, also reduces thiamine availability? Alcohol blocks thiamine no matter how many or how few drinks one has. With regular social drinking, symptoms simply take longer to present themselves.

Similarly, the standard American diet, which is generally very high in carbohydrates, is an enormous but wholly unrecognized impediment to thiamine sufficiency. The more carbs one consumes, the more thiamine one needs to metabolize them, and unfortunately, most dietary carbs don't come with sufficient thiamine to balance the scales. The best source of whole-food-based thiamine is pork, followed by salmon, whole grains, brown rice, and certain vegetables (cauliflower, oranges, potatoes, asparagus, and kale). Many fortified and/or enriched grains and other food products also have thiamine, but often come with added sugars and anti-thiamine factors, effectively negating the benefits of intake. Finally, coffee and tea also diminish thiamine availability, and once again, the more one consumes the greater the potential for deficiency. When these factors combine, as is so often the case, there's a very real risk of low thiamine.

Dr. Lonsdale has spent much of his long and illustrious medical career trying to educate medical professionals about the importance of thiamine as a critical nutrient in mitochondrial function, but only recently has the profession begun to realize that his message is both important and increasingly relevant.

Thiamine Equals Energy

Now that we've established that thiamine deficiency symptoms are in close alignment with those of our sensitive patients, including many symptoms of the illnesses that trigger sensitivity, let's explore the underlying mechanisms of autonomic dysfunction, particularly as related to thiamine, the mitochondria, and oxidative metabolism.

The most important thing to understand about thiamine and health is that thiamine is absolutely essential for the production of cellular energy, and cellular energy is essential for everything else, so when thiamine is low, the cells don't have enough energy to do the things they need to do. Eventually, this leads to illness, and how these symptoms are expressed varies greatly from one individual to another.

Every cell in the body and the brain requires energy to function. The bulk of this energy is synthesized in tiny organelles within the cells called mitochondria via a process called oxidative metabolism. We have trillions of mitochondria working arduously to convert the derivatives of macronutrients (proteins, fats, carbohydrates) and micronutrients (vitamins and minerals) from the food we eat into adenosine triphosphate (ATP), the molecule of energy our cells use to survive. Through oxidative metabolism, we get around 36–38 units of ATP per cycle. This is in comparison to 2 or so units of ATP produced by extra-mitochondrial processes of energy generation, which also happen to require thiamine to work effectively. With such an enormous difference in ATP production, it's easy to see how low thiamine would impact health. The body simply wouldn't have the energy to perform optimally.

When cells have insufficient ATP, all sorts of compensatory reactions are turned on. All of these reactions are beneficial in the short term as they keep us alive during periods of inadequate energy resources. In the longer term, however, they create all sorts of problems. Think about inflammation, one of the main responses the body uses to fight illness. It's an energy-intensive process. It takes energy to initiate the appropriate amount of inflammation in response to an acute injury or illness. It takes energy to regulate that response so that it's not too much or too little, too soon or too late; and it takes energy to shut everything back down once the threat has passed. If the individual doesn't have enough energy, if there's insufficient thiamine and thus poorly functioning mitochondria, the inflammatory reaction might not match the need; that is, it might be too weak or too late. It might be too strong and completely unregulated and/or it might persist for too long because there's not enough energy to activate the anti-inflammatory cascades and return the body to a non-inflammatory state.

A recent example of poor energetic capacity leading to dysregulated inflammatory cascades is COVID. On the severe end of the spectrum, the cytokine storm associated with acute COVID (but also with other serious viral infections, or even injury or trauma), is a manifestation of the relationship between insufficient mitochondrial capacity and a dysregulated inflammatory response. With the cytokine storm, the immune system goes all-in to fight the illness or injury, but there's not enough energy to regulate the response or to tamp it down when the threat is quelled. Similarly, Long COVID represents the slow-burn version of the same problem. At its root is the poor energetic capacity and the inability to fully clear the virus and resolve the inflammatory process.

Many modern illnesses are attributed to excessive inflammation. Everything from cardiovascular to autoimmune disease carries a heightened inflammatory component. The common response of physicians to these disease processes is to squelch the inflammation by prescribing anti-inflammatories, effectively overriding the body's natural, albeit excessive. response. This might be a necessary short-term approach, but in the longer term, the problem of insufficient energetic capacity remains and will continue to worsen if not addressed. An alternative approach would include supporting the mitochondria and their ability to produce energy. Here again, thiamine rules.

Thiamine is unique among the other nutrients required for mitochondrial function because the enzymes it supports sit atop the pathways that allow components of proteins, fats, and carbs into the mitochondria, there to be converted into ATP. Thiamine is a gatekeeper to the entire process, so when thiamine concentrations are low, the macronutrients cannot be metabolized into the components that will enter the mitochondria and produce ATP. Instead, they are diverted toward less efficient metabolic pathways that produce far less energy than the mitochondria could, and they do so at a much higher cost.

A way to conceptualize this process is to imagine the mitochondria as mini-factories whose primary task is to extract energy from the food we consume. In this model, proteins, fats, and carbs are the raw materials that must be converted into the end product, ATP. The machines responsible for this work, the enzymes, require vitamins and minerals in order to operate. This is their fuel. When the factory machines don't have enough fuel, they don't work. When the first machines on the line are broken, it doesn't matter that the other machines work, because all the raw materials will sit idly at the gates, waiting to be processed. This is what happens when thiamine is lacking: the machines responsible for preparing the raw materials for entry into the factory don't work well; the main machine that opens the door to the factory doesn't work well; and the machines within the factory, which are also thiamine-dependent, don't work well either.

To help control the buildup of raw materials, the factory activates subsystems, generators, if you will, that are capable of processing some of the materials into product. As one might expect, these subsystems burn dirtier and produce far less product than the primary factory. Since energy is the product, the more one has to rely on these subsystems for energy the less energy one has to function—and so begins the decline.

While any nutrient deficiency would cause problems in the energy factory, slowing processing at the juncture where that nutrient is required, thiamine is uniquely consequential. It's involved in each of the macronutrient pathways that lead to the mitochondria and it sits at the entry gates. It also determines whether or not glucose enters the mitochondria, and influences how fats and proteins are metabolized and eventually become ATP.

Thiamine governs the oxidative component of oxidative metabolism. It influences whether and how oxygen is used in the metabolism of glucose. When thiamine is low, molecular oxygen is not used effectively. This leads to a state of what is called pseudo-hypoxia; pseudo because there's no obstruction blocking the intake of oxygen, so there's technically plenty of oxygen floating around. It's only because there's not enough thiamine that the oxygen can't be used. This manifests as something commonly referred to as air-hunger. Those who experience air hunger are typically low in thiamine. It should be noted that riboflavin deficiency may also cause air-hunger, as it too is cofactor to the gatekeeper enzyme.

Modern dietary practices assume that with any given food there are always enough vitamins and minerals to keep the mitochondrial machinery active, but that's not always the case. Sometimes there are far more raw materials than there is fuel to process them (high-calorie malnutrition); at other times, components of the foods we eat or the medications we take contain anti-thiamine factors, so even though we've consumed enough of the nutrient and should not be deficient based upon intake, we can yet be deficient because other substances have blocked or deactivated the vitamin.

Another potential anti-thiamine variable is life itself. A severe stressor or illness can simply overwhelm our thiamine intake and thus our capacity to produce energy. Again, COVID is a prime example, but any illness or significant stressor (death, divorce, loss of a job) has the capacity to tip one into deficiency, especially if one's nutrient intake was marginal to begin with.

For women, the increased energetic demands of pregnancy pose a significant risk of developing thiamine deficiency, a risk magnified exponentially with hyperemesis (nausea and vomiting, i.e., "morning sickness") and a risk often ignored by current medical practices. The RDA for thiamine during pregnancy, established decades ago, is wholly insufficient for the increased energetic demands of pregnancy. Once vomiting sets in, the potential for thiamine deficiency increases significantly.

Metabolic Fatigue and Autonomic and Cerebellar Dysfunction

When one becomes deficient or even simply skirts deficiency of thiamine, metabolic fatigue sets in. Metabolic fatigue is the slowing of metabolic function, and the inability to consistently produce enough energy to meet the demands of daily living. With insufficient energy, physiological activities that were once automatic and highly regulated become less so over time. The autonomic system (ANS) and cerebellum are areas of the brain that are noticeably affected by low thiamine and highly susceptible to it.

The ANS controls aspects of bodily function that must happen automatically, like breathing and heart rate, heart rhythm, and blood pressure, digestion, and sexual arousal. It responds to signals from the environment, sends them to the brain to be translated, and then back to the organs or tissues for a response. Part of the system is hardwired, with communications sent from the brain to the organs and tissues via nerve conduction, but part of the system is soft-wired with hormone-based communications.

The whole process is lightning fast and beyond cognition, such that when an immediate threat presents itself, the ANS will have begun activating patterns well before we are cognitively aware of the danger. The raised hairs on the back of our neck, the increased breathing and heart rate, and the general sense that something is "off" are part of the ANS fight-or-flight response activated through the sympathetic nerves in the ANS. When the threat has passed, the parasympathetic system kicks in to slow everything down and return the body to balance. This part of the ANS is referred to as the rest-and-digest or breed-and-feed system.

Both the sympathetic and parasympathetic portions of the ANS operate automatically and depend upon vast and consistent quantities of ATP to do so. When oxidative metabolism and energetic capacity are limited, the balance between sympathetic and parasympathetic activity becomes skewed. Here, three patterns emerge: sympathetic dominant, parasympathetic dominant, and oscillating.

When the sympathetic system is dominant, the individual may experience a constant state of fight or flight, with agitation or anxiety and overreaction to stressors being the dominant presentation. Here, excessive vasoconstriction is the underlying theme. In the heart, this means increased heart rate or blood pressure. In the gut, it means slowed digestion and impaired gut motility. Symptoms such as gastroparesis and constipation may present, and because of slower motility, bacterial and fungal overgrowth are common. With excessive sympathetic activity, it's difficult to empty the bladder, as the sphincter contracts tightly. This is called neurogenic bladder, but in reality, it's often a component of a constellation of symptoms wherein the brain has insufficient energy to manage the balance between sympathetic and parasympathetic activity. In the nerves, because of the reduced parasympathetic activity, small-fiber neuropathies are common. Muscles may twitch and tremor or contract tightly, including the eyelids. In the skin, goosebumps and/or excess sweating may be present.

In contrast, a more parasympathetic-dominant presentation might include excessive or inappropriate vasodilation and the opposite pattern of symptoms emerges; that is, difficulty constricting vessels or contracting muscles. Heart rate and blood pressure are lower, gut motility is increased, bowel and urinary incontinence may develop, and neuralgia—intense nerve pain and muscle pain and weakness—are common. Sweating is absent and heat intolerance may develop.

The oscillating pattern, in which many people find themselves, is the fluctuation between too much stimulation and not enough. These are ill-timed and poorly managed autonomic responses. No matter the pattern, when autonomic symptoms arise, one should consider the possibility that poor energetic capacity underlies these symptoms, which inevitably means thiamine ought to be addressed. While thiamine isn't the only nutrient required for energy production, it is the most critical and most frequently missed.

Since autonomic messages are regulated both through central and peripheral nerve conduction and via hormone release, individuals with ANS symptoms will also have endocrine-related signaling issues; e.g., too much too soon, too little too late. The signaling issues are the tip of the hormone iceberg (see chapter 20). The first steps in steroid hormone synthesis begin in the mitochondria, so poorly functioning mitochondria in the various endocrine glands will reallocate resources to those hormones involved in survival processes (cortisol and the mineralocorticoids) rather than to those involved in sex and reproduction. In other words, everything is a mess, but the mess can be fixed, or at least managed, if one supports mitochondrial function by addressing the root causes of mitochondrial dysfunction.

Another region of the brain noticeably affected by low thiamine is the cerebellum, the cauliflower-like tissue located at the back of the brain. It consumes an enormous amount of ATP. Among its primary tasks is the management of motor control; think balance, and the rate, rhythm, force, and accuracy of motor movements. Individuals with low thiamine have difficulty controlling motor movements. This is most commonly observed with either gait disturbances—how one walks (ataxia), or abnormal eye movements (nystagmus). Regarding the gait, think drunken sailor with reduced speed and smaller but wider steps that are highly variable and sometimes asymmetric. Muscle atrophy and weakness are common. The patterns can be subtle at first but become more noticeable over time. With nystagmus, the eyes bounce back and forth or up and down. Again, this can be subtle at first, but is easily observed and is a clear indicator of low thiamine. Videos of the various patterns of ataxia and nystagmus are available on YouTube and provide an easy resource for testing oneself at home.

The cerebellum is also involved with similar functions relative to cognitive and affective balance. It regulates the force, rhythm, and accuracy of our thoughts and moods. Does our response to a situation meet the demands or the tenor of the situation, or, like the dysautonomic responses, is it too much or too little, too soon or too late? When one finds oneself unusually reactive cognitively or emotionally, it might be time to look into thiamine.

Diagnosis of Thiamine Deficiency

It would be wonderful if tests for assessing thiamine were readily and accurately available, but unfortunately, this is not the case. The main reason for this is that thiamine, like magnesium, is primarily an intracellular nutrient. What this means, using magnesium as an example, is that most of the magnesium in the body resides *within cells* and does not float around in blood or serum for easy measurement. This means that our usual measurement of magnesium (and thiamine) is not very accurate.

Getting an accurate assay requires special testing from a specialty laboratory, and at this time, this is not easily available. To my knowledge, the only lab currently running this test, by special request, is Vitamin Diagnostics. This testing involves a two-step process from blood, measuring first ETKA (erythrocyte transketolase) and then measuring TPPE (thiamine pyrophosphate effect), in which after ETKA is measured, a specific amount of thiamine is added to the specimen, and the ability of the red blood cells to utilize that thiamine is then measured.

For academic and research purposes, it would be helpful if this test was more readily available. For the moment, it might be empirically necessary to provide a trial of thiamine treatment and see how the patient responds to it, with the diagnosis of thiamine deficiency a reasonable assumption based on the patient's symptoms, diagnoses, and medications.

Treatment of Thiamine Deficiency

Since my practice consists of primarily very sensitive patients, I have found that quite a few patients need to start treatment with very low doses and slowly work up to higher doses as they begin to tolerate thiamine better over time. A typical starting dose for many patients is 100mg of thiamine hydrochloride, but for my sensitive patients, I will suggest they try just a few "sprinkles" of thiamine, as they open the capsule and use a few granules. If that is well tolerated, then I suggest more measurable amounts, such as ¼ of a capsule, then ½, then 1 whole capsule. If that's well-handled, or the original 100mg well tolerated, I suggest slowly bumping the dose up to 100mg twice daily, then 200mg twice daily.

If this is well tolerated, I encourage patients to try a better-absorbed formulation of thiamine, TTFD (thiamine tetrahydrofurfuryl disulfide), again starting at 50mg once daily and slowly increasing the dose, as tolerated to 200mg twice daily, or then doubling that as well. The TTFD penetrates the blood-brain barrier and provides increased amounts of thiamine for the brain, where it is especially needed.

On page 139 of Marrs and Lonsdale's book, we see an intravenous protocol to provide not only thiamine but other helpful cofactors. If IV treatments are available, this gets around the possible problem of poor nutrient absorption faced by many of our patients.

Magnesium is an important cofactor of thiamine in many of the biochemical reactions so critical to mitochondrial energy production, and 250–500mg of magnesium daily would be necessary to take along with the thiamine itself. Chandler Marrs has shared with me that it is not uncommon, once thiamine deficiencies have been alleviated, to find that other vitamin deficiencies become more noticeable and other B vitamins, especially B2, B6, B9, and B12 may be needed for supplementation as well. Similarly, other minerals like calcium and potassium are often required. For individuals with POTS, migraines, and long term SSRI use, sodium and phosphate are often lacking as well.

Conclusion

While many other nutrient deficiencies play a role in our patients with extreme sensitivities and chronic illness, the special importance of thiamine deficiency has been highlighted as a major missing puzzle piece that I believe is just beginning to be revealed as a central concern to be looked for and addressed in all of our patients.

As we begin to appreciate the role that the autonomic nervous system plays here, along with the limbic system, in all of our sensitive patients, we can readily understand that the replacement of thiamine deficiency is yet another modality that will help our patients to move toward healing.

DR. CHANDLER MARRS received a BA in philosophy and then spent many years in the tech industry before returning to academia for a master's in clinical psychology and a master's and PhD in experimental psychology with an emphasis on neuroendocrinology. She spent decades in health research, has written hundreds of articles, and has edited and published the online journal *Hormones Matter* since 2011. Together with Dr. Derrick Lonsdale, she co-authored the groundbreaking book *Thiamine Deficiency Disease, Dysautonomia, and High Calorie Malnutrition.* You can contact her at chandler@hormonesmatter.com.

Chapter 19: The Genetics of Sensitivity

Bob Miller, CTN

Dr. Nathan's Introduction

In chapter 13, Greg Nigh introduced us to several SNPs that were essential to sulfur metabolism and could contribute to sensitivity. Here, Dr. Miller deepens our understanding of how genetic predispositions can affect sensitive patients in a variety of ways. He will begin with a basic understanding of what SNPs are and then goes into detail about some of the specific biochemical pathways that appear to be the most important for our understanding of inflammation and sensitivity. This presentation requires some in-depth discussion of enzyme biochemistry, which will be of great value for medical practitioners. For those readers for whom biochemical pathways are not a common topic of conversation, I encourage you to get as much from this chapter as possible. Bear in mind that when patients are really struggling and operating at survival level, attending to treating the triggers of these conditions (e.g., mold and Lyme) and the limbic, vagal, and mast-cell dysfunction they create, comes first. In my experience, the information Dr. Miller provides allows us to help our patients optimally once the primary triggering issues have been addressed, at which time this information becomes invaluable.

✿ ✿ ✿

As this book has shown, there are multiple environmental factors that many people respond to more strongly than others. We often hear from patients in our clinic who have mold in their homes that one person is greatly impacted by it while another barely notices. One person can get Lyme disease and do very well with treatment, while someone else, despite getting the best treatment, both medical and holistic, suffers for years without finding relief. In some individuals, the mast cells are ready to fight when needed, but in others, as Beth O'Hara points out in chapter 4, the mast cells become extremely overactive and cause serious problems.

Additionally, some individuals can comfortably spend any amount of time around cellphones and Wi-Fi, while others are very sensitive and feel their impact. We're now going to examine the possibility that genetic factors might make some individuals more sensitive than others, but first let's explore elementary genomics.

Functional Genomics 101

At the moment of your conception, when the sperm and the egg got together, you became a combination of your mother's DNA and your father's DNA. Locked in at conception, that never changes. If we were to test your DNA after you passed from this earth, it would be the same as it was at the moment of your conception. I'm sure you've seen photos in which DNA looks like a twisted ladder; each rung on the left gets the DNA from the mom, and each rung on the right gets DNA from the dad. It's a complex subject, but we can simplify and say that DNA makes proteins, of which enzymes are an important example. Enzymes (which are proteins composed of amino acids) take a substance, add something else to it, and make something new. Then another enzyme comes along and repeats the same process. It's amazing that the fats, carbohydrates, proteins, the water we drink, the air we breathe, and the sunlight we're exposed to get made into our hair, skin, nails, blood, neurotransmitters, and energy to fuel us. The purpose of your DNA is to make these proteins, which include enzymes. Sometimes we get what are called SNPs (single nucleotide polymorphisms) in which the instructions to make the enzymes might not be totally efficient. This results in an enzyme that can be less than optimal in its function. It is called homozygous when we get a SNP from both parents, and heterozygous when we get a SNP from one parent.

It's estimated that a heterozygous SNP may reduce the efficiency of the enzyme by 25%–35%, while a homozygous SNP can make the enzyme even less efficient. In our clinic, we look only at what we call functional genomics. We don't examine or interpret mutations that are related to disease. Functional genomics simply looks at where genetic mutations, or SNPs, may result in less-than-optimal antioxidant production, more-than-excess free radicals, less-than-optimal detoxification, or in the proper transport of nutrients. By examining the DNA and looking at functional genomics, we can determine if it's to an individual's advantage to take nutrients that support antioxidants, support one's ability to neutralize free radicals, support detox pathways, or support the transportation of key nutrients throughout the body. This is not a diagnosis of disease or a treatment for disease, but rather a *supporting function*. This support of function can be done by actually giving a person some of the nutrients, herbs, or plant sources that support an enzyme's function. It's very important to bear in mind that genetic mutations create a *potential* for suboptimal function, but SNPs are never a given or a diagnosis.

Underactive vs Overactive – The Enzymes and Toxins that Stimulate Inflammation

I'm perennially amazed at how our body has mechanisms to build, function, and protect itself. When we're faced with a virus, bacteria, parasite, or pathogen of any kind, the body has powerful mechanisms to launch a fight against it and kill it or remove it. Without this process, life couldn't exist—we would be overcome by invading organisms.

In many people who've become sensitive, however, we have observed that many of their defense mechanisms are *overactive*. There's a delicate balance between underactive and overactive. If our immune system is underactive, we're overtaken by pathogens; if it's overactive, we can be harmed by increased inflammation and the formation of free radicals. We often cite the simple analogy of *Goldilocks and the Three Bears*: "Not too hot, not too cold, not too hard, not too soft—just right!" Our body is very similar. We need a proper balance for many functions. Unfortunately, environmental factors, amplified in those with genetic weakness, are pushing us to a pro-inflammatory state that creates a fertile ground in which sensitivities emerge.

Our chapter will focus primarily on chart #1, which shows where environmental factors can overstimulate our body's defense systems. At the very top of the chart you'll see TNF-a, which stands for tumor necrosis factor alpha. This creates what are called inflammatory cytokines. Cytokines fight pathogens. During acute inflammation, this cytokine is produced by white blood cells called macrophages and monocytes. TNF-a is responsible for a diverse range of signaling events within cells; these events can lead to necrosis (the death of most or all of the cells in an organ or tissue due to disease, injury, or failure of the blood supply) or apoptosis (the death of cells that occurs as a normal and controlled part of an organism's growth or development).

This protein is important when we need to fight infections and cancers; however, if it's overactive, it can stimulate other enzymes and result in inflammation in the body. From a functional genetic standpoint, there is an important TNF-a SNP (RS1800629). This is an interesting SNP because when there is a mutation (from one or both parents), the TNF-a may be overactive or sometimes what is called gain of function—in other words it *over-responds*.

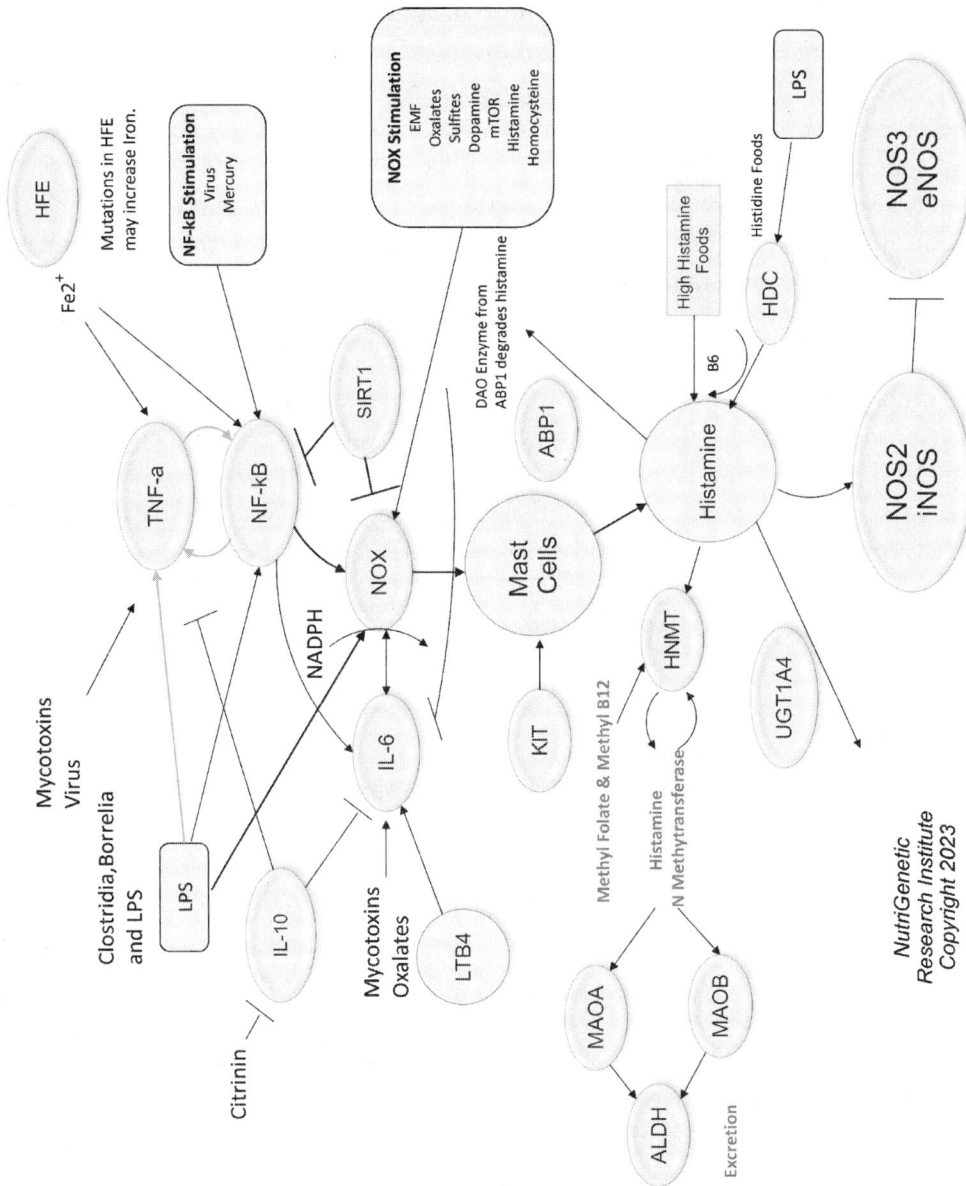

NOX Stimulation
EMF
Oxalates
Sulfites
Dopamine
mTOR
Histamine
Homocysteine

NF-kB Stimulation
Virus
Mercury

HFE

Mutations in HFE may increase Iron.

Fe^{2+}

SIRT1

TNF-a

NF-kB

NOX

NADPH

IL-6

IL-10

LPS

Mycotoxins
Virus

Clostridia, Borrelia
and LPS

Citrinin

Mycotoxins
Oxalates

LTB4

DAO Enzyme from ABP1 degrades histamine

ABP1

Mast Cells

KIT

High Histamine Foods

Histidine Foods

LPS

HDC

B6

Histamine

NOS3
eNOS

NOS2
iNOS

HNMT

UGT1A4

Histamine
N Methytransferase

Methyl Folate & Methyl B12

MAOA

MAOB

ALDH

Excretion

*NutriGenetic
Research Institute
Copyright 2023*

Chart #1

Looking at chart #1, you'll see that mycotoxins (from mold), clostridia (bad gut bacteria), *Bartonella* (a coinfection of Lyme disease), lipopolysaccharides (gram negative bacteria), pesticides, and mercury will stimulate TNF-a. Consequently, when we're exposed to these toxins, often several of them at the same time, TNF-a may be activated; however, if a patient has the mutated SNP, there is the potential that it would be *overactivated*. If TNF-a is responding normally, and we are exposed to several of these toxins or pathogens (or any one in excess), there's potential that TNF-a becomes overactive even without a mutation.

Iron is a very important mineral. Without it we couldn't carry oxygen through our blood attached to hemoglobin, but excess iron can be inflammatory and may stimulate TNF-a. There are genetic mutations on what is called the HFE gene that create the potential for more iron absorption from the diet than in someone who doesn't have this mutation. Note on the chart that excess iron stimulates TNF-a. Two of the common genetic mutations in HFE are HFE H63D and HFE C282Y.

As you see in chart #1, TNF-a stimulates and activates the NF-kb pathway. Note too that NF-kB is also stimulated by iron and lipopolysaccharides, but look closely and you'll see that NF-kB also stimulates TNF-a, and consequently, we can have a feedback loop that keeps us becoming more and more inflamed.

The Pathway of Continual Inflammation

You'll also see in chart #1 that NF-kB will stimulate an enzyme called NOX (or NADPH oxidase). Once again, NOX is our protector from pathogens, viruses. and bacteria, but when overstimulated and overactive it can become harmful.

The NOX enzyme will stimulate the production of superoxide and stimulate mast cells when exposed to pathogens or other substances such as sulfites or homocysteine. You'll also note that the NOX enzyme is stimulated by IL-6, another cytokine.

Interleukin 6 plays an important role in the body. When faced with pathogens, we need IL-6 to create superoxide and stimulate mast cells and histamine production to kill the pathogens, but IL-6 can also be stimulated by multiple environmental factors. These factors are listed in chart #2, "Environmental IL-6 Stimulation," while chart #3, "Potential Endogenous Mediators / IL-6 Stimulation," illustrates potential endogenous stimulators of IL-6. Each of these can stimulate interleukin 6, which will then stimulate the NOX enzyme and begin the process of stimulating mast cells and histamine.

Environmental IL-6 Stimulation

> Mold/Mycotoxins
> Lyme Disease (lipopolysaccarides)
> Lipopolysaccarides (lead amplifies)
> EMF - Radon
> Air Pollution - Particulates
> Smoking
> Sodium Sulfate - Coffee
> Lead, Mercury, Aluminum
> Glyphosate
> Omega 6's (Canola Oil)
> VOC's Volatile Organic Compounds
> Pesticides
> Any mTOR stimulator

Chart #2

Once again, however, when *overstimulated* IL-6 becomes a problem. IL-6 is created by the IL-6 enzyme, and just like the other enzymes we've discussed, there are genetic mutations that can cause IL-6 to be overactive.

Potential Endogenous Mediators IL-6 Stimulation

> Histamine - Dopamine
> Angiotension II
> NOX (NADPH Oxidase)
> Bradykinin
> Obseity - Hyperglycemia
> High Homocysteine
> Oxalates - C. Diff
> Estriol
> Hydrogen Peroxide
> Over Exercise
> Virus
> Anxiety

Chart #3

To learn more about IL-6, I encourage you to watch the interview with Dr. Jill Carnahan on YouTube regarding IL-6. Go to YouTube, search "Jill Carnahan IL-6," and it will pop up. Dr. Jill's and my nearly two-hour conversation illustrates both the advantages and disadvantages of IL-6. The video will give you a good understanding of how it can be helpful or harmful, what overstimulates it, and the steps you can take to reduce it if it's overactive.

The NADPH Steal

There's a very important substance in the body called NADPH. It's a critical player in making the important gas called nitric oxide, which supports circulation and many other critical body functions. It's also needed to help recycle a vital antioxidant called glutathione. If glutathione isn't "recharged" or "recycled," we have limited ability to process toxic substances and neutralize free radicals. NADPH is a unique molecule because it can wear two hats. It can help make crucial substances for our health, but it can also be used to make free radicals to kill pathogens. I am not aware of any other substance in the body that can perform such opposite functions. There are multiple pathways and enzymes that make NADPH, and mutations in some of these enzymes may reduce the pool of available NADPH.

The NOX enzyme uses NADPH to create inflammation. When the NOX enzyme is overstimulated by IL-6 and/or NF-kB or other environmental or internal factors, there is potential for NADPH to become overused and depleted.

In our educational program for health professionals we have coined the phrase the "NADPH Steal." This is where the NOX enzyme uses NADPH *excessively*, consequently depriving the body of NADPH for other important functions. If NADPH isn't available to help recycle the master antioxidant glutathione and make nitric oxide, this can lead to higher levels of inflammation and suboptimal detoxification.

SIRT 1, HEME Oxygenase, and IL-10 – Critical for Lowering Inflammation

As you've just learned, environmental toxins and genetic mutations have the potential to increase inflammation while the body works at killing pathogens. The body is amazing in that it has other enzymes whose function is to *reduce* the inflammation being made so the body won't be damaged. What a fascinating balance! And SIRT1 is one of those enzymes.

As we age, we also experience progressive organ dysfunction. Recently, molecules called sirtuins have emerged as having the potential to slow aging and decrease age-related disorders. Sirtuins are a family of proteins that regulates your cellular health. They play a critical role in regulating cellular homeostasis (keeping the cell in balance). The sirtuins manage everything that happens in your cells; however, sirtuins can only do their job if they are made properly (no genetic mutations) and there is adequate NAD+ (nicotinamide adenine dinucleotide), which is a coenzyme found in all living cells.

To date, seven sirtuins (SIRT1 to SIRT7) have been identified. Sirtuins research has focused on aging and metabolic activity, and there are now about 12,000 papers on the subject.

Referring to chart #4, you'll see that SIRT 1 suppresses, or holds back, the NOX enzyme and NF-kB, potentially keeping them from creating too much inflammation such as what occurs in some autoimmune diseases like rheumatoid arthritis. As shown in the chart, SIRT1 not only inhibits the NOX enzyme and NF-kB but supports the production of an important antioxidant called superoxide dismutase (SOD). The role of SOD is to neutralize a nasty free radical called superoxide. Superoxide can be created as we make energy within the cell, and it may be stimulated by EMFs (cellphone, Wi-Fi, etc.); it can also be created if glutathione is not recycled properly, and by NOS uncoupling, a subject we'll discuss later. SIRT 1 is considered an important enzyme for your health and longevity as it also stimulates the eNOS enzyme to make nitric oxide, which is critical for good circulation to the muscles and organs.

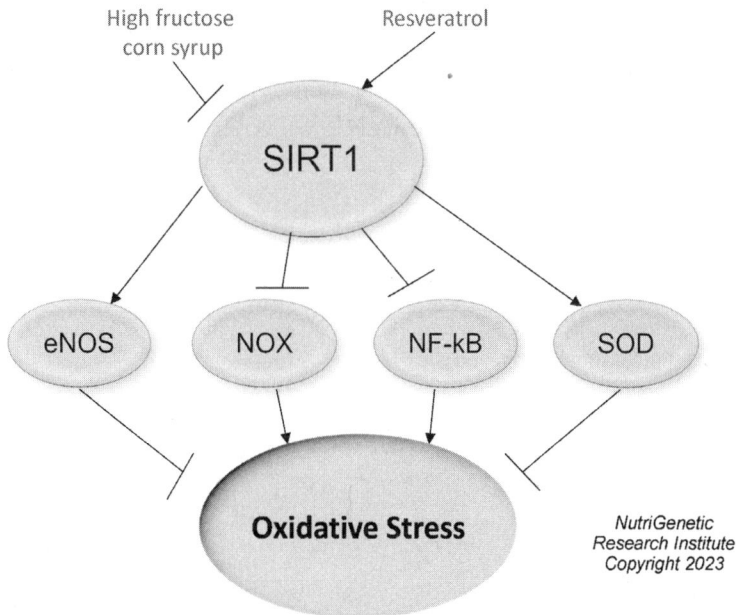

SIRT1 support eNOS for good circulation and SOD to neutralize the free radical superoxide, and inhibits NOX and NF-kb that create oxidative stress. High fructose corn syrup inhibits SIRT1 and resveratrol may support SIRT1.

Chart #4

The scientific community has identified that mutations in SIRT1 (rs12778366) might decrease SIRT1 activity, hence decreasing our ability to control the inflammatory process. Also, studies have shown that high-fructose corn syrup inhibits SIRT1. Sadly, more and more processed foods contain high-fructose corn syrup. In our clinic, we've observed that especially those with genetic mutations in SIRT1 (rs12778366) have started to feel better when they eliminated the use of high fructose corn syrup as much as possible. Additionally, some papers show that resveratrol may boost SIRT1 activity. Since SIRT1 is NAD+ dependent, in some instances, supplementing with nicotinamide riboside may also help boost SIRT1.

And finally, some studies show that intermittent fasting may boost SIRT1 activity. Potential Action Steps to support SIRT1:

- Try to avoid or significantly reduce high-fructose corn syrup, especially if there are mutations in SIRT1.
- Consider supplementing with resveratrol if advised by a health professional.
- Consider intermittent fasting if advised by a health professional.
- Consider gentle supplementation with nicotinamide riboside if advised by a health professional.

The body is so complex that although we have enzymes like TNF-a and NF-kB that create inflammation, properly functioning SIRT1 calms them. An enzyme called HEME oxygenase (see chart #5) will also slow down NF-kB, NADPH oxidase, and IL-6.

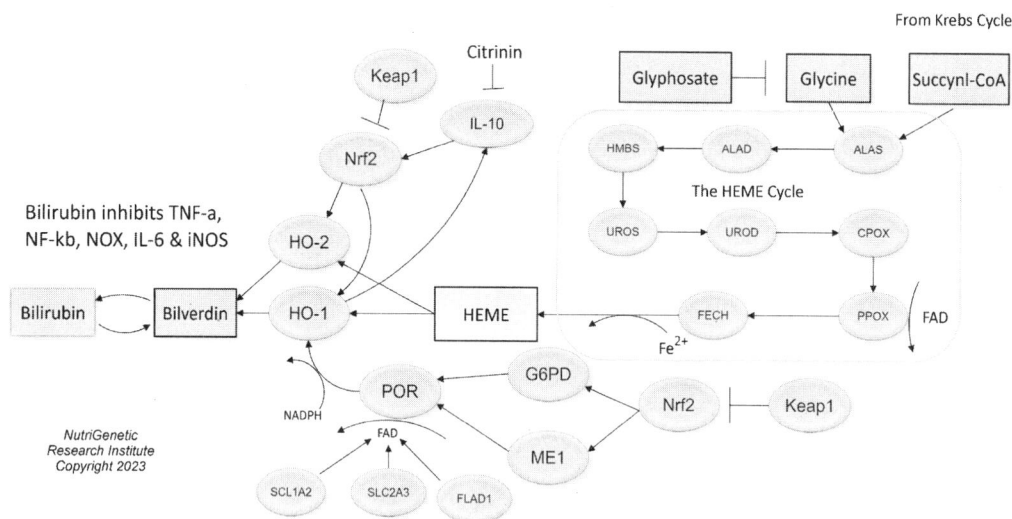

Chart #5

Once again, mutations in HEME oxygenase can cause these enzymes to be less than effective. There is also an enzyme called Nrf2, which plays many roles in the body and is related to making, using, and recycling our antioxidants, and is involved with all of our phase 1 and 2 detoxification, lipid metabolism, and many other processes. Nrf2 also stimulates HEME oxygenase, and mutations in NRF2 can make this less than optimal, consequently not adequately stimulating HEME oxygenase.

To date, one of the most interesting mutations we are finding in those who are overly sensitive is mutations in something called KEAP1. Understanding KEAP1 can be a little complex because it *degrades* Nrf2. When KEAP1 senses inflammation, it stops degrading and allows Nrf2 to perform its many functions. Interestingly, there is a mutation in KEAP1 (rs9676881) that is a *gain of function,* meaning that the activity of KEAP1 might be stronger. If Keap1 becomes stronger it might not stimulate Nrf2 as quickly as it needs to, thus allowing more inflammation that's not properly neutralized (see chart #6).

As a clinical observation only, we are discovering that when people inherit a homozygous (from mother and father) on the *gain of function KEAP1,* these individuals struggle more than most with sensitivity to mold, Lyme disease, and other infections, and thereby experience severe health challenges.

Finally, there's an interleukin called IL-10. Unlike other interleukins that are pro-inflammatory, IL-10 is anti-inflammatory. IL-10 supports NRF2 and inhibits IL-6 and TNF-a.

The mycotoxin citrinin inhibits IL-10. Consequently, citrinin-inhibiting IL-10 might be another cause of runaway inflammation.

To summarize, if someone has environmental factors that stimulate TNF-a and NF-kB, and/or has mutations in TNF-a that make it overactive, or has mutations that cause iron to become elevated and then has weakness in either SIRT1, HMOX, and IL-10, you could have the perfect storm that creates a cascade of inflammation that impairs energy production and makes excessive inflammation in the body. This sets the table for limbic and vagal dysfunction and for mast-cell activation, which are some of the primary triggers for the creation of sensitivity in our patients.

Now let's examine how this inflammatory cascade wreaks havoc in your body.

Mast Cells and Histamine

Again referring to chart #1, note that the NOX (NADPH Oxidase) enzyme stimulates mast cells (see chapter 4 on mast-cell activation). Here I'll simply mention that mast cells are a type of white blood cell intended to protect us. If, however, they become overactive, they can create excess inflammation in the body. From a genetic standpoint, an enzyme called KIT stimulates the mast cells, and there are multiple KIT SNPS that can make mast cells overreactive. One of the main substances that mast cells create in an effort to kill off pathogens is histamine, which plays an important role in the body and can help us in many ways. Excess histamine can, however, cause allergic reactions that can affect the eyes, nose, throat, skin, and lungs. It can cause inflammation in the body and might contribute to allergies and asthma. Other symptoms of high histamine include reactions to fermented foods (which contain large amounts of histamine), over-reaction to mosquito bites, excess itching, hives, sensitivity to heat, and worsening of seasonal allergies.

To help us deal with histamine, we have an enzyme called HMNT (histamine N methyltransferase) that helps degrade histamine. Here again, there can be genetic mutations in the HMNT enzymes that don't allow the histamine to be degraded effectively. Mutations in rs11558538, rs758252808 and rs745756308 can reduce the effectiveness of HNMT to clear histamine from the body.

Additionally, the body makes an enzyme called diamine oxidase to help degrade the excessive histamine that can be present in our food. Here again, there are genetic mutations that can impair the body's ability to make the DAO enzyme.

Consequently, if there is suboptimal production of DAO, eating a low-histamine diet (primarily non-fermented foods) and/or taking the DAO enzyme with foods can be helpful. There are many resources on the internet, and books that can help you find a list of the high-histamine foods that could be harmful if you appear to be reacting to some foods.

There's also an enzyme called HDC (histidine decarboxylase) that will use the amino acid histidine (high in beef and pork) to create more histamine. We believe that mutations in the HDC can cause this gene to be overactive and make more histamine, but this has not been clearly proven.

In our clinic we commonly see people who are struggling and who present with many mutations with the histamine-degrading enzymes that create higher levels of histamine in their bodies. Histamine can create more problems than just allergic reactions and a runny nose; it can impact the gastrointestinal system and the circulatory system and increase the stress-inducing neurotransmitter glutamate.

You'll see in chart #1 that in addition to HNMT, the HNMT enzyme makes N-methyl histamine. The MAOA and MAOB enzymes then need to take this N-methyl histamine and degrade it further. If there are mutations in MAOA and/or MAOB and not enough of a substance called FAD (made from B2, Riboflavin), which is used by the MAOA enzymes, the N-methyl histamine can become very pro-inflammatory and actually *suppress* HNMT and create problems that are worse than the original histamine!

Perhaps this has happened to you. You might have learned that you have genetic mutations in MTHFR or just decided to take methyl folate or B12 and had a reaction to these supplements such as agitation and inflammation. What potentially could be happening is that (as you'll see in the chart) folate and B12 stimulates the HNMT enzyme. If the activity of MAOA or MAOB is weakened, this is one reason why taking methyl folate or methyl B12 can be detrimental. Consequently, before taking either of them, you might need to support the MAO enzyme with riboflavin (the cofactor for MAO) to support MAO, or break down histamine with diamine oxidase enzymes, or reduce your intake of histamine-rich foods, or take supplements that stabilize the mast cells that create histamine as a first step prior to being able to successfully take methyl B12 and/ or methyl folate or SAMe.

To learn more about histamine metabolism, watch the video that Dr. Jill Carnahan and I made on histamine on Jill's YouTube channel. Just go to YouTube and search "Dr. Jill Carnahan Histamine" and our forty-five-minute interview will be available for viewing. In this presentation we show charts and graphs of just how histamine is made and then metabolized.

Histamine Stimulates iNOS

In chart #1 you'll notice that histamine also stimulates the iNOS enzyme. To fully understand this we need to understand nitric oxide, a gas that dilates the blood vessels and has many benefits throughout the body. Three scientists won a Nobel Prize in 1998 for their research on the circulatory benefits of nitric oxide. An enzyme called NOS3, or eNOS, makes the nitric oxide that's beneficial to us. You may have heard of individuals with heart problems carrying nitroglycerine with them. Nitroglycerin and its relatives are metabolized to yield nitric oxide, which relaxes the smooth muscle and blood vessels in your body. There are also many nutritional formulas on the market that are designed to boost nitric oxide.

There's another enzyme called NOS2, or iNOS, that, when activated, makes a lot of nitric oxide when the immune system has a virus, bacteria, or pathogen to fight. Just like the other enzymes we've been discussing, however, *iNOS can be overactive.* You'll see in chart #5 that many environmental factors can cause the iNOS enzyme to become overactive; of special note are high-fructose corn syrup, BPA from plastics, and EMFs. These are all relatively new triggers that we were not exposed to just a few decades ago. Additionally, there are genetic mutations that can cause iNOS to be overactive, including mutations in NOS2 (C-1026A) (rs2779249) and NOS2 (S608L) (rs2297518).

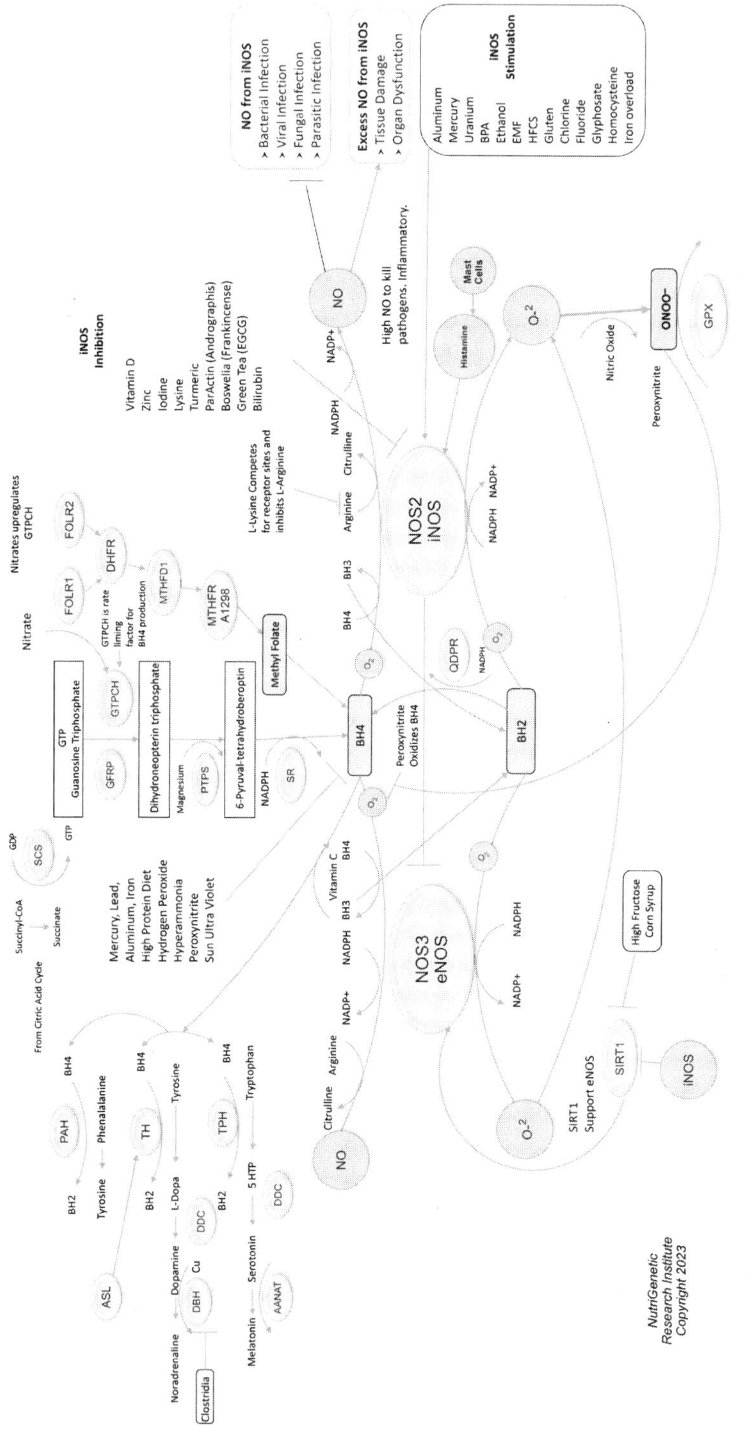

Chart #6

NutriGenetic
Research Institute
Copyright 2023

NO from iNOS
> Bacterial Infection
> Viral Infection
> Fungal Infection
> Parasitic Infection

Excess NO from iNOS
> Tissue Damage
> Organ Dysfunction

iNOS Stimulation
Aluminum
Mercury
Uranium
BPA
Ethanol
EMF
HFCS
Gluten
Chlorine
Fluoride
Glyphosate
Homocysteine
Iron overload

iNOS Inhibition
Vitamin D
Zinc
Iodine
Lysine
Turmeric
ParActin (Andrographis)
Boswellia (Frankincense)
Green Tea (EGCG)
Bilirubin

High NO to kill pathogens. Inflammatory.

Nitrates upregulates GTPCH

L-Lysine Competes for receptor sites and inhibits L-Arginine

GTPCH is rate liming factor for BH4 production

Nitrate

FOLR1   FOLR2
DHFR
MTHFD1
MTHFR A1298

Methyl Folate

GTP Guanosine Triphosphate
GFRP   GTPCH
Dihydroneopterin triphosphate
Magnesium
PTPS   SR
6-Pyruval-tetrahydrobeopterin
NADPH

BH4

Peroxynitrite Oxidizes BH4

BH2

QDPR
NADPH   O₂⁻

Peroxynitrite Oxidizes BH4

NADP+   NO
NADPH   Citrulline
Arginine

NOS2 iNOS
NADPH NADP+

BH3
BH4

Mast Cells
Histamine

O₂⁻   ONOO⁻   GPX
Nitric Oxide
Peroxynitrite

Succinyl-CoA   GDP
From Citric Acid Cycle   SCS   GTP
Succinate

Mercury, Lead, Aluminum, Iron
High Protein Diet
Hydrogen Peroxide
Hyperammonia
Peroxynitrite
Sun Ultra Violet

Vitamin C   BH4
BH3   BH4

NOS3 eNOS
NADP+   NADPH
NADPH

Citrulline   Arginine
NO

O₂⁻   SIRT1
SIRT1 Support eNOS

High Fructose Corn Syrup

iNOS

Noradrenaline
ASL
DBH   Cu
Dopamine   DDC
BH2   L-Dopa
Tyrosine   BH4
PAH
BH2   Phenalalanine
Tyrosine   TH
BH4
Clostridia
Melatonin   Serotonin
AANAT   5 HTP   DDC
BH2   TPH   BH4
Tryptophan

Though there's much debate about EMFs (cellphone, wireless, etc.), there is growing evidence that EMFs could be responsible for increasing inflammation in the body and stimulating the NOX enzyme to make the free radical superoxide. To learn more about EMFs, go to YouTube and watch my interview with Dr Jill Carnahan (and see chapters 9 and 10). To access our interview, search "Dr. Jill Carnahan, EMF" and watch episode #54, in which we show the peer-reviewed literature on how EMF stimulates the creation of free radicals in the body.

Easily implemented action steps:

- Don't charge your cell next to your bed while sleeping.
- Try to keep cellphones off your body as much as possible.
- Use speaker or wired headsets.
- Try not to be near Wi-Fi generators.
- Consider turning off Wi-Fi at night.
- Try to use wired computers as much as possible rather than wireless.

We have made a serious error in using plastics in so many areas of our lives. They're everywhere, and sadly, as they're dumped into the environment, they don't fully degrade. Our waterways and oceans are being polluted with plastic residue, and the impact may be significant. BPA is an endocrine disruptor. Sadly, we now find male frogs with ovaries, and changes to the aquatic population as a result of BPA usage (see chapter 11 for more details).

Evidence shows that BPA can interfere with the endocrine function of hypothalamic-pituitary axis, changing the secretion of gonadotropin-releasing hormone (GnRH) in the hypothalamus, and promoting pituitary proliferation. Such actions may affect puberty and ovulation, and may even result in infertility.

Easily implemented action steps:

- Drink out of glass or stainless steel containers.
- If you microwave, use microwave-safe containers.
- Consider reverse-osmosis water rather than buying plastic bottles of water. (This can save you money, too!)

You'll also notice in the nitric oxide chart, #5, that there's a substance called BH4 (tetrahydrobiopterin), which is needed to help make nitric oxide. If, however, the iNOS enzyme is running too fast for too long we can run out of the BH4, and rather than making nitric oxide we make a free radical called superoxide. This is referred to as NOS uncoupling. Between histamine stimulating the iNOS and the other environmental factors, and for some individuals with genetic gain-of-function mutations, this iNOS can be overactive and can also suppress the eNOS. This often manifests as cold hands and feet, or a predisposition to varicose veins or spider veins. If this continues long term, there are many conditions that can result as an upregulation of the iNOS.

To learn more, watch the video with Dr. Jill Carnahan called the "Carnahan Reaction," so named because Dr. Carnahan appears to have this pattern. In the video we carefully go through all the environmental and genetic factors that can cause the iNOS enzyme to be upregulated. Just search "Dr. Carnahan iNOS" and interview #82 will pop up. In seventy-five minutes, we show charts and the peer-reviewed literature that make the case for NOS uncoupling and the "Carnahan Reaction."

Platelet Activation

As you know, floating in our blood are platelets. They move harmlessly through the bloodstream until we experience a cut or injury, whereupon the platelets stick together and form clots to stop the bleeding. This is a critical part of our survival; without it we would bleed to death with the slightest injury. We need to be careful, however, that the platelets don't get "activated" excessively. This can not only cause clots or raise the risk of cardiovascular disease, but activated platelets may also stimulate RANTES, sCD40L, and VEGF, all of which may be harmful to the body.

Excess iNOS can stimulate platelet aggregation. Another pathway that we won't cover in this chapter is the biochemistry of how arachidonic acid may also activate platelets. To learn about this entire pathway, I encourage you to watch the video with Dr. Jill Carnahan called "Genetics of Platelet Activation." We walk through all these pathways and delve into the arachidonic acid pathway of platelet activation.

The reason this could be so important to you is that these reactions can create RANTES, which may be a contributing factor to sensitivity in many individuals who are seriously reacting to mold, Lyme, EMF, virus, etc. Before we get into RANTES, let's investigate how omega 3s can be a critical part of keeping those platelets functioning normally.

Your Balance of Fats is Critical

I'm sure you're aware that omega 3 fish oils can be very beneficial for us. As you'll see in chart #7, consuming healthy fats and using them will make something called protectins and resolvins, which are beneficial to the cardiovascular system, reduce inflammation, and can slow the activation of platelets and the inflammation that activated platelets causes.

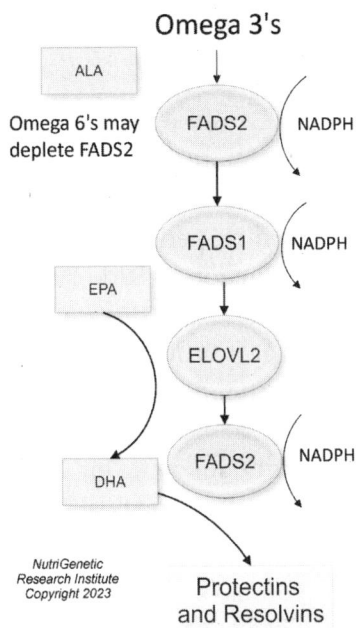

Omega 3's

ALA

Omega 6's may
deplete FADS2

FADS2 — NADPH

FADS1 — NADPH

EPA

ELOVL2

DHA — FADS2 — NADPH

NutriGenetic
Research Institute
Copyright 2023

Protectins
and Resolvins

Chart #7

Enzymes called FADS (fatty acid desaturase) and ELOVL2 are responsible for transforming the omega 3s from your diet, or taken in the form of fish oils, into those protections and resolvins. There can, however, be mutations in the FADS1 and FADS2 enzymes that can inhibit the omega 3s from making anti-inflammatory substances.

Additionally, the standard American diet that used to be equally balanced between inflammatory omega 6 oils and the omega 3s is now 20:1 (bad to good). If our diet is higher in pro-inflammatory fats along with genetic mutations that can impair the body's ability to make these protectins and resolvins, the result can be an inability to hold back the inflammation and platelet activation. Consequently, making sure that your diet is rich in omega 3s and low in omega 6s can be an important part of balancing inflammation in your body. There are many good websites, books, and dieticians that can help you learn whether you have the right balance of fats. Vegetable oils are often high in the bad fats, while fish, especially salmon, is high in omega 3s.

Arachidonic acid-derived prostaglandins not only contribute to the development of inflammation as intercellular pro-inflammatory mediators but also promote the excitability of the peripheral somatosensory system, contributing to worsened pain.

Online, you can order a test called Omega Quant, which simply entails a drop of blood that will show you how you're doing on omega 3s, omega 6s, and arachidonic acid.

RANTES (Regulated Upon Activation of Normal T-Cells Expressed and Secreted) or CCL5

RANTES is a powerful pro-inflammatory mediator of the cytokine (CC chemokine family). RANTES regulates the mobilization and survival of immune inflammatory cells from the bloodstream into tissues and other areas of injury and infection. Once again, this is a good thing when used properly, but if it's excessive it can be a problem. Research shows that sustained production of RANTES is associated with several detrimental effects such as atherosclerosis, liver disease, viral infection, and many other illnesses. Research is also finding that treatments that interfere with RANTES are associated with improved outcomes in patients with chronic inflammatory conditions.

As you'll see in chart #8, RANTES is stimulated by activated platelets. Research demonstrates that excess iNOS activity along with inflammation of other pathways (from arachidonic acid) will activate the platelets; and finally, the upregulation of IL-6 that we discussed earlier, as well as the release of aldosterone, can also stimulate RANTES.

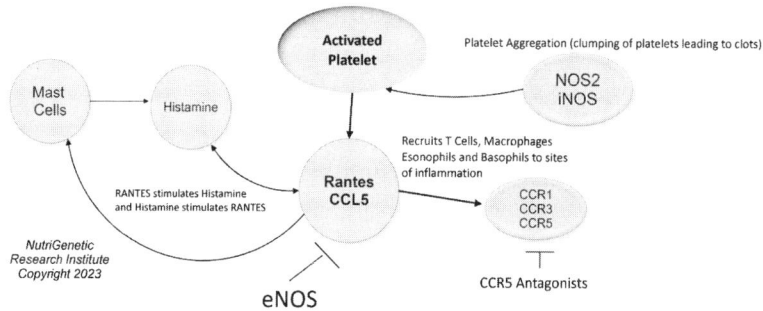

Chart #8

Sadly, RANTES will also stimulate mast cells and histamine and can create a loop of inflammation in the body. This is a complex phenomenon, and the best way to understand it is to watch the video that Dr. Jill Carnahan and I made on her YouTube channel called "Platelet Activation and RANTES." In it you'll see how everything we've discussed in this chapter goes together and culminates in the excess RANTES. We've been observing very high levels of RANTES in patients with Long Haul COVID-19, chronic Lyme, severe mold exposure, and in some patients with autism.

In Conclusion

Most people who are struggling with extreme sensitivity might have overexposure to the environmental factors listed in this chapter, and possibly have genetic weakness that encourages the production of additional inflammation or have a limited ability to neutralize free radicals. As we do our health coaching with individuals who are really struggling with Lyme, mycotoxins, or other environmental insults, we've discovered that a trend is emerging.

In patients who've become unusually toxic and/or sensitive, we usually find some combination of upregulation of TNF-a and/or weakness in HEME oxygenase, increase of function in Keap1, weakness in Nrf2, weakness in SIRT1, upregulation in mast cells, inability to degrade histamine, and gain of function on iNOS. It's usually some combination of these factors that sets the stage for becoming sensitive to everything. If you'd like to see whether you have a genetic predisposition to any of these up- or downregulations described feel free to reach out to our clinic via the contact information at the end of this chapter.

I trust this information was eye-opening. To close with a phrase that I like to use with many of my health coaching clients, I have four important words for you: "It's not your fault." Unfortunately, many people have been made to believe they're imagining things, haven't enough willpower, aren't praying hard enough or meditating enough, or have done something wrong, and are made to feel guilty for their health challenges.

If you're one of those struggling individuals, I hope this explanation helps you understand that *it's not your fault,* and if you can find and remove the triggers or environmental toxins, compensate for genetic weakness, or make dietary or lifestyle changes, you're likely to be able to regain the health that you so fervently seek.

Bob Miller, CTN, is a Traditional Naturopath who specializes in the field of genetic-specific nutrition. He earned his traditional naturopathy degree from Trinity School of Natural Health and is board certified through the ANMA. In 1993, he opened the Tree of Life practice where he has served as a traditional naturopath. For the past several years, he has focused exclusively on functional nutritional genetic variants and related research. Bob lectures nationally and internationally at seminars to educate health-care practitioners about genetic variants and nutritional supplementation for achieving optimal health, and holds live webinars for health professionals. In 2016, he created an online certification course on genetic nutrition, which is now training more than 900 health professionals in the program.

In 2015, to support his growing genetic research efforts, Bob founded and personally funds the NutriGenetic Research Institute to study the relationship between genetic variants and presenting symptoms. This research led to several awards from ILADS.

Bob has created eighty-eight nutritional supplement products exclusively for health professionals. The products he formulated are based on his genetic research and are designed to support function that may be impaired by genetic weakness.

Bob is the founder and president of Functional Genomic Analysis, an online software program that organizes and analyzes genetic SNPs for functional health professionals (https://www.functionalgenomicanalysis.com).

He contributed the chapter "How Your Genetic Makeup May Affect Your Ability to Detoxify" in Dr. Neil Nathan's book *Toxic.* You can contact Bob's clinic at www.tolhealth.com.

Chapter 20: Hormonal Dysfunction and Sensitivity

Neil Nathan, MD

The majority of patients who've become sensitive also complain of symptoms related to hormone imbalances. Looking at the causes of sensitivity, this should come as no surprise. Most notably, as we emphasize throughout this book, mold toxicity, other environmental toxicities, and Lyme disease with its coinfections directly affect the pituitary gland (our "master gland") and its ability to regulate hormones. The main hormones thus affected are those of the adrenal gland, thyroid gland, sex hormones, and, to a certain extent, insulin, as it relates to hypoglycemia.

While this chapter is not intended to review this information in depth (that could be another book), I do think it's important to point out the areas most likely to be involved and how to diagnose and treat these hormonal imbalances. This overview will help both the practitioner and patient to keep in mind, throughout treatment, that evaluating the patient's hormones can be extremely helpful.

To complicate this subject, fluctuating toxin levels cause fluctuating hormone levels, so remember that it's not possible to provide perfect balance in our treatments; we're essentially trying to hit a moving target, so our aim should be for "reasonable" balance with better control as our goal once the triggering conditions have been resolved. As a basic principle here, leaving patients in a state of extreme hormonal deficiency is not helpful for healing. Any improvement in hormonal function will help the patient to not only feel better but to heal more efficiently.

Adrenal Dysfunction

Deficiencies of the adrenals are the most common hormonal deficiencies in our patients. This should not come as a surprise, since, in simple terms, the adrenal is the gland that deals with stress. Getting sick and suffering with sensitivities that engender anxiety, depression, fatigue, and cognitive impairment all put a strain on the adrenals.

In the first stages of illness, we might see an outpouring of adrenal hormones to help the body deal with these stressors. As the illness persists, the body becomes unable to produce adequate amounts of these hormones, and our ability to cope with stressors decreases accordingly. Sometimes we refer to this as "adrenal burnout."

The adrenal gland makes three main groups of hormones, and a deficiency of any one of them will contribute to worsening our patients' symptoms and their proclivity to develop sensitivities. These three groups are DHEA (dehydroepiandrosterone), cortisol, and the mineralocorticoids. Let's discuss each separately, remembering that a patient might have a deficiency of one, two, or all three.

DHEA

DHEA is the main hormone made by the adrenal glands. Biochemically, the body makes a series of hormones from DHEA, including testosterone, progesterone, and estrogen. When the body initially faces a stressor, it might make more of this hormone to help us cope better. After a while, the gland's ability to make DHEA decreases, and the majority of our patients who've been ill for any length of time become DHEA deficient.

Symptoms of that deficiency primarily involve decreased energy, fatigue, depression, decreased libido, and the sense that "I just don't feel right." Since these symptoms, especially fatigue, are so common in our sensitive patients, raising the level of DHEA can have a significant effect on those symptoms. DHEA is easily measured with a blood test of either DHEA (unconjugated) or DHEAS (S=sulfate), the storage form of the hormone. DHEA is readily available through health-food stores or via the internet, and taking it in appropriate doses can be quite helpful. Side effects are possible, though relatively infrequent and usually related to taking too high a dose. These include acne and excessive growth of facial hair. A typical dose for women is 10mg once daily, and for men, 25mg once daily, but it's best to check blood levels to be sure we're getting the correct dose. Its use is contraindicated in hormonally sensitive cancers such as breast and prostate cancer.

I've found that the vast majority of my chronically ill patients have developed a DHEA deficiency, and many will respond to DHEA supplementation with a noticeable increase in energy within four to six weeks of starting it.

Cortisol

Cortisol is another adrenal hormone that's critical to helping the body cope with stress. Symptoms of cortisol deficiency include fatigue, exhaustion, tiredness, a tendency to the expression of allergies, abnormal hair growth, and a tendency toward miscarriage.

Cortisol is typically made in a diurnal pattern; that is, it's primarily manufactured while you sleep, peaking at about eight in the morning and slowly dropping off during the day. A single measurement of blood cortisol might not reflect the full picture of how a patient's cortisol level fluctuates throughout the day. In the past, when it was less expensive and more readily available, I found the cortrosyn stimulation test most accurate for measuring cortisol. For quite a few years now, I've found that the measurement of cortisol in saliva, done multiple times during the day, is a better and easier way to determine how well the adrenal glands are producing cortisol.

If testing determines a low cortisol level, we can supplement it with pharmaceutical hydrocortisone acetate. In small doses, this has been quite effective in improving energy levels and immune function in patients who were compromised. William Jefferies, MD, an endocrinologist, wrote the classical book *Safe Uses of Cortisol*, which provides excellent guidelines for how to prescribe and use these medications safely and effectively.

Mineralocorticoids

The mineralocorticoids are a third group of hormones made by the adrenal glands. These hormones raise blood pressure when it's low, helping to regulate it properly. Symptoms of mineralocorticoid deficiency include low blood pressure, with prominent dizziness or lightheadedness upon standing or sitting up (caused by further lowering the blood pressure), referred to as *orthostatic hypotension*. Other symptoms include exhaustion and fatigue.

Think about it this way: If you had low water pressure in your home and tried to take a shower, the water would come out as a trickle. Low blood pressure is like that, meaning that your blood pressure is a bit too low to meet your body's circulatory needs and doesn't adequately perfuse your body. With blood flow that's not quite adequate, it's easy to see that this would predispose to fatigue and dizziness.

I encourage patients to obtain a series of blood-pressure readings. If they routinely run 110/70 or less, and report dizziness and/or lightheadedness when they stand or sit up, a trial of the medications Florinef or Mitodrine should be considered. It's also a good idea to measure blood pressure while both lying flat for five minutes and then sitting up, to see if there's a drop of 10–20 mm in BP, which would confirm the diagnosis orthostatic hypotension.

A patient can have a deficiency of one, two, or all three of these adrenal hormones, and since they're relatively easy to test for, diagnose, and treat, all patients with chronic illness should have adrenal evaluation included in their evaluation. While this might not cure the underlying condition that's creating these deficiencies, often the patient will feel much better and have more energy to pursue more definitive treatments.

Thyroid Deficiency

The essence of thyroid hormone function is about the regulation of metabolism. Therefore, deficiency of that hormone, termed *hypothyroidism,* creates a sluggish overall chemistry that affects every part of the body. Excesses of hormone, called *hyperthyroidism,* speeds up metabolism, creating the classical symptoms of palpitations, increased heart rate, elevated blood pressure, and anxiety. For our purposes here, the majority of patients who've been chronically ill typically have low thyroid function, so that will be our focus.

Symptoms of thyroid deficiency include fatigue, exhaustion, constipation, temperature dysregulation (usually low body temperature, feeling cold all the time), hair loss, dry skin, cognitive impairments, menstrual abnormalities, weight gain, and loss of the outer eyebrows.

For decades, patients have arrived at my doorstep with the certainty that they have low thyroid, but had been told repeatedly by their family physicians, internists, or endocrinologists that, based on testing, they do not.

The standard test for hypothyroidism has long been the measurement of TSH (thyroid stimulating hormone), the pituitary hormone that regulates the production of thyroid hormones. Many physicians are under the impression that this test, alone, can accurately determine who has a low-functioning thyroid gland. Unfortunately, as our clinical experience accumulates, we've come to realize that the TSH does not give a complete picture of thyroid production and balance. To accurately assess this system, we need to measure not only the TSH but also both T3 (triiodothyronine) and T4 (thyroxine). In addition, many patients with subtle, but clinically significant, deficiencies of thyroid hormone need to measure their Reverse T3 (RT3) to get a full overview. With this more complete picture, we've discovered that many patients who were told that their thyroid was "normal" do indeed have thyroid dysfunction, and they improve with the proper treatment.

Here's how the production of thyroid hormones works: The thyroid gland receives a message from the pituitary in the form of TSH to stimulate the thyroid to make more thyroid hormone. First, the thyroid gland produces T4, the inactive form of thyroid hormone, which in turn must be broken down (by the removal of an iodine molecule) to T3, the active hormone. When this system is not working well, the thyroid gland produces Reverse T3, which inhibits the normal conversion of T4 to T3. Over time, RT3 accumulates and further prevents this conversion. It's not uncommon for patients to present with the classic signs of thyroid deficiency with a normal TSH and even a normal T4, but have a low T3 and high RT3. This means that "normal" testing for thyroid will suggest normal function, but by looking further, we often find that the body is not functioning properly and requires thyroid supplementation to resume true normalcy.

Since the major thyroid-hormone replacement provided by family physicians and endocrinologists is only T4 (Synthroid or Levothyroxine), many physicians are unaware that this will only further cause the buildup of RT3 and make it even more difficult for their patient to convert T4 into the active hormone T3. For these patients, T3 in the form of commercially available Cytomel, or compounded sustained release of T3, or Armour thyroid (a combination of 20% T3 and 80% T4) is needed to provide the proper hormone replacement. Over time, the use of T3 will take the pressure off of the buildup of RT3, which can normalize thyroid hormonal conversion. I've treated several thousand patients in this manner with excellent results, so I'm convinced that this is the future of thyroid medicine.

As you can see, this form of thyroid treatment is a form of "rebooting" to get the thyroid gland back to normalcy. It was first popularized by Dennis Wilson, MD, and is sometimes referred to as "Wilson's Syndrome," (which must be distinguished from a rare copper-accumulation condition called Wilson's Disease). This treatment is not yet common practice in conventional medicine, and patients who seek this approach will need to find physicians trained in functional medicine to get the proper treatment.

To provide additional perspective here, the most common cause of hypothyroidism is referred to as *Hashimoto's thyroiditis,* an autoimmune condition that begins with an inflammation of the thyroid gland that often produces initial symptoms of hyperthyroidism, but as the disease progresses, the thyroid gland burns itself out and becomes hypothyroid. The inflammatory immune dysregulation produced by mold toxicity and Lyme disease is a frequent cause of autoimmunity, so anyone with an autoimmune process should consider evaluation for those conditions. We have found that if caught early, their autoimmune condition might be able to be reversed. The longer it persists, untreated, reversal becomes less likely.

You can see that *both* by predisposing to autoimmune illness and by creating dysregulation of the HPA axis and pituitary gland, chronic inflammatory illness might need to be addressed, and, conversely, by correctly rebalancing the thyroid gland, we can help our patients improve their functioning while we address the underlying causes of their illness.

Sex-Hormone Deficiencies

Estrogens

The ovary makes a variety of estrogens that have different physiological functions, even though inadequate production is often referred to simply as "estrogen deficiency." When a woman starts to go through the process of menopause, the first thing that happens is that the ovaries begin to make less progesterone. This leads to an imbalance called "estrogen dominance," in which the menopausal woman has relatively more estrogen than progesterone. By providing additional progesterone at this point, the hormonal balance can be stabilized. After a while, the ovaries start to make less and less estrogen(s), and this initiates full-blown menopausal symptoms. Some women don't have much difficult with these symptoms, which can be minor, but others experience a profound disturbance. A variety of toxins and infections can affect the pituitary gland's ability to regulate these hormones, so some women can experience menopausal symptoms (estrogen deficiency) long before they would have been expected to do so. In addition, zearalenone, as a mycotoxin, specifically interferes with estrogen metabolism and can set off some of these problems.

Symptoms of estrogen deficiency include hot flashes, night sweats, insomnia, mood swings, depression and/or anxiety, cognitive impairment, fatigue, vaginal dryness, and decreased libido. It's important to understand that the brain and vaginal area have estrogen receptors, and when those receptors don't receive the stimuli they're used to (from the proper amount of estrogens in the body), they respond by letting the body know that they're not happy. The heart also has estrogen receptors, and I see a few women every year who have palpitations or cardiac arrhythmias that resolve when they're given the proper dose of estrogens. Women who have suffered migraine headaches sometimes discover that without adequate estrogens they have a recurrence or worsening of migraines until the proper hormone balance is achieved.

Unfortunately, when it became clear that synthetic, horse-urine-derived estrogens (Premarin) caused a marked increase in breast cancer, many women assumed that all estrogens were bad. Understandably unwilling to risk breast cancer, they were afraid to take any estrogens, and many have suffered greatly. It does not appear that taking bioidentical, or "natural," estrogens subjects women to these same risks, and many women would benefit from the judicious use of bioidentical hormones. For our population of sensitive patients, this is even more relevant.

Though one might think this discussion is confined to women in their mid-forties or older, I've increasingly seen younger and younger women, some in their twenties, with clear symptoms of estrogen deficiency, which is confirmed by laboratory testing.

They respond to bioidentical hormones with immediate improvement, and I think we need to be more aware that sex-hormone deficiencies are more prevalent in younger patients than we realized.

I do recommend that anyone contemplating hormonal treatment begin with measuring all three estrogens: E1 – estrone; E2 – estradiol; and E3 – estriol, as well as progesterone, testosterone, and DHEA, to understand the bigger picture. I've found the Genova Hormonal Assay test the most accurate for helping determine these hormonal needs. Another useful test to include in this evaluation is sex hormone binding globulin (SHBG), a protein that, as its name suggests, binds estrogen and testosterone in the blood. If SHBG is elevated, even if blood tests reveal normal hormonal levels, these hormones may be so tightly bound to this protein that it's not actually available to be used by the body as it normally would be. Thus the body might behave as if deficient in those hormones due to what is actually a relative deficiency. All prescribed treatments should, of course, be provided only by trained health-care providers.

It's particularly relevant to our discussion of chronic inflammatory illnesses that mold toxicity and Lyme disease affect pituitary function directly and are a common cause of these imbalances. When the underlying cause is treated, normal hormonal balance can resume, but sometimes the system needs to be "rebooted" by giving the correct hormones and reminding the body of the balance it requires. There's a complex interwoven relationship between estrogens and thyroid hormones, and both hormonal dosages might need to be adjusted to provide balance. Both hormones can also be influenced by adrenal hormones, so we need to take all of these factors into consideration to help the body find its proper comprehensive hormonal balance.

Progesterone

While estrogen receives most of the attention as the most important of women's sex hormones, it functions in close relationship to progesterone. Many women who undergo hysterectomy are offered estrogen alone as their hormone replacement, the mistaken concept being that since a woman no longer has a uterus, we needn't worry about helping slough the lining of that uterus that builds up with every monthly period. True, an important function of progesterone is, indeed, the need to remove the built-up uterine lining each month, but this would be a short-sighted understanding of the complete role progesterone plays in health.

Progesterone is an important precursor for other hormones, especially adrenal hormones. It helps calm the nervous system (a deficiency of progesterone can contribute to anxiety and insomnia); it stimulates new bone growth (important for those women who are at risk of osteoporosis); it improves libido, and, especially important, it regulates the sensitivity of estrogen receptors. After a hysterectomy, if progesterone levels are low, which is almost universal, progesterone should be part of a hormone-replacement program. For all women contemplating bioidentical hormone replacement, estrogen and progesterone should be used together in the proper balance.

Testosterone

Since testosterone is the quintessential male sex hormone, we'll focus our discussion on testosterone deficiencies in men. Please keep in mind that women can also be deficient in this hormone, and might need to take small doses to restore optimal health.

Men also make estrogen and progesterone, but in far smaller concentrations than women do. Once again, the balance of these hormones is what's important.

Symptoms of testosterone deficiency include fatigue, decreased stamina, decreased libido, erectile dysfunction, muscle weakness, depression, mood swings, hot flashes, palpitations, insomnia, inability to concentrate, and antisocial tendencies.

As men age, they're prone to the equivalent of the female menopause, appropriately referred to as "male menopause." If a patient has the pertinent symptoms, measuring testosterone levels becomes important to determine how to approach treatment. We not only need to know the amount of testosterone in the bloodstream but also need to measure SHBG (sex hormone binding globulin). As we discussed with women and estrogen, SHBG binds to testosterone, and a high level of SHBG will prevent adequate testosterone from reaching the tissues, causing a low "free" testosterone, which is now measured more frequently as well.

Once it's clear that a testosterone deficiency exists, we need to keep in mind the age of our patient. Taking testosterone, by cream, patch, orally, or injection, can send a message to the brain that will turn off testosterone production, since the body now gets the feedback that it has all the testosterone it needs, so why bother making any more? In younger men, this can cause a prolonged turn-off of the production of testosterone, and it can be hard to get it back to normal. In younger men we often use the medication Clomid (clomiphene citrate) to stimulate the pituitary's production of LH (luteinizing hormone), which in turn stimulates the testes to make testosterone. In this way we don't engage the negative biofeedback loop that occurs when taking testosterone turns off testosterone production.

Another important factor when evaluating testosterone levels is to consider estrogen levels in men as well. As men get more obese, fat cells, called adipocytes, begin to produce more of an enzyme called aromatase. Aromatase enzymes convert testosterone into estrogen, which can change the hormone balance and affect all of the functions of testosterone. We can treat this by using small doses of aromatase inhibitors to prevent the conversion, lowering the levels of estrogens and making testosterone more available to the body.

It's clear that testosterone is important in male health, not just in the treatment of decreased libido or erectile dysfunction. Unfortunately, some athletes have abused the use of testosterone and its precursors, and the FDA has made testosterone a *scheduled* drug, placing it in the same class of prescription as narcotics. This has made it somewhat more difficult for physicians to prescribe testosterone, but that doesn't change its importance or the need for it in those who are medically deficient.

Hypoglycemia

Many of our hormones interact closely with each other in a carefully orchestrated process. While insulin is not an adrenal hormone, its production is directly impacted by adrenal-hormone function. Many of our patients with chronic inflammatory illnesses have developed hypoglycemia, or low blood sugar.

Hypoglycemia is caused by an excessive release of insulin from the pancreas in response to consuming carbohydrates (especially sugars). In normal individuals, as soon as your body recognizes that you've has eaten carbohydrates, as the blood-sugar level starts to climb, the pancreas is signaled to release just the right amount of insulin to bring the blood-sugar level back to normal (which typically would be 80–90 mg/dL). A patient with hypoglycemia has what I call a "trigger-happy pancreas," releasing an extra amount of insulin as soon as the climb in blood sugar begins, which lowers the blood sugar to levels that produce symptoms until the body can right its chemistry and bring that blood sugar back into balance.

Symptoms of hypoglycemia include fatigue, brain fog, palpitations, anxiety, and sweating. You can see how these symptoms could interface with the symptoms of sensitivity and worsen them. Typically, these symptoms occur three to five hours after a meal (occasionally sooner), and the patient may be aware that the symptoms are often associated with hunger.

The diagnosis of hypoglycemia is straightforward. After not eating or snacking following the evening meal, the patient has their fasting blood sugar measured first thing in the morning, then consumes 50gm of sugar in a drink called Glucola. The blood sugar is then measured every hour for the next four to five hours. Occasionally, patients who have relatively severe hypoglycemia can, as a result of the hypoglycemia created during the test, display intense sweating and palpitations, which will end the test early. It's helpful to correlate symptoms with the blood-sugar levels measured during the test. It can be of additional value to measure insulin levels at baseline and at one and two hours as well, to confirm that the patient is making excessive insulin.

Interpreting the test correctly is important. Many conventional physicians are under the impression that it's not true hypoglycemia unless the blood glucose level is measured at less than 50 mg/dL. This misconception has resulted in a significant under-diagnosis of this condition. As I've emphasized throughout this book, we all have different body chemistries. I've seen hundreds of patients exhibit the classical symptoms of hypoglycemia when their blood sugar levels were 70mg/dL and certainly when they were lower than that. The improvement in these patients when they treat their hypoglycemia is immediate and obvious, which further confirms the diagnosis.

The treatment of hypoglycemia is fairly simple, and it usually results in rapid improvement of some symptoms, so delaying treatment makes little sense. Since ingesting carbohydrates is the key trigger for hypoglycemia, limiting carbohydrates with a high-protein, low-carbohydrate diet is essential. Again, because we're all different in our biochemistry, the amount of carbohydrate that will trigger (or successfully treat) hypoglycemia varies, usually ranging from 20–60gm of carbohydrate consumed per day.

It's also helpful for patients to snack on high-protein foods between meals, to keep their blood-sugar levels up and not trigger additional hypoglycemia by eating carbohydrates. High-protein snacks could include luncheon meats, cheese, or nuts. The use of chromium, often in the form of chromium picolinate, 200mcg twice daily, helps stabilize blood-sugar levels. Additionally, the use of coconut oil, often combined with MCT (medium chain triglycerides) oil to provide ketone bodies as an alternative fuel for the brain when levels of brain-sugar drop, has been found very useful. For many patients, there's a noticeable improvement in energy and cognition within a few days of beginning treatment.

My take-home message is that hormonal dysfunction is extremely common in our sensitive patients due to the underlying conditions that's triggering this sensitivity. We need to be aware of this and look for hormonal deficiencies early in the course of treatment so they can be corrected. By doing this we can not only make our patients more comfortable, relatively quickly, but also improve their chemistry so healing is enhanced and progress can be more rapid.

Chapter 21: Emotional, Energetic, and Spiritual Considerations for the Sensitive Patient

Neil Nathan, MD

I'm about to embark on a potentially difficult subject that might be particularly important for the sensitive patient. When patients appear to be "stuck" in their treatment, when they're doing everything you've asked them to do and aren't making progress, it becomes clear that there's a blockage or impediment to progress somewhere. I have found, as have my colleagues, that when this occurs, we need to look at areas that are not in the physical plane—the focus of our treatment suggestions thus far—but in other realms. This means we need to see if our patient is open to exploring issues that might arise in the psychological/emotional realm, or the spiritual realm, or in an obstruction to the flow of energies through their body.

For most patients, these are issues that can't be addressed on their first visit, and often not for a year or more. It takes an accumulation of trust, which must be earned, for someone to decide that they feel safe enough with you to begin this exploration. Often, this represents the art of medicine. It takes an astute, compassionate, empathetic healthcare provider to build this trust space. Even then, one must be aware of that moment when a patient appears, sometimes for the first time in years of visits, open and vulnerable to the possibility of broaching these discussions. When that door opens, we can, with great care and tact, review with our patient our lack of progress, and suggest that perhaps there's another area preventing them from moving toward healing. At those moments, I ask them if they suspect that there's some emotional issue, or spiritual concern, or perception of energy blockage, that they wish to explore.

Part of being ill for a long period of time often creates a situation in which a patient begins to define themselves by their illness; e.g., "I have mold toxicity," "I have Lyme," "I have Chronic Fatigue," or "I have MCS." In doing so, they unconsciously lock themselves into a self-definition that will put limits on their ability to heal, because "If I am not that, who am I?"

Whatever you're experiencing and whatever diagnostic labels have been given to you, please don't let that define you. You are always more than that: you're a human being whose birthright is to be capable of love and well-being—and that's what you must own if you're going to heal.

With that in mind, if, over time, trust has been solidified between patient and health-care provider by mutual respect and concern, most patients are then open to that discussion. If I broach the subject prematurely, or if they're not ready, it will push them even further into denial and amplify their defenses against those considerations.

If, however, we correctly perceive that the door to this discussion has opened, now is the time for us to explore these areas. For our most sensitive patients, I've found it very likely that these issues are indeed present, and that by beginning this phase of exploration and treatment, we can finally move past the area of blockage and move toward healing.

Emotional or Psychological Issues

It is not commonly recognized that emotions, when unable to be expressed, are stored in the tissues of the body, most notably the muscles and fascia (the connective tissue that covers the muscles). When questioned, most patients believe that their emotions are stored in the brain as memories. While the brain does store memories, the actual storage site for the energies of our emotions is usually localized to the musculoskeletal system. If a patient has had injuries or infections that involve particular areas of the body, emotional energies tend to be stored in those more vulnerable tissues.

Massage therapists, acupuncturists, osteopaths, and chiropractors have long noted that when they release the tension from certain tissues, a patient may have a profound emotional reaction. In acupuncture, for example, when emotional releases occur with the expert placement of a needle, you might reflect on the phrase "It hit a nerve." Experienced practitioners know that being supportive during these reactions, and allowing them to release those emotions unhindered, is the most effective way to facilitate healing. The deeper the emotional release the more likely a permanent release of tension from those tissues. Following an intense emotional release, patients usually report feeling entirely much better.

Of course, our patients usually have very good reasons to have emotions that they weren't in a position to release. As Dr. Porges describes in chapter 3, throughout our lives we are exposed to situations in which we correctly feel unsafe. One of our protective mechanisms is to literally shut down (in a state of near paralysis), so that whatever we are experiencing emotionally, be it sadness, fear, anger, rage, despair, anxiety, or terror, we don't allow ourselves to release it because it's not safe to do so. It might be months or years before we feel safer, but the emotional energies stored in our tissues accumulate and directly produce increased muscular tension and pain. As our muscles tighten to hold in these emotions, they compress their own blood supply and lymphatics, so that the blood and lymphatic flow through those tissues decreases, adding to the pain and tension. This in turn creates the blockage to movement and energy flows, and blockage of biochemical reactions (a buildup of lactic acid in the muscles, for example) that add to the difficulties of healing.

The idea that the mind, body, and spirit are one is now accepted to the point that it's almost become cliché. Often, those who embrace this concept don't stop to recognize how profound a truth it is. The physical body, the energy flows of the body, the emotional openness of the body, and the spiritual path of the person who inhabits that body are indeed one. I've encountered no medical condition in which this unity is missing. For example, when considering an illness that you might think is purely physical, like pneumonia, while the infection of the lungs, with its concurrent symptoms of cough, production of phlegm, fever, chills, and shortness of breath are most obvious, these are always accompanied by other concerns. Being unable to breathe comfortably is frightening to everyone, and with that fear come worries such as: "Do I need antibiotics? Should I go to the ER? Could I infect my loved ones? What if I should stop breathing? What if I can't go back to work and I lose my time off? Will it leave scarring and lead to a more chronic condition?" With pneumonia, then, comes anxiety, fear, and frustration.

If left to fester, like the infection, these emotions can embed themselves in the muscles that mobilize the ribs and the diaphragm, and can lead to a more chronic condition if not dealt with. From an energy standpoint, the diaphragm occupies a key place in the body as a regulator of energies that move between the upper and lower halves of the body, and a diaphragmatic issue can interfere with those flows and ultimately create dysfunctional movement of energies throughout the body. From a spiritual perspective, questions arise: "Why me, God?" or "If there was a God they wouldn't have done this to me, since I've long prayed for healing."

You can see that what appears to be a simple pneumonia could in fact have profound effects for all systems of the body, and most often we're unaware of the implications for healing. We are prone to simply wanting to take an antibiotic and some cough syrup, and when we get better, just go back to life as we knew it. Osteopathic physicians have long recognized that for more complete healing and to prevent a recurrence, manipulations of the diaphragm, ribs, and other related tissues can be needed and very helpful. Similarly, acupuncturists have found that treatments provided when the cough has resolved can also prevent recurrences by reestablishing the normal flows of energy disrupted by the infection.

Complicated? Yes, but when dealing with complicated medical issues demonstrated by our sensitive patients, we have to bring a more comprehensive perspective to the table to find out where our patients are stuck.

The holding of emotions in our musculoskeletal system can take two different patterns. One is that of an acute traumatic event—an episode of injury, or abuse, or surgery, or childbirth, in which something frightened us and put us in a position where it wasn't safe to release the emotions generated by the traumatic event. In treatment, when those tissues are worked on and those muscles release their tensions, the emotions stored there are released as well, and often the memory of that specific trauma comes to the surface, even if long-buried.

Another pattern is that of attitudes instilled in childhood that have no specific focal point, but rather years of suppression of emotion. If you grew up in a family that valued stoicism, being "strong," and were told (often nonverbally) that "big boys don't cry," and you tried to be the best son or daughter you could and followed the family tradition, it is common that your emotions accumulated gradually, with no clear causal event. When their muscles are treated and release their tensions, these patients can have a deep emotional release but have no clear memory of any event that provoked their emotions.

Again, Dr. Porges makes it very clear that the accumulation of stressors that lead to the perception that you're not entirely safe triggers dysfunction in the polyvagal and limbic systems that leads directly to a marked increase in sensitivity. Initially this sensitivity is protective in nature: Your nervous system is simply monitoring the stimuli in your internal and external environment for safety. If it feels you're not safe (remember, this is neurological, not psychological), it essentially shuts you down so you'll become aware that you aren't safe and will protect yourself by avoiding that stimulus. Over time, this protective mechanism becomes overprotective, hyperreactive, and hypervigilant. It's now part of the problem, but don't forget that it's intended to be protective, and that that protection worked well for many years—until it didn't.

If our sensitive patients are unable to take or respond to the treatments we offer, eventually we might need to look at possible emotional impediments to healing. It is common for my patients to be aware of childhood traumas and tell me: "Oh, I've had lots of therapy and I've worked through all of that." Perhaps, and perhaps not. Initially reluctant to go back to these difficult times, it might be necessary if we're going to make progress.

For an example of how long-held emotional energies can impact the healing process, look at Lisa's case in An Overview of the Sensitive Patient. Lisa had made good progress with her treatment of *Bartonella* and mold toxicity, but was treading water until the vague memories of childhood abuse began to make themselves known after Lisa received chiropractic bodywork. As with most patients, while worried about what she might learn as she pursued those memories with a therapist, the memories finally became clear, and after Lisa had released long-repressed feelings about her abuse, she was able to make excellent progress and heal completely. Wheelchair-bound and unable to leave her home because of her extreme chemical sensitivities, she was now able to travel anywhere and resume activities that had been unthinkable at the start of treatment.

There are many types of treatment that can be helpful here. To get at deeper, more repressed, emotional material, if a patient is willing, I have found Reichian therapy or similar body therapies especially effective. Reichian therapy was developed by Wilhelm Reich, MD, a psychiatrist who was a contemporary of Freud's. Reich discovered that by studying a patient's muscular tensions and then releasing those tensions using a combination of bodywork and breathing, the patient could access repressed emotions and release them. There are many variations of this, including Heller bodywork.

Hypnosis can be used to access some of these memories. A process called Voice Dialogue, a variation of Gestalt Therapy developed by Hal Stone and Sidra Winkelman, allows patients to talk to the various aspects of their personality (e.g., the Hurt Child, the Judge, the Critic, the Rebellious Teenager, etc.) to learn when and how these emotions may have been stored, which facilitates their release.

Any type of bodywork done by an empathetic, compassionate therapist can focus on areas of muscular dysfunction that, when released in a place of safety, can lead to this same emotional release.

Simple "talk therapy," in which a patient just talks about their day and their concerns, is not likely to produce the desired effect, as it will often reinforce the defense mechanisms that have enabled the storage of emotions. We need to help release these emotions by going to their source—the muscles and fascial layers that hold them, and perhaps the events that triggered them.

Impaired Flow of Energies

In the context of the physical body, the word "energy" is remarkably difficult to define. I've tried, and discussed this in more detail in my book *Energetic Diagnosis*. The body has lots of different energies, all merging with one another in a complex dance that animates us. The most obvious energies are electrical: those of the heart and brain, which we measure medically with ECGs and EEGs, and which we can treat by applying electrical energies to the body, such as in cardiac resuscitation. We also have electromagnetic energies coursing through us. The cells of our body energy are piezoelectrical currents, which play a huge role in our functioning, though we don't have the ability to measure them with precision in a clinical setting, as we would like. The flows of blood through arteries and veins, the flows of the lymphatic systems, and flows of cerebrospinal fluid all generate a current, and with it an energetic movement that needs to be smooth and coordinated throughout the body. Any impingement upon those structures interferes with that flow and will cause symptoms and disease.

The measurement of these energies is still in its infancy—but that doesn't mean they're not important to our health. Acupuncturists can feel the "pulse," which is a measurement of many different energies, and can feel when these are too strong or too weak or deficient. Then, with needles or acupressure, they can improve the weak flows and diminish those that are too strong, to move the body toward balance.

Osteopathic physicians can feel these energies directly, as Dr. Van Deven describes in chapter 16. Using well-defined osteopathic techniques, we can access this information and balance those energies.

A variety of medical devices can measure the imbalance in energy flows and can restore that balance. Examples of this include frequency-specific microcurrent (FSM) and a number of medical instruments including the LENS and EAV (Electroaccupuncture according to Voll) and biofeedback devices such as ZYTO.

Equally important, but not yet within the purview of the medical field, are energies that are being hijacked by other people, currently referred to as energy vampires by the psychiatric profession. Helping a patient to become aware that their personal energies are being drained by others, which can include associates, colleagues, or most commonly family and friends, can be very important in their healing. There are energetic connections among all of us, referred to as "energy cords," in which we are, or were, connected to people or objects that were important to us. If they have harmed us or hurt us, even if this was long in the past, the cords can still be open and active, draining our energies. Working with a therapist to discover these cords and remove them can be very helpful for our patients who are unable to respond to the usual treatments.

Working with an energy healer can be extremely valuable in this instance; finding those who are truly gifted in this arena might not be easy, but it's worth the effort.

Spiritual Dysfunction

Spirituality means so many different things to different people that definitions won't be helpful here. The majority of Americans consider themselves "spiritual," but have little clarity as to exactly how.

Spiritual energy is what sustains us, moves us, and gives meaning and purpose to our lives. I have come to understand that without that central flow of energy, it's difficult to heal from any medical condition, and anyone without that base is at risk for becoming ill. We can discuss this core energy from many vantage points, including religious credos, a belief in the Divine, God, or Unity, but I'll come to this subject from a nonreligious perspective. The best way I've learned to do this is to ask my patients, as I ask you now: "What gives your life meaning and purpose?"

For some, this immediately brings to mind their religious affiliations and connections. For others, it's their relationships, friendships, community activities, work, hobbies, artistic endeavors, or their connection to the natural world. Whatever provides meaning should be honored, cherished, and nurtured. This is the fuel that moves us, gets us up in the morning with enthusiasm to face another day. With fifty years of medical experience behind me, I've come to understand that this energy, which I call spiritual energy, is the essence of our lives.

If we lose contact with this spiritual focus, we get lost in the seas of a complex world. The gritty details of life begin to overwhelm us, and we lose sight of ourselves, our essence, what makes us, us. When asked about the meaning and purpose of their lives, a surprising number of my sickest patients admit that they just don't know anymore. When I get that response, I know that I must bring this to their attention so they can begin to get back on track to find themselves again. When a patient says, "I don't know," I respond, "Well, what *used to* give your life meaning?" They often recall loving to play a musical instrument, or paint, or go fishing, or take a walk in the woods, or go to church or synagogue, or participate in community activities, or go bowling on a team, or read, or… you get the point. Then, I suggest that they find some time to try to do whatever they loved once again. That's a good starting point. For others, things have changed and they need a new starting point. At least we've begun the discussion. Hopefully, a seed has been planted that will encourage them to really think about their lives in a broader context.

I consider the spiritual dimension one of the most important areas to explore in our patients who've been unable to progress, and at the same time a realm that our medical education rarely trains us to address at any level. As long as we come to the table with an open, compassionate, and nonjudgmental perspective, welcoming our patient to explore this area using their own language, and supporting and encouraging them to pursue these ideas in their own unique way, we can help them heal. It can be of value for the patient to consult with their own clergymen or rabbis, or to find a therapist who can help them clarify their thinking and belief systems. Prayer, in whatever form it takes, can be a wonderful opportunity for a patient to accept that they need help and to reach out for it.

For sensitive patients who haven't been able to improve with the treatments they've tried, a willingness to look deeply into the possible roles of emotional, energetic, or spiritual issues that might be an impediment to healing could be the next step in allowing them to move forward and to be able to become more response-able to treatment.

Chapter 22: Carbon Monoxide as a Sensitizing Agent

Neil Nathan, MD

We've been aware of carbon monoxide (CO) poisoning for more than a century. Carbon monoxide is an odorless gas produced by the incomplete combustion of any fuel; poorly ventilated gas stoves, gas or oil furnaces, space heaters, fireplaces, and cars running in closed garages are all possible sources of exposure. Because CO is an odorless, tasteless, and invisible gas, it can be hard to know if you're being exposed to it. As our awareness of this problem grows, the use of carbon monoxide detectors in our homes is increasing, and they can be lifesaving.

Acute toxicity can be obvious, as in the case of a person found lying unconscious on the floor of a garage with the car's motor running. Chronic exposure is much less evident, and discovering this possibility sometimes requires detective work.

A review of the symptoms of chronic carbon monoxide poisoning reads very much like the symptoms we discussed for mold toxicity, Lyme disease, mast-cell activation, and porphyria.

A multisystem list includes:
- Fatigue
- Weakness
- Nausea
- Confusion
- Dizziness
- Chest pain
- Headache
- Extreme sensitivity to stimuli

Especially important to this discussion is that carbon monoxide amplifies a person's sensitivity to light, sound, touch, smells, and tastes.

A more detailed discussion of this subject can be found in the article "Background on Sources, Symptoms, Biomarkers and Treatment of Chronic Carbon Monoxide Poisoning" by Albert Donnay, MHS, available at www.mcsrr.org.

Making the diagnosis of CO poisoning can be difficult. When a person who suspects exposure presents at an emergency room, the standard procedure is to test the patient's carboxyhemoglobin level. If this test is performed days after exposure, however, it becomes inaccurate and might not pick up the toxicity the patient has been exposed to. Another test that can point to this diagnosis is a blood test for venous blood gases (called PvO2). Measuring carbon monoxide in exhaled breath could be used to make the diagnosis, but the technology isn't readily available.

Complicating the possibility of exposure to CO is that the body is capable of making it: Stress can stimulate the production of an enzyme called heme oxygenase-1 (HO-1), which breaks down heme from heme proteins, creating a variety of metabolites that can include carbon monoxide. You can see how this might relate to porphyria, in which the breakdown of heme is similarly disordered.

My take-home message: In a patient who's become extremely sensitive to everything—light, touch, sound, smell, and taste—with the accompanying hypervigilance and anxiety, carbon monoxide poisoning should be considered as a possible source.

Shortly after the publication of my book *Toxic,* I was gratified when a physician wrote to me that after reading the chapter on carbon monoxide, he realized that one of his patients might have such an exposure, and when tested, did indeed have that diagnosis, which was then successfully treated.

The treatment of this acute condition primarily entails breathing 100% oxygen through a nasal canula from an oxygen tank or oxygen concentrator at a rate of 6–10 liters per minute for two hours a day. Healing often requires three to four months of treatment. Unfortunately, it can sometimes be difficult to provide this for patients' home use because the medical prescription for oxygen requires that strict, specific criteria be met to allow distributors of oxygen devices to do so. Patients who might benefit from this treatment often don't meet these requirements.

Albert Donnay did a study of thirty-four patients with ME/CFS (myalgic encephalomyelitis/ chronic fatigue syndrome) and noted improvement in all who were treated with oxygen in this manner. Of those patients, 25% reported marked improvement in all their sensitivities, and 38% reported improvement specifically in their chemical sensitivities.

William Rea, MD, a pioneer in the treatment of patients with multiple chemical sensitivities, found that the daily use of oxygen in his clinic was of great benefit. I too have seen a number of patients with extreme sensitivities improve with oxygen treatments. This might require the use of a ceramic mask (rather than the usual plastic mask, which can be reactive for sensitive patients) and nonallergenic tubing to conduct the oxygen from the tank to the mask.

The possibility that chronic CO toxicity might play a role in the development or exacerbation of intense sensitivities clearly needs to be explored in greater depth.

What I hope I've conveyed in this brief chapter is the need to consider carbon monoxide poisoning as a contributing factor in the evaluation and treatment of sensitive patients. Treating it may be of great benefit to quiet some patients' overly reactive nervous systems so that healing can move forward.

Chapter 23: Secondary Porphyrias in Sensitization

Neil Nathan, MD

When physicians hear the word "porphyria," our first thought is of rare genetic conditions. I can't recall ever having seen a case in my fifty-plus years of medical practice. In this chapter, we'll explore what's called *secondary* porphyria; i.e., porphyria triggered by a nongenetic source.

I've studied porphyria for decades. Over those years, many physicians have suggested that porphyria is more common than is currently appreciated. Accordingly, I delved into it and periodically tested some of my patients for it. A larger percentage than I anticipated tested positive, but then I got mired in the difficulties of treatment and integrating those treatments into the larger therapeutic plan. Feeling overwhelmed, I abandoned the subject, but found my interest rekindled every few years.

My interest was most recently piqued by reading *Porphyria: The Ultimate Cause of Common, Chronic and Environmental Illnesses* by Steven Rochlitz, PhD. I'm grateful to Dr. Rochlitz for his extensive work on this subject and for helping me to grasp enough of it that I feel I can broach the subject here. What follows should by no means be taken as gospel, but I believe it's important to include this information in our understanding of the conditions that can contribute to causing ultrasensitivity in our patients, but I still haven't figured out how to integrate it into the bigger picture. Despite that, as we strive to help our patients, I think this subject deserves its own chapter, and I hope that others will do a better job of integration than I have.

Porphyria is a very complicated subject, and I'll try make it understandable (with simplifications) and help put our understanding into perspective. Efforts to diagnose and treat porphyria have waxed and waned, probably due to its unique complexity and the fact that the treatment of porphyria is in some ways the complete opposite of the treatment of some of the causes that trigger it.

First of all, what is porphyria? Our bodies can only use the red blood cells we make for about ninety days, and then we have to recycle them to make new ones. One of the central components of red blood cells is heme (think *hemoglobin*). For a variety of reasons, if the liver isn't working properly and is genetically predisposed to an insufficiency of certain enzymes, the liver might not be able to make an adequate quantity of the enzymes required for heme to be properly recycled. Consequently, we get a build-up of some of these break-down products, called porphyrins. There are eight named porphyrins that we can measure, and when porphyrins accumulate in the body, we get porphyria.

There are a number of rare genetic types of porphyria that are well described in the medical literature, all of which take their names from those eight porphyrins that can accumulate in the body, depending on which enzyme is genetically lacking to properly metabolize any given porphyrin. Having never seen a case, I won't discuss them here; however, the occurrence of secondary porphyria, meaning a porphyria that's created by an infectious process or toxin and interferes with the breakdown of hemoglobin, may be more common than is generally understood. The important point here is that porphyria contributes to triggering sensitivity, hence its relevance for us.

What are the symptoms of porphyria? They're global, and it will be obvious to the reader that they're similar to those of mold toxicity, Lyme and its coinfections, mast-cell activation, and PANDAS. Like those conditions, porphyria sets off a series of inflammatory biochemical reactions that can affect virtually every system of the body.

The symptoms that most strongly draw my attention to porphyria as a contributing factor to chronic inflammatory-type illnesses and sensitivity are those that are psychological in nature. These include intense anxiety, depression, and panic, along with severe nausea and vomiting. When these symptoms follow closely on the heels of a patient's taking a new supplement or medication, and this reaction lasts longer than two or three days (a typical Herx-like reaction), it suggests to me that we might have triggered a porphyric reaction caused by or secondary to the ingestion of that medicine.

Other symptoms of porphyria include:
- Palpitations
- Weakness
- Unusual neurological symptoms
- Paresthesias
- Peripheral neuropathy
- Abdominal pain

- Constipation and/or diarrhea
- Nausea and/or vomiting
- Allergic reactions
- Asthma
- Shortness of breath
- Chest pain
- Insomnia
- A wide variety of skin rashes
- Dizziness
- Increasing intolerance to medications, supplements, stress, light, sound, heat, cold, fragrances, and electromagnetic frequencies

In my experience, the basic issue here is that, like mast-cell activation, secondary porphyrias are most commonly triggered by mold toxicity and Lyme disease, especially *Bartonella*, but can also be triggered by viral infections, chlamydia and mycoplasma infections, and other toxins.

This means that it's crucial not to lose sight of the need to treat the primary trigger, or cause, of porphyria, while also not ignoring its biochemical effects, which might need to be addressed to quiet the intense reaction. We might not be able to treat the underlying cause unless the porphyria (the excessive amounts of porphyrins in the body) is treated first or concurrently. Unlike the other conditions we might be working with here, like mold or Lyme or mast-cell activation, the chemistry of porphyria is distinctly different and can be at odds with the treatment of those conditions.

This means that I often find myself struggling to find the correct balance of what to treat, how, and in what order. The most obvious example is that treatment of porphyria requires a higher carbohydrate intake. When we treat mold or candida, we typically limit carbohydrate intake to 60gm or less daily. It's fascinating that some patients find they feel "awful" until they raise their carbohydrate intake to 80–100gm, which makes me wonder whether these patients have a mild degree of porphyria. I haven't yet studied this in depth, but I think it's worthy of research.

An acute flare-up of porphyria, which looks like a prolonged Herx reaction (lasting from one to three weeks or longer) might respond well to daily use of 500cc of intravenous dextrose in a 10% concentration (D10W).

In my experience this is the single most useful modality for settling down a flare-up of porphyria. Often, one or just a few intravenous treatments will produce a significant and rapid improvement in symptoms, greatly shortening the usual length of a porphyric reaction. Since it's not always easy for my patients to get this intravenous treatment, they can also try taking dextrose (glucose) tablets to see if it aborts their reaction. The mechanism of this appears to be that the IV dextrose affects the liver by stopping the production of heme (and therefore of its breakdown products), and blocking the effects of a chemical made by the stomach called PGC-1 alpha, thus ending the production of excess toxic porphyrins.

Since the treatment of mold toxicity and Lyme or *Bartonella* usually involves limited carbohydrates, and the treatment of porphyria is to markedly increase carbohydrate intake, you can see that these approaches are diametrically opposed and difficult to coordinate. Orchestrating the treatment requires the use of careful clinical judgment, increasing the carbohydrate intake when a flare-up of porphyrins is suspected, and resuming a low-carbohydrate approach when that's settled down. At present, from my perspective, this implies the need for excellent guesswork and is thus inherently problematic.

Another simple treatment of a porphyria attack (and a way to quiet it) is to increase the blood level of carbon dioxide. There's good evidence that a low CO_2 level (hypocapnia) prevents the body from using oxygen properly by depleting glutathione, which then depletes 2,3 DPG (diphosphoglycerate) in red blood cells. This appears to be able to be reversed, to an extent, by rebreathing techniques such as breathing into a paper bag, or using shallow-breathing techniques developed by Dr. Konstantin Buteyko. *The Oxygen Advantage* by Patrick McKeown goes into these breathing techniques in easily understood detail.

A low sodium level, or hyponatremia, is common with porphyria, and taking a small amount of salt under the tongue might help with an attack; however, in some patients, this can trigger an attack, so the patient must approach this intervention carefully.

Since the function of liver enzymes is essential to alleviate porphyria, supplements that assist this process, such as milk thistle and charcoal, which can adsorb excess porphyrins, can be helpful. In *Porphyria*, Steven Rochlitz provides a more extensive list of supplements and therapies that are of potential benefit to our patients. Another of the complexities in treating patients with porphyria is the biochemical individuality that each patient brings to the table. The list of possible substances that have been shown to trigger a porphyric reaction is very long, and it's important for patients to realize that they might react only to a few, They'll have to evaluate how they personally react to each specific material to learn how to work with this type of sensitivity. Unfortunately, this requires a great deal of trial-and-error effort, with the constant threat that if they stumble on a triggering substance, they could be ill for days or weeks afterward.

In the world of Lyme treatment, the most common trigger for porphyria has sometimes arisen from treating *Chlamydia pneumonia* with antibiotics. Charles Stratton, MD, an infectious disease specialist at the medical school of Vanderbilt University, has discovered that killing *Chlamydia pneumonia* with antibiotics or the supplement NAC (N-acetyl cysteine) triggers a porphyric reaction that's not uncommon. Since the antibiotics used here are so similar to those we use in the treatment of *Bartonella*, you can see that we might inadvertently trigger a porphyric reaction in susceptible patients. Dr. Stratton has an excellent website, www.cpnhelp.org, which reviews this in detail and provides suggestions for treatment. Also, Dr. Stratton notes that patients with secondary porphyria might need additional vitamin B-12 and folic acid to treat it and to prevent recurrences.

I think of the interventions described above as fairly simple, and I encourage patients who have porphyria to try them to see what quiets their inflamed systems. Since renewing my interest in porphyria, I've checked twenty of my most sensitive patients with a Labcorp urine porphyrin test, and fifteen have come back positive. This would seem to confirm the assertion that the prevalence of porphyria in patients with marked sensitivities triggered by chronic inflammatory conditions might be far more common than we had realized. Admittedly, this is a small sample, but hopefully others will start looking at this as well. For anyone who collects a urine porphyrin sample, be sure to wrap the specimen in aluminum foil as soon as you collect it. and put it in the refrigerator until it can be brought to the lab for analysis. Protecting the specimen from light until it can be analyzed is important, since some porphyrins break down in the presence of light. Remember too that porphyrins can be fleeting or transitory in the body, like the mediators of mast-cell activation, so the results will be more accurate if the patient can collect their urine during a severe flare-up or when they feel their absolute worst.

I'm still trying to integrate the treatment strategies for porphyria into my treatment plans for patients with mold toxicity, Lyme, *Bartonella*, and mast-cell activation, and I find this quite a challenge. Each patient needs to be treated individually, and I don't have any clear rules or any kind of algorithm to follow. Because the patients we're discussing tend to be extremely sensitive and toxic, each treatment modality needs to be assessed separately so we can be sure that it's safe and helpful before we move on to the next component of treatment.

I hope I've conveyed the need to consider the diagnosis of porphyria in the evaluation of our sensitive and toxic patients as a possible contributing factor. Treating it could then be of great benefit for some of these patients, quieting their overexcited nervous systems so they can move forward in their healing process.

Chapter 24: Long Haul COVID and COVID Vaccines as Sensitizing Factors

Greg Nigh, ND, Lac

Dr. Nathan's Introduction

The COVID pandemic has profoundly changed our world in ways we could never have imagined. COVID is still with us, and, in addition to the illness and suffering it created, has left a deep lingering fear and mistrust. One underrecognized result of COVID is that the intense inflammatory response it engendered has contributed to increased sensitization in those exposed to the virus and to the vaccines provided for its treatment. This should come as no surprise given the limbic issues of fear and isolation and the influence of inflammation on sensitivity. In this important chapter Dr. Nigh helps us understand the effects of COVID in detail.

○ ○ ○

The COVID-19 pandemic has changed our world in ways we could never have imagined. COVID is still active, and, in addition to the suffering and countless deaths it caused, has left us feeling deep fear and mistrust. An underappreciated result of COVID, given the intense inflammatory response it engendered in our patients, is that it significantly increased the sensitivity of those exposed to the virus and innoculated with the vaccines. Given the limbic issues, the isolation, and the direct influence of inflammation on sensitization, this comes as no surprise. In this important chapter, Dr. Nigh helps us understand and appreciate how COVID contributes to these processes.

There is no question that there's been a dramatic increase in the number of individuals who experience extreme sensitivities and reactivity to a wide range of triggers. It's unlikely that there's any sole underlying cause for this debilitating condition. That said, with extremely rare exceptions, babies are not born into this world with those sensitivities already in place. These reactions are acquired over time, and it's only through educated guessing (and testing, as indicated) that we come to a clearer understanding of the underlying drivers. For so many people, this reactivity progressively expands and escalates over time, leaving many as prisoners of their own homes, afraid to venture out into a world that seems rigged to cause misery at the slightest provocation.

In the most basic analysis of what's causing this growing problem, it seems obvious that we need to account for all kinds of exposures that lead to this hyperreactive state. The kinds of exposures to account for is vast: heavy metals and other environmental pollutants; food additives and genetic modifications to our food; the ocean of wireless signals we are all now immersed in; the ubiquitous messaging from most media outlets promoting fear and insecurity, etc. Each of these, and many other exposures, has consequences that impact our physiology from the subcellular level all the way up to the whole organism.

Given what appears to me to be a rapid increase in the number of patients who present with extreme food and environmental reactivity, I think it prudent that the review of possible contributing factors include something newly introduced in the past few years, an exposure now common to hundreds of millions of people in the United States and billions globally—SARS-CoV-2 vaccinations. I'll focus primarily on the mRNA vaccines distributed by Moderna and Pfizer, as those are, by a large majority, the type deployed for use in the US and contain the vaccine technology I'm most familiar with.

Before diving into the details of the vaccinations, I want to offer a few observations about the heightened reactivity I'm seeing clinically. My impression is that it is *predominantly* rooted in the "tone" of the autonomic nervous system (ANS). I wrote about this in some detail in the chapter on sulfur metabolism (chapter 13). Given that reactions to a wide range of exposures can start within minutes or even seconds after that exposure, it seems unfeasible to me to attribute these reactions to immune activation. Immune cells may become activated later, and cytokines surely rise around that immune activation, but I believe the ANS is the switch that's getting flipped first. For more and more individuals, the ANS, with its increased sympathetic signaling, establishes an exquisitely sensitive security system such that even the most benign of breaches sets off a full-scale alarm cascade in the body.

Further, three important underlying factors predispose toward this sympathetic dominance and quick trigger in the ANS. The first is toxicity, which can come from a wide range of sources: pollutants, food additives, medications, EMFs generated by wireless communication, etc. The second is inflammation, which often follows on the heels of toxic exposures but can also stand on its own. A significant body of literature demonstrates that inflammation strongly drives sympathetic signaling in the ANS, so chronic underlying inflammation will predispose in that direction. Finally, a history of trauma, especially complex trauma, establishes within the ANS a strong predisposition toward sympathetic activation and an exaggerated stress response (fight, flight, or freeze), which often occurs for the individual even when no source of threat is apparent.

This latter topic, concerning the history of trauma, is far too complex for me to go into thoroughly. I will say, though, that individuals with a history of complex trauma who have not sought out and pursued ANS-regulating therapies will very likely have a challenging time getting their extreme exposure sensitivities under control (see chapters 1, 2, and 3 for more on this subject).

The Relevance of COVID-19 and mRNA Vaccination to Hypersensitivities

In considering the impact that natural infection, COVID-19 disease, and COVID-19 mRNA vaccinations might play in driving these hypersensitivity reactions, there are two general considerations: The first has to do with the direct impact of these events on physiology; the second has to do with the feed-forward effect those physiological changes can have on the recipient's mental/emotional state. Let's first consider the physiology; I'll start with the mRNA injections.

There are many important components of these injections. The mRNA is packaged within a sphere called a lipid nanoparticle (LNP). These LNPs are fats that have a positive charge, also called *cationic lipids.* The scientific literature on cationic LNPs goes back over a decade. *Not found naturally in the human body,* they have long been recognized as toxic to humans, partially because we have no innate enzymes that break down cationic lipids. Thus they persist.

What do they do while they're in the body? They are inherently inflammatory. As long as they're present, they provoke an inflammatory response. In fact, that was the desired feature of these LNPs during the design of these vaccines. Whereas prior vaccinations used aluminum or other irritants as what are called *adjuvants,* or *immune stimulants,* to enhance response to the vaccine material, the mRNA vaccines used the cationic LNPs to play a dual role: they protect the mRNA from degradation, and they provoke an inflammatory response. How long do these LNPs persist in the body after vaccination? We can say with confidence that no one knows. One comprehensive review correlates the inflammation and cellular damage that can be caused by exposure to both the spike protein and LNPs to fourteen general categories of adverse event types reported following mRNA vaccination, encompassing several dozen specific conditions. These include gastrointestinal, neurological, cognitive, and hypersensitivity reactions.[1] It's shocking that there are currently no studies published that attempt to determine how long after injection the LNPs persist in the various organs of the body. The paper just cited notes, though, that as these LNPs chemically degrade in the body over time, those degradation products would also be expected to provoke inflammation, though this has not been studied either.

Another central component of the mRNA injections is the genetically modified mRNA itself. It's intended to induce our cells to produce SARS-CoV-2 spike proteins. This protein is inherently inflammatory, and in fact researchers have put forth a compelling case that it's the spike protein itself that drives the large majority of the symptoms attributed to COVID-19.[2] It is this protein that the injected mRNA provokes cells to produce. Studies have shown that our cells continue to produce spike proteins up to sixty days after a second mRNA injection.[3] It could be longer; we don't know.

It's important to note, however, that the mRNA being injected is not identical to the RNA of SARS-CoV-2. It's been genetically modified in some very significant ways. These various modifications, while dramatically enhancing cellular production of the spike protein, also enhance the inflammatory potential of the injections. I will briefly discuss two of these modifications.

The first involves the replacement of a nucleotide in the virus called *uridine* with a synthetic form of that nucleotide called *methylpseudouridine*. Normally, free RNA within cells is a danger signal and is degraded quickly to prevent problems. With the methylpseudouridine substitutions, however, the RNA evades our cellular surveillance and thus enjoys a significantly extended lifetime during which to create more inflammatory spike proteins.

A second genetic modification applied to the mRNA being injected is called GC enrichment. This, again, is a method of substituting nucleic acid bases in order to dramatically extend the lifespan of the mRNA, prevent its degradation, and dramatically increase spike-protein production. These genetic changes help explain why spike-protein production can continue for several months after vaccination.

Both the LNPs and the spike proteins are inflammatory, and both can persist in the body for at least a few months after vaccination and possibly for much longer. How might this inflammatory package make its way to the brain and induce inflammation and hypersensitivity there? Actually, this is not a mystery. Each step along the way has been documented in the published literature, though no one has tied these steps together to offer a science-based explanation for the increase in symptoms related to brain/nervous system inflammation associated with the injections.

Briefly, a portion of the material injected into the deltoid via vaccination migrates to lymph nodes under the arm. From there, it follows lymphatic channels to the spleen, an organ of major importance for the immune system. When immune cells of the spleen take up the mRNA and start making spike proteins, they generate very small lipid spheres called *exosomes*. These contain spike proteins, mRNA coding for spike-protein production, and other types of RNA to compel cells to initiate an inflammatory response. The exosomes ultimately migrate along the vagus nerve and travel from the spleen to the brain. At that destination they're taken up by cells called *microglia*. Once the exosomes are taken up by microglia, they initiate spike-protein production and activation of the inflammatory cascade in those cells.[4]

Microglia inflammation is associated with a wide range of neurologically based conditions, from Alzheimer's and Parkinson's to anxiety, depression, ADHD, and aggressive behavior. It's important in this regard to note that microglia activation also activates the sympathetic nervous system. This is in addition to other pathways of sympathetic activation potentially induced by the injected material, including suppression of innate immunity with resulting reactivation of latent infections; activation of immune cascades that result in inflammatory cytokine production; disruption of multiple cancer surveillance networks operational within cells; interference with prion-protein regulatory systems; and many others.

If microglia become activated, then the sympathetic nervous system is activated, which means that the parasympathetic nervous system in general, and the parasympathetic signals flowing through the vagus nerve in particular, are suppressed. Suppression of vagal parasympathetic activity leads to a range of hypersensitivity reactions, including enhanced perception of pain, heart irregularities, systemic inflammation, blood sugar dysregulation, and increased risk of inflammatory and noninflammatory bowel disorders, among many others.

The media has suggested that all of these sequalae can follow natural infection with SARS-CoV-2. Unfortunately, it's now very challenging to do any large studies to determine if there's a difference in these sequalae in vaccinated vs. unvaccinated individuals, because virtually all vaccinated individuals have now had COVID-19, more than once for many. If someone develops anxiety and panic attacks after they received vaccination and also was naturally infected, there is no way to determine the cause of the anxiety and panic. I think there are good reasons to believe that both natural infection and vaccination could lead to these complications, but I suspect that vaccination will have more risk associated with it overall.

As early as August 2020 it was recognized that severe COVID-19 illness was driven in part by autonomic dysregulation.[5] Individuals in the highest risk groups for severe COVID-19 illness (e.g., those with hypertension, heart disease, and diabetes) were already known to have autonomic dysregulation associated with those illnesses. COVID-19 appeared to heighten the degree of that dysregulation and so amplify several lethal manifestations of the disease such as low blood oxygen and the immune over-activation known as the *cytokine storm.*

The sympathetic activation induced by COVID-19 illness can persist for weeks after a positive PCR test for SARS-CoV-2. It's important to note, however, that in a study of young, healthy individuals, those with prior infection had a suppressed pain response rather than a heightened one.[6] I believe that COVID-19 illness in those who are already chronically ill will have more persistent sympathetic activation. Spike protein has been found to be expressed in a type of circulating immune cell as many as sixteen months after infection.[7] The persistence of spike-protein production for nearly a year and a half following natural infection is suspect, though. The virus-derived mRNA coding for this protein should have been degraded within weeks or possibly a few months. It's plausible that spike production lasting this long is driven by the genetically modified, long-lived mRNA associated with these injections. The authors in the cited study did not control for vaccinated vs. unvaccinated subjects.

I should make a final comment about what is now widely referred to as Long COVID. This refers to a constellation of symptoms following either natural infection and illness or following injection with one of the gene therapies. Symptoms can include fatigue, brain fog, neuropathic pain, orthostatic hypotension, dizziness, and even episodes of fainting (known medically as *syncope*). It's been proposed that COVID-19 illness can induce a persistent autonomic dysregulation that can result in an episodic reduction in sympathetic signaling in the vagus nerve. The consequent unchecked parasympathetic firing leads to the symptoms of Long COVID.[8] You can readily see how this could lead to either triggering or to worsened sensitization. Both of our authors, Annie Hopper (chapter 1) and Ashok Gupta (chapter 2) have observed significant improvement in patients with Long COVID who used their methods of limbic retraining, which adds weight to these observations.

One mechanism through which COVID-19 is suggested to lead to Long COVID is via a very high production of a group of molecules called *catecholamines*. These include epinephrine (aka "adrenalin") and norepinephrine. One study has gathered evidence that the mRNA injections currently in use can also trigger this excess of catecholamines in the body.[9]

Whatever its underlying cause(s), Long COVID represents an extension of the autonomic dysregulation that can be induced by either natural infection or injection. For this reason it could be expected to contribute to development of hypersensitivity reactions for all the reasons described throughout this chapter.

Mitigating Vaccination-Induced Autonomic Dysregulation

Mitigating the impact of these injections on the nervous system has an overlap with mitigating the impact of spike proteins and the inflammation it induces, but these aren't synonymous. The Front Line COVID Critical Care Alliance (FLCCC) has done an excellent job of maintaining and updating their website with protocols for both preventing and treating COVID-19, as well as a protocol for treating Long COVID and vaccine injuries. It can be found here: https://covid19criticalcare.com/treatment-protocols/i-recover/. I find their recommendations valuable, but I would add a few to their list of first-line therapies.

Monolaurin

This is a constituent of coconut oil. There is a great deal of research into monolaurin's antiviral properties. Interestingly, it has this property in part because it acts as a detergent. Viral particles can have lipids as part of their membrane, which is necessary for the particles to fuse with and infect cells. Monolaurin dissolves that lipid membrane, leaving viruses unable to infect cells. The value of this detergent property is with respect to clearing those cationic lipids out of the body, clearing the fats used to deliver the mRNA, and to agitate the immune system. I believe that the presence of those lipid nanoparticles might be driving as much of an inflammatory response as the spike proteins are.

Low-dose Lithium Orotate

Lithium is most widely known as a drug used to treat bipolar disorder. The form given is lithium carbonate, and the dose is commonly 300mg taken three times daily. Lithium can also be taken in an organic form called lithium orotate, and this therapy typically uses much smaller doses. A common dosing strategy would be 5mg one to four times daily. Lithium dosed this way has a wide range of positive effects that are directly relevant to the type of nervous-system inflammation that could underly injection-induced hypersensitivities.

Vagus Nerve Therapies

Dysregulation of the parasympathetic signaling via the vagus nerve is a primary contributor to the hypersensitivity an increasing number of patients experience. There are very clear pathways and mechanisms through which synthetic mRNA and LNP injection could contribute to that dysregulation in a significant way. In addition to electrical stimulation of the vagus nerve using medical devices designed for that use, there are other home therapies that can be important components of an overall treatment program. These include, for example, Safe & Sound Protocol (SSP), which is based on Polyvagal Theory as developed by Dr. Stephen Porges. I have all of my patients consult with Maria Zilka, the nutrition therapist I work with, who provides guidance about and access to the audio files that make up the SSP. She has developed a program using SSP in conjunction with breathwork and somatic therapies, all of which work to establish normal parasympathetic tone in the vagus nerve and throughout the body (see chapters 1, 2, and 3 for more on this subject).

Conclusion

Generalized hypersensitivity is surely a condition with multiple contributing causes. I'm not suggesting that COVID-19 vaccination with either a synthetic mRNA or DNA product is sufficient to trigger a debilitating hypersensitivity, but a substantial amount of evidence suggests that these injections could play a significant role in destabilizing the autonomic nervous system and the immune system. Viewed in combination with the myriad other potential underlying factors described in this book, therapies to mitigate the impact of these gene therapies should be implemented, when applicable, with patients who suffer from this challenging condition.

DR. GREG NIGH is a naturopathic physician and licensed acupuncturist in practice at Immersion Health in Portland, Oregon. In addition to his clinical specialty in naturopathic oncology, Dr. Nigh has coauthored several published or in-review articles on the potential negative health consequences of the mRNA therapies currently in use. This includes the first peer-reviewed comprehensive review of the possible risks associated with these gene therapies, "Worse Than the Disease? Reviewing Some Possible Unintended Consequences of the mRNA Vaccines Against COVID-19," published in the *International Journal of Vaccine Theory, Practice, and Research* in May 2021. He continues to research, publish, and speak about the potential for both short- and long-term harm caused by these gene therapies.

References

1   Mouliou, Dimitra S., and Efthimios Dardiotis. "Current Evidence in SARS-CoV-2 mRNA Vaccines and Post-Vaccination Adverse Reports: Knowns and Unknowns." *Diagnostics* 12.7 (2022): 1555.

2   Cosentino, Marco, and Franca Marino. "Understanding the Pharmacology of COVID-19 mRNA Vaccines: Playing Dice with the Spike?" *International Journal of Molecular Sciences* 23.18 (2022): 10881.

3   Röltgen, Katharina, et al. "Immune imprinting, breadth of variant recognition, and germinal center response in human SARS-CoV-2 infection and vaccination." *Cell* 185.6 (2022): 1025-1040.

4   For references describing this process, see Seneff, Stephanie, et al. "Innate immune suppression by SARS-CoV-2 mRNA vaccinations: The role of G-quadruplexes, exosomes, and MicroRNAs." Food and Chemical Toxicology 164 (2022): 113008.

5   Del Rio, Rodrigo, Noah J. Marcus, and Nibaldo C. Inestrosa. "Potential role of autonomic dysfunction in COVID-19 morbidity and mortality." *Frontiers in physiology* 11 (2020): 561749.

6   Stute, Nina L., et al. "COVID-19 is getting on our nerves: sympathetic neural activity and haemodynamics in young adults recovering from SARS-CoV-2." *The Journal of physiology* 599.18 (2021): 4269-4285.

7   Patterson, Bruce K., et al. "Persistence of SARS CoV-2 S1 protein in CD16+ monocytes in post-acute sequelae of COVID-19 (PASC) up to 15 months post-infection." Frontiers in immunology (2022): 5526.

8   Dani, Melanie, et al. "Autonomic dysfunction in 'long COVID': rationale, physiology and management strategies"; *Clinical Medicine* 21.1 (2021): e63.

9   Cadegiani, Flavio A.; "Catecholamines Are the Key Trigger of COVID-19 mRNA Vaccine-Induced Myocarditis: A Compelling Hypothesis Supported by Epidemiological, Anatomopathological, Molecular, and Physiological Findings"; *Cureus* 14.8 (2022).

Part IV

Treatments for Sensitive Patients

Chapter 25: Low Dose Immunotherapy (LDI) in the Treatment of the Sensitive Patient

Ty Vincent, MD

Dr. Nathan's Introduction

When I first began to see patients with multiple chemical sensitivities, one of the first tools I found useful was LDA (low-dose allergy treatment). While often effective (perhaps 50% of MCS patients responded to it well), it usually took three years or longer to achieve success, and many patients couldn't tolerate their reactions to the treatment. Unlike the sublingual use of LDI, it required subdermal injections every seven weeks, which was also an issue for some patients. When Dr. Vincent developed LDI, I recognized immediately that I had long agreed with his observations, and his approach truly revolutionized our ability to modify the LDA technology to be more comfortable, more individualized, and more effective. Since it begins with extremely low dilutions of the antigens used in treatment, it's ideal for working with the unusually sensitive patients we encounter. Dr. Vincent's descriptions of its effectiveness are not exaggerated, and the observations and results he derived from his pioneering role in developing this process reflect my own experience.

✿ ✿ ✿

It's obvious that our immune system is critical to survival, as evidenced by how badly things go when the immune system is disabled in conditions such as AIDS, genetic immunodeficiency, or the use of various immunosuppressive drugs. We become susceptible to life-threatening infections and certain types of cancer, and we don't live very long without our immune system.

Those examples involve a failure of immune defense, which is what most people think of when discussing the immune system. They think it's there to defend us against enemies both foreign and domestic. When you fail at defending against microbes from the outside world, you get infections. When you fail to defend against your own cells that misbehave, you get cancer, and certain types of cancer involve the interplay between your own cells, certain viruses or bacteria, and your immune system.

What people don't appreciate is that "defense" is the smaller part of what your immune system does for you. A far more expansive role involves *tolerance.* There are many more things in your world, both internal and external, that are harmless or even beneficial to you, and they shouldn't be attacked. Your immune system must comprehensively identify and catalog all of those harmless things, and choose to tolerate rather than attack them.

Tolerance is an active process, not a passive one. People tend to think it's the default situation: your immune system doesn't attack anything unless it has a good reason, and it simply accepts everything else with a sort of indifference. That's not the case. The burden of illness related to loss of immune tolerance is enormous and is increasing steadily. As with the concept of defense, we can think about tolerance in terms of the outside world and our internal milieu. If you lose tolerance for something in your external environment we call it allergy; and if you lose tolerance for something inside your body it manifests as something we would call autoimmune or inflammatory.

There are many different autoimmune disorders, including Hashimoto's thyroiditis, rheumatoid arthritis, and ulcerative colitis. There are also many chronic inflammatory conditions that are immune-mediated and represent a loss of self-tolerance, but they're not usually thought of as autoimmune conditions. The immune system resides diffusely within you, all over your body; therefore, when your immune system attacks *you* inappropriately, the symptoms can include just about anything and involve any part of you.

Chronic medical problems in these categories are due to immune-system hypersensitivity, and they collectively represent a massive burden of disease and cost to the public and our health-care system. The dramatic increase of immune-related illnesses we've seen in recent decades can be ascribed to the combination of insufficient nutrition and the myriad foreign chemicals in our everyday lives.

The work of Weston Price, DDS, in the 1930s (see his *Nutrition and Physical Degeneration,* 1937) showed that indigenous populations all over the world who were eating their natural native diets were completely free of these disorders. In fact, they didn't even have doctors or dentists because none were needed. It was only after the introduction of processed foods into our diet and various chemicals into our environment that chronic illnesses became an issue for humans. This includes tuberculosis, classically viewed as an infection process. Those eating their natural diet almost never developed symptoms of TB, while those who ate a processed diet suffered from active tuberculosis and even died at a significant rate. My work with LDI has shown me that many illnesses we've understood to be infections are actually the result of immune dysregulation and hypersensitivity responses.

The explosion of noxious chemicals in our world over the past century has compounded this problem in devastating fashion. Chemicals might be tested for whether they cause cancer (and only a small percentage are even tested for that), but they're not tested for immunological or endocrine effects. If you search, you can find studies showing that many common chemicals do in fact cause hormonal effects or disruption. Finding research into immune system effects is harder, but there's ample evidence that man-made chemicals cause immune-system effects as well. It seems obvious that having thousands of foreign chemicals in your body would interfere with something so fragile and complex as the human immune system. All of us are polluted with countless chemicals, no matter how hard we try to avoid them and live "clean."

The fact that these illnesses rarely cause death greatly increases the overall burden of illness. People may die fairly soon from serious infections or cancer, but when it comes to hypersensitivity disorders, people will live with those for decades. These disorders amount to many years of suffering and seemingly endless medical expenses. If you do survive cancer or infection, then you're done with those problems, but the chronic immune-reaction conditions just keep on going unless you can reprogram the immune-system response.

Low dose immunotherapy (LDI) can provide a way to restore immune tolerance for those target antigens involved in a person's illness. Antigens can be foods (plants, animals, fungi), inhalants (pollen, mold, dust mites, etc.), chemicals, your own internal molecules, such as hormones or collagen, or any microorganism within your internal microbiome or the outside world. If you restore normal immune tolerance for the antigens involved, you can completely stop the disease process. This works for allergies, autoimmune diseases, and immune-mediated chronic inflammatory disorders.

Unfortunately, once a person has developed a chronic immune issue, detoxifying chemicals or heavy metals and drastically improving the diet and nutrient status might do little or nothing to improve their immune/inflammatory problems. Becoming as "healthy" as possible doesn't tend to reverse this sort of disease process. It usually requires some sort of therapy that directly reprograms the immune response in an antigen-specific manner. This could be because a healthy immune system can still be misdirected and attack the wrong things. It isn't a matter of making the immune system "stronger" or "weaker"; it must be redirected or reprogrammed instead.

There are numerous techniques designed to correct inappropriate immune reactions to specific antigens. They vary in mechanism, delivery, administration, cost, complexity, and success. Most of these methods use only those antigens to which the patient tested allergic, which means they actually have to test for every relevant thing. LDI uses broad mixtures of things together and doesn't require any preliminary testing. LDI doses can generally be taken much less frequently than other methods, and typically costs far less.

With conventional allergy shots, sublingual immunotherapy (SLIT), and oral immunotherapy (OIT), the doses begin at a moderate dilution and then escalate steadily to larger and larger amounts of exposure. This forces what we refer to as "adaptation" of the immune system; it must become more accustomed to those antigens along the way and extinguish the immune reactions somewhat forcibly. These methods all have the potential to trigger severe immune reactions against the doses themselves in patients who are highly allergic. LDI uses dilutions that are much further out and effectively retrains "tolerance" for all the antigens used. That's why we use such broad mixtures of antigens and don't rely on any sort of testing; it doesn't matter if you promote tolerance to something the patient already tolerates. There's also no risk of the patient's having a severe reaction directly to those doses. The concept employed by LDI was initially developed by an allergist named Franklin, working in London in the 1950s. He was treating food and environmental allergies with broad mixtures of highly diluted antigens, and working out the protocol for dilution and dose timing. The process was modified somewhat by another British doctor, who tried to make it more profitable and proprietary; he told everyone that a small amount of the enzyme *beta glucuronidase* had to be added to each antigen dose in order for the therapy to work. To be clear, *this was not and is not true.*

There were many other dogmatic rules and practices mandated in the use of what was then called enzyme potentiated desensitization," or EPD. There were fixed dilutions that had to be the same for each patient; doses had to be given at least seven weeks apart; the antigens had to be kept cold at all times, and there was a very restricted diet for the patients to follow for three days around the time of every dose. None of these rules proved real or relevant once I started to experiment with them. I gave doses with no beta glucuronidase, and doses that had been drawn up and left out at room temperature for two months, and they worked just the same.

EPD was brought to the United States in the 1990s and used in the same way initially. Dr. William Shrader spearheaded its use in the States and suggested that the doses could be given via intradermal injection (prior to that, they had been excoriating a small patch of skin and placing some antigen onto the raw area for exposure to immune cells within the dermis). This worked just as well. All of the other dogmatic rules were continued, even after Doctor Shrader remade the mixtures in the U.S. through domestic pharmacies and renamed the technique low dose allergy therapy, or LDA.

The implementation of this therapy remained fairly consistent for more than forty-five years. It was primarily used to treat allergies; mixtures were produced containing foods, inhalants, and chemicals in three separate combinations. There were also several bacterial mixes. used to treat a small number of autoimmune conditions. There were two strengths of the food mixture, but only one strength for the others.

I learned LDA from Dr. Shrader in 2007. It worked very well in most cases—80% or better for those with clear allergies and certain autoimmune disorders. I began to experiment with breaking the LDA rules after the first couple years, and found that most of them were totally unnecessary. Also, beginning in 2009, I began to experiment with using different antigens in the same manner. I acquired mixtures of *Candida* and other yeast species, and a mix of *mycobacteria* early on, and found that both could be useful in inflammatory bowel disease cases. Also, I found the yeast mixture useful for many people with various complex chronic illnesses. I then began to use self-derived samples from patients to make "autologous LDI" antigens for them, which proved extremely effective in certain situations.

I acquired more and different microbes to use as antigens, and discovered effective treatments for more and more autoimmune and inflammatory conditions. I found that we could drastically modify the way this therapy was implemented, breaking almost all the LDA rules. I had to devise a new way to apply the therapy, experimenting systematically with dosing at progressively stronger dilutions until a response point was found for each individual. I developed the concept of "booster doses," and also proved that you can give doses on variable time schedules. I decided to call this new and expanded form of therapy low dose immunotherapy in order to clearly distinguish it from LDA.

Other practitioners began to take notice when I found that we could treat chronic Lyme disease using LDI with a high success rate, completely changing the paradigm for how we think about that condition. In 2015 we created a cooperative practitioner network so we could try to train other practitioners in how to use this therapy and supply them with the same antigen mixtures I use. That way we could have some consistency among different practitioners while sharing knowledge and experience. Since 2015 we've had well over 200 practitioners worldwide take up LDI in their practices, though to my knowledge, only a fraction of them have truly used it correctly and effectively.

It's complicated to use this therapy successfully because every patient must be treated in an individualized manner; we have to find the optimal specific dose for each different antigen mixture a person might need. Intellectually challenging, it requires the processing of a lot of information, and a wholly different level of communication with our patients that isn't time-efficient for a practitioner who also has a busy clinic practice. LDI is the only thing I've done in practice since the end of 2016, working from my home in Kona, Hawaii, and helping people all over the world through the mail and the internet. I've found that I get much better results doing all the communication directly with patients and focusing all my attention on this one thing. That said, some other practitioners have clearly mastered this treatment as well and use it with great skill.

The application of LDI starts with a thorough patient interview. The most important information relates to any and all symptoms the patient has, specific allergic reactions that are known, the circumstances surrounding onset of any unexplained chronic symptoms, responses to prior treatments that were tried, and current functional status. Laboratory testing is rarely helpful. Tests that measure antibodies or some other sort of immune response to any organisms are meaningless; cultures or other tests that look for the presence of GI organisms, oral flora, *Borrelia*, or other microbes are generally unhelpful too.

Understanding the difference between an infection and an immune response against a microorganism is critical in understanding how LDI works and the underlying process. For example, you can find Borrelia, the bacteria implicated in Lyme Disease, in virtually all adults on any given day if you run the right tests. Therefore, having the organism in your body isn't the same as having a disease or infection; finding *Borrelia* in your body doesn't mean you have Lyme disease, because they are essentially normal flora. It doesn't matter at all whether you have positive antibodies indicating Lyme either; that result has no correlation with whether you have the illness. Lyme disease is a prominent example of this concept, and one of the most controversial now, but there are many other examples.

A Case of Acute Lyme Disease

I had been using LDI to treat chronic Lyme patients for a year or so when a ten-year-old boy came in with symptoms of acute Lyme disease. We virtually never saw acute Lyme in Alaska (where I first practiced), presumably because we had no ticks there. The boy had been on vacation in Oregon until a couple of days prior, playing in a yard where they found a dead deer (no signs of injury or foul play). Within a few days of that exposure, he developed a classic erythema migrans ("bull's eye") rash on one arm (no tick or other blood-sucking arthropod was ever seen), fever, exhaustion, sweating, sound sensitivity, and widespread pain in his joints and muscles.

He presented to our office and we initially gave him antibiotics, thinking that acute Lyme should still be treated as an infection. His condition became much worse over the following days, presumably from a Herxheimer reaction, so we stopped the antibiotics on day three and gave him an LDI dose of Lyme 10C ("Lyme" is the antigen mixture, and "10C" is the dilution). That caused no change in his symptoms, so three days later he was given Lyme 9C (which is a hundred times stronger in relative concentration). By the next day his symptoms had virtually disappeared, and he even went to school.

Those symptoms all began to return by one to two weeks, which suggests the improvement had been due to that LDI dose and not just his disease process naturally ending. He was then given Lyme 8C (another hundredfold increase in concentration from the 9C, now 10,000 times stronger than his initial 10C dose), and his symptoms went away again. This time they stayed gone for more than a month. That Lyme 8C dose was repeated every six to seven weeks until, over time, the benefits lasted longer and longer. As time went on, the patient's doses were lasting more than six months, but his symptoms would still return eventually. That's because the immune system has a stubborn memory. The same aspect of the immune system that allows your measles vaccine to provide lifelong immunity also means that your immune-related problems can return at any point if you endure some event that aggravates your immune system or stresses you severely.

Starting with only two new antigen mixtures in 2009, ten years later I had accumulated more than a hundred. I've been able to determine antigen-disease relationships for a number of autoimmune or chronic inflammatory conditions, antigenic links that were never known before. I've demonstrated that alopecia areata is linked to *H. pylori*, sarcoidosis is caused by mycobacteria, psoriasis is an immune reaction to fungi that normally live on your skin, and osteoarthritis is a true autoimmune disease because it responds to an LDI mixture of human collagen. I have also developed numerous antigen mixtures that have yet to show any promise for any conditions at all—you win some, you lose some. I have autoimmune type 1 diabetes, and have so far failed to find an LDI antigen after more than eight years of trying. I still think I'll figure it out.

Treating allergies is much more straightforward than treating unexplained chronic symptoms or most autoimmune conditions. In the case of allergy, you already know which antigens to use. If someone sneezes and their nose runs around cats or dogs, you know they're allergic to those animals. If someone throws up or gets a rash whenever they eat chicken, you know they're allergic to chicken. We use broad mixtures of airborne allergens, foods, chemicals, essential oils, and some other odd things to treat most types of allergy. This way we promote tolerance to that whole category of things at once, and the cross-reactivity of antigens means that many other things are covered well that aren't specifically in the mixtures. If someone is allergic to some specific thing not represented in our mixtures, we can make a custom antigen dilution for that item by simply diluting a sample like we would with anything else. Anyone can do this if they acquire an antigen sample and the necessary supplies.

When someone has nonspecific symptoms like fatigue, insomnia, anxiety, brain fog, headaches, migratory body pains, neurological issues, and various GI symptoms, they could be reacting to just about any sort of antigen. There are also many non-immune causes for those same symptoms. When someone comes in with that type of symptom picture, the odds of LDI fixing it are less than 50%. There are just too many possible causes, most of which have no immunological basis. When someone has allergies and knows exactly what triggers their symptoms, our success rate is better than 90%. Success rates vary for named autoimmune conditions depending on the disease process.

Corn allergy has become a major problem for an increasing number of people. It's worth discussing here because it causes massive problems and it behaves somewhat differently from other food allergies. The number of chemicals, food additives, personal-care products, and other everyday items that contain some amount of corn or corn-derived substances is truly vast, and people who become highly sensitive to corn can react to all manner of things. They have to purge most things from their homes and most foods from their diet. They have to acquire food from sources that are proven corn-free, and that's a small percentage of sources.

Some patients I've seen didn't know they were allergic to corn when they came to me. I might suggest it because they seem to have frequent and fluctuating symptoms with no clear and consistent specific triggers or exposures. They feel like they're "reacting to everything." People can be so sensitive that they react to the smell of popcorn from more than twenty feet away. For others, their skin might develop a rash on contact with corn, or they might have to eat substantial quantities of corn before they elicit a reaction. How sensitive they are in that regard guides where we begin with the Corn LDI dose dilutions.

We often use isolated corn antigen alone to start with, because many people with corn allergy will have a much greater sensitivity to corn than they do to their other food allergens. It's also hard to know whether reactions to other foods are only due to a corn reaction from something in that food or a direct reaction to that food itself. Many people cross-react with all sorts of corn-derived chemical products too. By getting the corn reaction under control first, we can then determine whether they do in fact have other specific food and chemical reactions.

This problem is becoming more and more common owing to two factors: First, the average human immune system is more and more damaged with each generation of exposure to all the toxic chemicals in our environment; second, corn is literally everywhere. To my knowledge, no one else had successfully tackled the problem of corn allergy before I worked out a way to treat it with LDI. We have a 90% success rate with it, and now that the Facebook/Meta group for corn allergy has discovered us, we see new patients with corn allergy every week.

We have a dilution of Corn by itself, and we have a mixture that contains all our other food antigens except Corn. We use that to cover the rest of the person's food allergies if their Corn dose is significantly different from what they need to correct the others. After using LDA for several years, I realized that those food and environmental mixtures had some serious limitations. They were at fixed dilutions, and people are more diverse than that. Some need different dilutions for different foods or inhalant allergens than others do, so the fixed-ratio mixtures couldn't cover all the allergies for those individuals. Basically, the therapy could not be tailored to the needs of different individuals.

I made my Food mixture from a collection of thirteen different sub-mixtures. Some are single foods like Corn, Egg, Soy, and Peanut. Others are collections such as Meats, Fruits, Shellfish, Dairy, Nuts, and others. I made the Environmental LDI mixture from collections of Molds, Mites, Animals, Weeds, Trees, Grasses, and others. This way, I can treat people with complex situations who need different dilutions for different sub-categories. We haven't had to do this for those with allergies to chemicals or essential oils—at least not yet.

When EPD and LDA were being used, it was very clear that celiac disease did not respond to this therapy. There were gluten-containing grains like wheat and barley in the antigen mixtures, but for unknown reasons they simply didn't work for the sort of immune-system reaction present in celiac disease. If someone had more typical allergy symptoms from eating wheat or other gluten-containing grains, LDA would work just fine, but those with the celiac disease manifestation had no success. When I made my Food LDI mixture, it too didn't work for those with celiac disease. I made an isolated LDI dilution from just wheat Gluten itself and tried that. Luckily, it worked extremely well, so now we can effectively treat celiac disease patients with the same success we have treating other food sensitivities.

These improvements in treating allergies are some of the advances I've made using LDI, beyond what was being accomplished with LDA or EPD. I have otherwise expanded the clinical application of this technique far beyond what was being treated with EPD and LDA earlier. I've found successful antigens for many other autoimmune disorders, including psoriasis, Crohn's disease, multiple sclerosis, alopecia areata, and many others. I've also demonstrated that this is the ideal approach for treating chronic inflammatory conditions like osteoarthritis, costochondritis, chronic Lyme disease, sarcoidosis, acne, and all sorts of other skin conditions.

Most autoimmune or inflammatory conditions are related to just one antigen, but some are more often multifactorial and require multiple antigens to achieve complete resolution. Eczema is one example in the world of "allergic" conditions; it's usually related to foods, but sometimes requires the addition of environmental or chemical antigens, and sometimes yeast or skin fungi. Crohn's disease and ulcerative colitis are often multi-antigen-reaction conditions, involving reactions to multiple gut flora and possibly to foods. Acne too is fairly often related to multiple antigens, and requires some combination of foods, skin bacteria, and hormones. Sorting things out with more complex conditions is more challenging and takes longer, but can still be done successfully by following a certain strategy.

The first phase of treatment with LDI is what I call the "titration phase." I've already chosen an antigen and starting dilution, and now the patient takes progressively stronger doses until they have an obvious and dramatic response. Hopefully this response is a positive one, but it's possible to overdose someone and make their immune issues temporarily worse. If that happens, we have to wait at least seven weeks for the immune system to reset itself and then back up to a weaker dilution. How far to back up is based on how long the patient's symptoms remained aggravated. The formula is to back up roughly 1C (a 100:1 dilution step) for every week of symptom aggravation, plus another 1C–2C just to be safe.

If there's no significant response by one week, then we go on to the next stronger dilution. If we're treating allergies, the patient has to do some relevant test exposures six to seven days after each dose and base its effect on that reaction each time. If we're treating some chronic condition, the patient just observes their symptoms for a week after each dose. If there's no significant change, we work through progressively stronger doses week after week until some meaningful response occurs. At that point, the pace and increment of dose adjustment changes. This process sounds complicated, but it simply requires good patient guidance, effective and timely communication regarding responses, and careful record keeping.

The second phase of treatment is the "fine-tuning phase." We make small adjustments to the dose until it yields 100% improvement for at least seven weeks at a time. Complete improvement means there are no more allergic reactions or no chronic inflammatory symptoms, whichever is related to the antigen being used. Some symptoms are multifactorial, so the patient won't see 100% success with any single antigen. Instead, they'll get partial improvement at a certain dose, and then, when they try the next-stronger dose, they'll have a symptom flare instead of further improvement. From that we can infer that the symptoms in question have more than one cause.

Once the ideal dose of an LDI antigen is found, that same dose is given repeatedly at least seven weeks apart. This is the "maintenance phase." It's ideal to wait until symptoms or reactions start to come back, and then give the dose again for each cycle. In that way, the person can allow the doses to space further and further apart over time. This is not necessary, as people can keep taking their dose every seven weeks forever if they desire, but it makes the treatment less expensive. Some patients eventually reach a point where they no longer need the doses at all for years. That can represent long-term remission, but we don't use the term "cure" when it comes to immune-mediated conditions. Our immune system has a stubborn long-term memory, and those same immune problems can return at any point if the person endures some stressful condition or event.

Those stressful situations, or catalytic events, as I call them, can happen to anyone at any time. They can initiate, worsen, or rekindle immune problems. Catalytic events can include pregnancy and childbirth (or miscarriage), vaccination, acute illness or infection, antibiotics use, physical trauma, surgery, or psychological stress. These things happen to people all the time and they can cause shifts in the person's LDI dose threshold or kick off totally new problems. Because of this, we have to continually monitor patients to make sure their LDI doses continue to work as they should and that we can make appropriate adjustments when necessary.

In summary, low dose immunotherapy is an effective, affordable, safe therapy that we can apply to virtually any disease process or symptom that's related to an aberrant immune-system response. We must identify the correct antigens involved with the symptoms and then strategically identify the proper dose of that antigen mixture for each individual patient. It's somewhat complicated, and the process involves a lot of engagement and communication between patient and practitioner. It's absolutely worth trying if the situation seems appropriate, because the results can be truly miraculous. Inflammatory processes and their resulting symptoms can stop quickly and completely when the dose is correct. Patients are usually very surprised when this happens, and feel like it's some sort of magic trick, but most "magic" is just science we don't yet understand.

Ty Vincent, MD, is an integrative physician who's been in practice since 2005. He completed medical school at the University of Washington, and a residency in family medicine in Anchorage, Alaska. Dr. Vincent is married, has nine children, and lives in Kailua-Kona, Hawaii. He works from home, helping chronically ill people worldwide via telemedicine consultation and sending low dose immunotherapy to their homes.

Dr. Vincent has gained additional training in acupuncture, Chinese medicine, environmental medicine, allergy and immunology, bio-identical hormone therapy, chelation therapy, hyperbaric medicine, integrative cancer therapy, Reiki, and nutritional medicine.

He has lectured nationally on the subjects of bio-identical hormone therapies, vitamin D, and low dose immunotherapy (LDI). In 2014, Dr. Vincent developed immune-therapy techniques for treating a large number of autoimmune diseases with a high degree of success and safety using LDI internal microbes. In September 2018, Dr. Vincent developed LDI for Allergens, which treats food, environmental, and/or chemical sensitivities and allergies. He is the author of *Thinking Outside the Pill Box: A Consumer's Guide to Integrative Medicine and Comprehensive Medicine.* He can be contacted at Global Immunotherapy: www.globalimmunotherapy.com

Chapter 26: Ketamine and the Sensitive Patient

Andreas Grossgold, MD, PhD

Dr. Nathan's Introduction

For some of our patients, ketamine has played a major role in reversing their sensitivities. Ketamine has proven to be a game changer, especially when the sensitivities are severe. Dr. Grossgold helps us understand ketamine's unique properties. He emphasizes that, used properly, by physicians who are practiced in its administration, ketamine is very safe and very effective. My own experience mirrors Dr. Grossgold's: ketamine has been particularly effective in treating sensitive patients.

✿ ✿ ✿

Introduction

The body is a battlefield where the immune system fights invading pathogens for territory and resources. Our army, the immune system, is well trained to combat infectious enemies. Most of the time, the immune system prevails before the enemy can even mount an attack. Other times, the invaders gain a foothold. The ensuing combat causes collateral damage that manifests as symptoms of illness.

One battle that has long gone misunderstood and underrecognized is against Lyme and other tick-borne diseases.* It's more complex and harder to treat than is generally thought. In addition, patients can develop post-treatment Lyme disease syndrome (PTLDS), a chronic pain disorder for which there's no gold-standard treatment. At times like these the immune system needs help; medications, supplements, antibiotics, and other therapies come in as special forces to assist. One, whose benefits are rapidly gaining attention, is ketamine.

I'm a navy physician; in combat, we use ketamine in emergencies and get great results. It's an efficient anesthetic and a potent anxiety reliever. I'm also an integrative clinician; at my practice, I've treated hundreds of patients with chronic diseases and multiple chemical sensitivities. All of them have been in different stages of emotional, physical, and neurological deterioration. I treat patients with chronic Lyme, myalgic encephalomyelitis/chronic fatigue syndrome (ME/CFS), multiple chemical toxicity, Long COVID syndrome, and more. Ketamine is one way I can get them from a stage of illness to a stage of wellness. It's a blessing. Patients benefit from better pain control for their physical illness, and get help with their emotional traumas, depression, anxiety, attention deficit, and PTSD.

Everyone needs help at times; our immune army is no exception. I hope this chapter will leave you feeling confident in your knowledge of ketamine, how it works, and how it can benefit you and those you love.

*In this chapter, for convenience, the term "Lyme" is broadly used to refer to disease caused by *B. burgdorferi* as well as other tick-borne infections such as *Babesia, Bartonella,* and *Ehrlichia*. Notes on specific pathogens will be called out as such.

Origins

In the 1950s, phencyclidine (PCP) was investigated as an anesthetic for surgery. While its anesthetic properties were sound, the intense delirium and side effects were highly undesirable, so a hunt was on for a compound that mirrored this anesthetic potency but minimized side effects. First synthesized in 1962, a PCP-derivative labeled CI-581 was found.

Its effects were unique to medicine. It produced a previously unseen state of altered consciousness called *dissociative anesthesia*. These effects came on rapidly, but weren't prolonged, so symptoms could be controlled with single or repeated administrations.

The chemical structure of this compound contained *ketone* and *amine* functional groups, and the names were combined to christen this new compound *ketamine*. Under the brand name Ketalar, ketamine hydrochloride was approved by the FDA in 1970. Ketalar was widely used as a field anesthetic for troops during the Vietnam War. It's still used for surgical anesthesia today because of its efficacy and wide margin of safety.

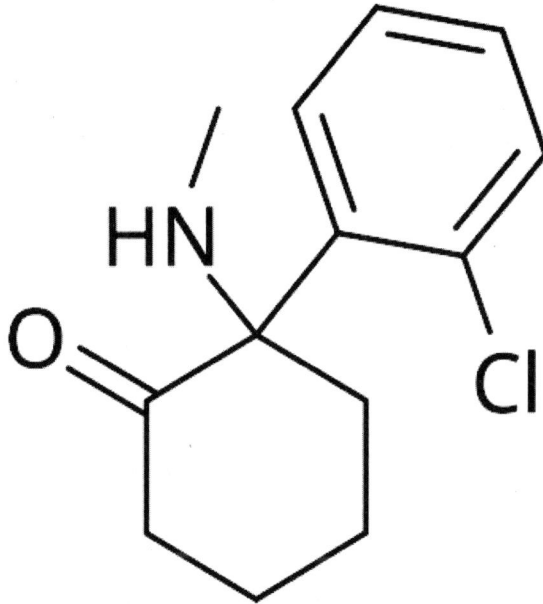

Chemical structure of Ketamine.

Forty years after its discovery, ketamine was investigated for its activity against depression. It revolutionized treatment for this disorder. Far from knowing ketamine's full range of applications, new uses and effects are continually being discovered. Many of these properties put it at the forefront of new treatment for chronic illness, specifically for patients with Lyme disease, and of particular benefit to patients who manifest severe sensitivities.

Mechanism of Action

Synaptic Transmission

To appreciate ketamine's uniqueness, we must first address the basics. In pharmacology, how a drug carries out its effects at the molecular level is called its mechanism of action. The brain communicates with itself and the rest of the body by special chemical messengers called neurotransmitters. Where the branches of two brain cells, or neurons,* meet is called a synapse. The discussion between two nerves begins with the initiator neuron synthesizing a certain neurotransmitter in its terminal. This is like thinking of what you want to say before you say it. Next, the neurotransmitter is packaged into small bubbles called vesicles, which are gathered near the end of the neuron (the pre-synaptic terminal). Once the neuron is excited by another nerve or stimulus, it spills the contents of the vesicles into the space between the neurons (aka the synaptic cleft).

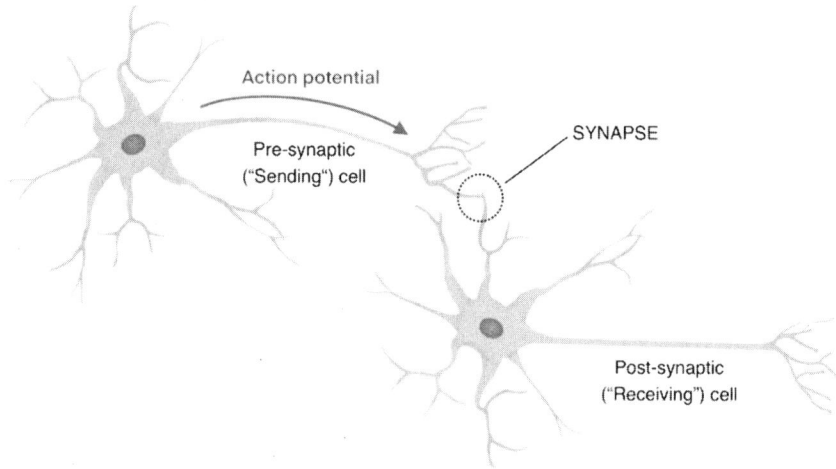

Across this cleft, the receiving neuron terminal (the post-synaptic terminal) is dotted with special proteins called receptors, each of which is specifically shaped to bind to a certain neurotransmitter. Once activated, these receptors transmit the correct message to the post-synaptic neuron and the message is received.[22]

Much like the words in a conversation, neurotransmitters can have an exciting or depressing effect on the listener. When a nerve wants things to increase or speed up, it releases an excitatory neurotransmitter. Likewise, it can send an inhibitory neurotransmitter to calm things down. This conversation can be altered by changing the amount of neurotransmitter released or by interfering with its receptor binding. This is how hormones and many medications work.

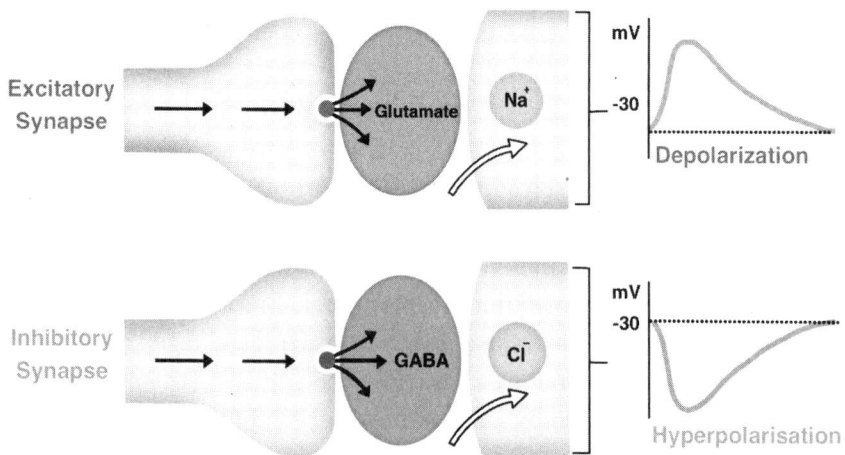

Ketamine, for example, is an antagonist, or blocker, of the N-methyl-D-aspartate (NMDA) receptor on neurons. NMDA receptors bind the neurotransmitter glutamate. Glutamate is important as it's the brain's primary excitatory (signal-increasing) neurotransmitter. Likewise, gamma-aminobutyric acid (GABA) is the primary inhibitory neurotransmitter in the brain, which will be discussed later.

As illustrated above, the presynaptic neurons synthesize, gather, and release glutamate to excite the other neuron. This is where ketamine comes in and blocks the receptor before glutamate can reach it to relay the signal. Since ketamine doesn't have the same excitatory effects, it inhibits the receiving neuron. Zooming out, this is how ketamine causes anesthetic, dissociative, and calming effects—by blocking excitation, it causes inhibition.

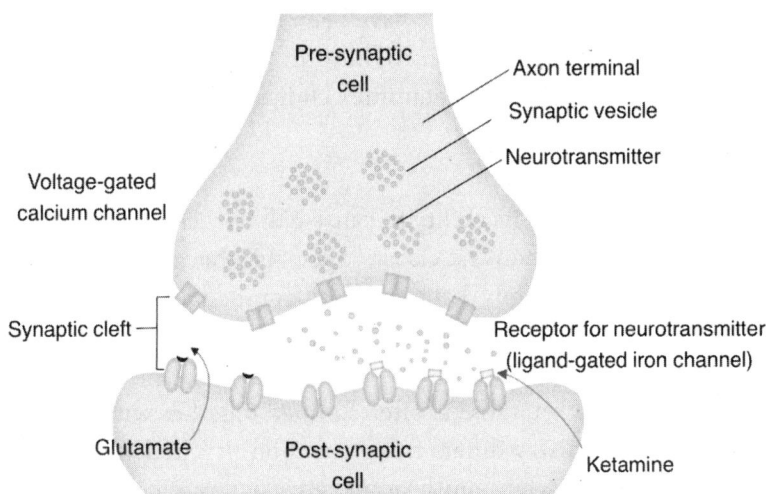

Courtesy of Andreas Grossgold 2023.

*While not technically the same, the words "nerve" and "neuron" are used interchangeably here.

Nightmare and Miracle?

The effect of ketamine on NMDA receptors is the best-understood action of ketamine. Research has shown the full mechanism of action is incredibly complex. While NMDA antagonism is its main job, it also interacts with GABA-ergic, opioid, monoamine, acetylcholine, purine, and adrenaline receptors, all while causing local anesthetic effects, which are summarized in the table below. Some of our readers might not want to review this in detail, but medical professionals should find this information of value.

Receptor	Type	Action	Effect
Cholinergic	Muscarinic/Nicotinic	Antagonist	Bronchodilation and muscle relaxation
Opioid	$\mu < \kappa < \delta$		Analgesia (weak)
Glutamate	NMDA, AMPA, Kainate	Antagonist	Sedation, anti-hyperalgesic, anticonvulsant, neuroprotection, antidepressant
GABA			Neurotransmitter inhibition
Catecholamine		Agonist	Cardiovascular stimulation
Adenosine		Agonist	Anti-proinflammatory

This wide breadth of activity makes ketamine's effects so difficult to fully explain that it has garnered the name "the pharmacologist's nightmare," but it's this very attribute that makes ketamine so useful. In the field of depression, ketamine has been called a wonder drug and even a miracle. Similar benefits have been noted for other conditions such as anxiety, and for patients with severe sensitivities. In this sense, anesthesia and depression are only the tip of the iceberg of ketamine's clinical applications.

Special K

To some, ketamine is known by its ability to cause hallucinations, and has also seen use as a street drug. Beginning on the West Coast, "Special K" became a widely abused party drug in the 1980s–'90s. Ultimately, ketamine was branded a federally controlled substance in 1999. The DEA now lists it as a Schedule III substance with low potential for abuse.

Because of this history, ketamine is often lumped together with other recreational hallucinogens, but its chemistry differs from common psychedelics. Most psychedelics* (MDMA/Ecstasy, psilocybin/mushrooms, etc.) act as *agonists* or "uppers." They bind serotonin, dopamine, and adrenaline receptors and boost their signal. Ketamine blocks a completely different receptor. How substances with different actions cause similar responses can be confusing, but here's a helpful metaphor:

Think of the mind like a room with a window: Ketamine relaxes and enlarges the window, allowing in more light. Common psychedelics increase the brightness outside, forcing more light through the same size window.[45] While the actions are different, both cause increased brightness in the room.

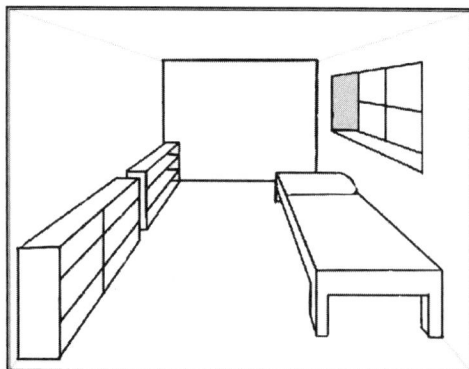

Courtesy of Andreas Grossgold 2023.

You might have heard horror stories about people getting caught in the "k-hole." At sufficiently strong doses, ketamine causes a dissociative high. The k-hole can be thought of as a state between intoxication and coma. Some describe it as an out-of-body or near-death experience. Hallucinations, confusion, and euphoria are common, but so are heart problems, brain damage, and seizures. This can actually cause PTSD instead of treating it.[21]

Here is where the line in the sand must be drawn. Ketamine as a recreational hallucinogen is not the same as its use medically. The doses, routes of administration, and effects are all different; however, ketamine is not always administered correctly.

What's the difference? First, any drug taken in excess or incorrectly can potentially cause damage. If patients experience the k-hole, they either took too much or too quickly. Our protocol starts with a minimum dose over a long infusion. Depending on our patient's response, the dose can be diminished, increased, or discontinued. This protocol is detailed later in the chapter.

*Psychedelics may have their own role in the future of medicine as well. This is discussed briefly at the end of the chapter.

Lyme Disease

How does ketamine specifically battle Lyme disease? Below is a list of symptoms of tick-borne diseases, each of which is treatable with ketamine.

Common Symptoms of Tick-Borne Diseases

- Depression
- Pain
- Headache
- Cognitive dysfunction (concentration, memory difficulty, and word recall)
- Low Blood Pressure (Hypotension)
- Fainting (Syncope)
- Anxiety
- Fatigue and malaise
- Mania, panic attacks, or delusion

Depression

Just as battlefields have multiple fronts, so do patients. We humans are made of mind-body-spirit, each of which is a frontline in the battle for health. When the mind is afflicted, the body can't fight infection well, which worsens outcomes. We see this clearly in depression, which is one of the most common symptoms of those with chronic illness, including Lyme disease, with rates as high as >90%. It's a heroic challenge for those affected, and an unwanted hindrance for those already sick. Fighting concurrent depression is key for defeating Lyme disease. This is where ketamine arrives.

Since its first investigation, ketamine has become a game-changer in the field of antidepressants.[10] One reason is its rapid onset. Current first-line antidepressants take two to four weeks to affect symptoms. Ketamine can start working in an hour. Its effects last for weeks and sometimes reduce symptoms of depression indefinitely.[28] The fast relief makes ketamine an ideal bridge therapy; infusions can effectively bridge the gap between changes of antidepressant medication by providing immediate relief during the down period. Additionally, ketamine treats disorders that coexist with depression, such as OCD, anxiety, and panic disorder.[36] The FDA realized this usefulness and approved esketamine (a ketamine enantiomer, or mirror image) nasal spray for treatment-resistant depression.[13]

How does this happen? It's said everything psychological is biological. Our thoughts and feelings have biochemical causes and repercussions. Depression is no different. The picture of depression's full effects is incomplete, but there are different theories. Each contains a partial aspect of depression's effect on the person. While not exclusive, these are the major schools of thought and ketamine's role in each.

The Monoamine Hypothesis

Monoamines are a well-known group of neurotransmitters that consist of serotonin, dopamine, adrenaline, and epinephrine. These compounds affect every facet of human activity. Monoamine levels are almost universally low in depression. Common antidepressants (Prozac, Paxil, Zoloft) increase the amount of available serotonin and sometimes norepinephrine; but the monoamines aren't the only neurotransmitters involved in depression. GABA and glutamate also play a key role. In contrast to glutamates' excitatory effects, GABA slows the brain, reduces anxiety, improves sleep, and calms body and mind. Unsurprisingly, GABA levels are also low in depression. This is where ketamine enters the picture. In addition to blocking glutamate, ketamine induces a compensatory increase in GABA. This was a revolutionary finding. By attacking depression through an entirely different hormone system than traditional antidepressants, ketamine produces remarkable results.

Inflammation

The link between depression and inflammation is well established. While important to healing, inflammation can cause unintentional damage and pain, hence the common use of anti-inflammatories. The immune system mediates inflammation through proteins called cytokines, which are linked to depression. Rates of depression are increased in patients with autoimmune disease and chronic infections, where inflammation runs high. Therapeutic injection of cytokines has even been shown to provoke depressive symptoms.[7] Ketamine decreases inflammation and controls cytokine levels. This alleviates patients' depression and benefits their overall health. Later in the chapter, I'll address these *anti-proinflammatory* effects of ketamine in depth regarding Mast Cell Activation Syndrome.

Neuroplasticity and Neurogenesis

It's sometimes assumed that the brain is stationary after infancy, with no growth or adaptation. While the brain certainly doesn't possess the regenerative ability of the liver, or retain its remarkable rate of growth during infancy, neuroplasticity (the brain's ability to change) does happen. The nervous system can change in response to its experiences, environment, and damage.[19,33] Depression can dampen this plasticity, which in turn decreases the mind's ability to fight depression. This worsens depression, which worsens plasticity, thus becoming a vicious cycle.

Depression lowers plasticity by decreasing pro-plasticity proteins. One of them is brain-derived neurotrophic factor (BDNF), which supports neuronal variation, growth, and protection.[3] BDNF is low in depression, Parkinson's, and other neurodegenerative diseases. Ketamine and traditional antidepressants increase BDNF levels to promote strength and response in synapses.

By activating GABA interneurons, ketamine increases glutamate levels (this is the opposite effect of what I previously explained; remember the pharmacologist's nightmare!) This increase activates AMPA receptors (a cousin of NMDA), which opens nearby voltage-gated calcium channels that lead to protein transcription, including BDNF. This increase is seen in the hippocampus, a brain structure key for learning and memory.

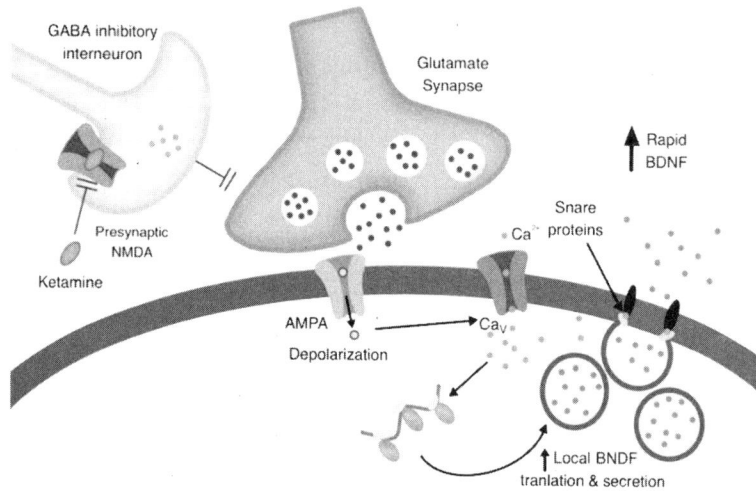

Courtesy of Andreas Grossgold 2023.

The increase in BDNF leads to strengthened neural connections, called long-term potentiation, which helps neurons grow new dendrites, which become new synapses. *Synaptogenesis* is huge for increasing the brain's plasticity gaining an edge in the battle against depression.[46]

Pain

Pain is a symptom of almost every tick-borne disease. It's reported by over 90% of those with Lyme.[29] Ketamine is used in both acute and chronic pain. It decreases pain levels and the use of addictive opioids.[1,27] One example is a case of post-treatment Lyme disease syndrome (PTLDS). Intractable pain was treated with IV ketamine to great success. There was a ~71% decrease in pain scores without increasing opioids and with decreased use of fentanyl.[20] Ketamine is also listed on the World Health Organization's list of essential drugs for refractory cancer pain.[42]

Antimicrobial

A recently discovered action of ketamine is suppressing the growth of pathogens. First investigated in the mid-2000s, ketamine has shown *in vitro* (in a test tube) activity against various bacteria, fungi, and parasites. Of note is its ability to inhibit growth of the spirochete *Borrelia burgdorferi*, the most common cause of Lyme disease, and fungi *Stachybotrys chartarum*, otherwise known as black mold, a common cause of mold toxicity.[4,11,14,38,41]

Pathogens Suppressed by Ketamine

Bacteria

- *Staphylococcus aureus*
- *Staph epidermidis*
- *E. faecalis*
- *S. pyogenes*
- *P. aeruginosa*
- *Borrelia burgdorferi*

Fungi

- *Candida albicans* (a pathogenic yeast)
- *Stachybotrys chartarum* (toxic black mold)

Parasites

- *C. elegans* (a roundworm)
- *ceylanicum* (hookworm)
- *suum* (a roundworm)

The table below summarizes the inhibitory effect of ketamine on *Borrelia burgdorferi*.

Percent Inhibition of *B. burgdorferi*		
Dilution of ketamine	**24 hours of culture**	**48 hours of culture**
1:10	100%	100%
1:20	100%	100%
1:40	100%	100%
1:80	100%	100%
1:160	86%–88%	74%–82%
1:240	41%–57%	
1:320	0%	0%

The mechanism behind this isn't fully understood, but it's known that glutamate and GABA are involved in how bacteria regulate their population density, alter their virulence, and govern formation of toxic biofilm. This represents a new prospect for treatment of chronic Lyme disease and mold toxicity. In addition to remitting common symptoms of pain and depression, ketamine could help defeat the infection.

Hypotension

Depending on the specific cause, low blood pressure appears in 40–70% of patients with Lyme. Often associated with autonomic nervous system dysfunction, it can lead to POTS (orthostatic hypotension syndrome), which occurs when the body doesn't compensate for the change in blood pressure between sitting and standing. With initial or prolonged standing, individuals affected can have lightheadedness and neurological symptoms. Ketamine can affect these symptoms through its cardiovascular effects. Acting on catecholamine receptors, ketamine increases how strongly and how fast the heart pumps. Unlike other agents, it does this while simultaneously not increasing resistance to blood flow in the rest of the vessels (called total peripheral resistance). This enhances the balance of transport and consumption of oxygen in the blood. Additionally, in a cohort study of adolescents with chronic pain, ketamine decreased pain score the most in those diagnosed with POTS.[39]

Seizures

According to the CDC, seizures are not listed as a common symptom of Lyme disease; however, due to increased recognition and correct diagnosis, these numbers are increasing. Reported surveys found rates of seizures ranging from 5–15% for common tick-borne illnesses. While uncommon, these symptoms can be debilitating.

Again, ketamine steps in as a common adjunct treatment for refractory *status epilepticus,* i.e., seizures that continue for longer than five minutes or that occur more than once within five minutes. Epilepsy is characterized by excessive neuron firing. As a treatment, ketamine might seem counterintuitive, as it can cause seizures during overdose, but common anti-seizure agents act by increasing inhibitory GABA levels. Ketamine does the same thing, while also blocking excitatory glutamate (again, the pharmacologist's nightmare!)[5]

Mast Cell Inhibition

As discussed elsewhere in this book (see chapter 4), Mast Cell Activation Syndrome (MCAS) is a complex illness often associated with Lyme disease and mold toxicity. In this condition, some factions of the immune army become agitated and cause friendly fire. Care for people with this syndrome can be challenging; anesthetics for simple procedures can induce mast-cell activation and symptoms.

Ketamine is a preferred anesthetic and narcotic for those with MCAS with low risk of worsening mast-cell activation.[30] The reason behind this is still not fully understood, but recent studies show that ketamine actively inhibits the release of inflammatory granules from the mast cells.[1] In addition, ketamine has remarkable systemic effects on the immune system and inflammation.

In the war of the immune system versus infection, cytokines are like bullets fired by white-blood-cells. The cytokines can damage infectious agents and regulate systemic (whole body) inflammation. This is necessary to stay healthy, but too much inflammation in the wrong area can cause damage. Ketamine inhibits production of these proinflammatory cytokines by interacting with the main white blood cells, monocytes, macrophages, and neutrophils. Ketamine also decreases white-blood-cell diapedesis (passage of blood cells through the intact capillary walls, typically accompanying inflammation) and phagocytosis (the engulfing of bacteria). These terms are fancy ways of describing how white blood cells chase down and eat pathogens. At first glance, this may appear to hinder the body's ability to fight an infection, but this level of inhibition is not enough to let a pathogen win, just enough to decrease unhealthy levels of inflammation. Finally, ketamine stimulates the release of adenosine, an anti-inflammatory protein.

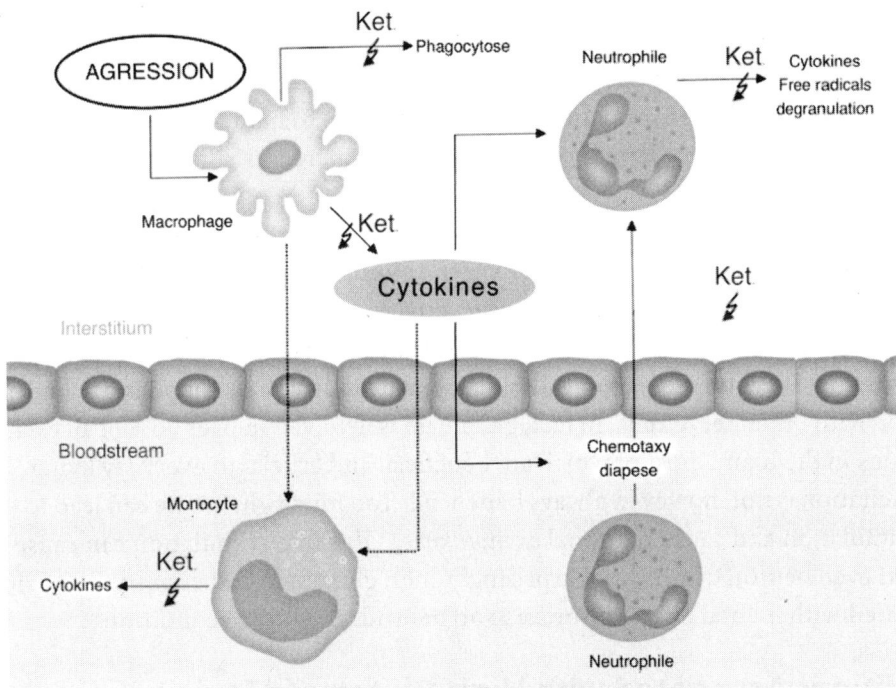

Courtesy of Andreas Grossgold 2023.

Ketamine is an *anti-proinflammatory*. This means it inhibits signals to the brain that would induce inflammation. This is different from the usual mechanism of anti-inflammatory medications.

For example, aspirin, ibuprofen (Advil), and naproxen (Aleve) are all nonsteroidal *anti-inflammatories* (NSAIDS), meaning they decrease pain and inflammation, but they work locally (like for a headache or toothache). Ketamine, on the other hand, works broadly and is an excellent regulator of excess **systemic** inflammation.[26] Think of it this way: NSAIDS are like using a towel to put out a fire on the stove. Ketamine is like unplugging the stove.

Ketamine sustains the positive effects of inflammation (like fighting infection and healing wounds), while softening the potentially harmful effects of whole-body inflammation. This is especially beneficial to those with MCAS, autoimmunity, and other systemic inflammatory syndromes.

Neuroprotection

We've established that ketamine can stimulate neuron plasticity and growth, which is good, but protecting what's already there is also necessary. Neuroprotection is exactly what it sounds like—protecting the brain and its neurons from damage that can come from overstimulation, inflammation, or lack of oxygen, to name a few causes. Ketamine can save injured neurons. It reduces cell injury and increases survival. One example is by battling *excitotoxicity*.

As described earlier, glutamate is the major neurotransmitter that carries excitatory signals in the brain. This is due to its sheer abundance and variety of receptors that respond to it. Most neurotransmitters interact with one or two receptors; glutamate can bind to four. Think of it as an activating master key that can fit into and work four different locks. This receptor assortment allows glutamate to have a major presence in communication with other nerve cells. In fact, glutamate is involved in over 90% of all excitatory functions in the brain, most of which are beneficial and crucial to everyday living.[1]

Excitation is not, however, always beneficial. Too much glutamate can lead to excessive stimulation and cause neuronal *excitotoxicity*. This overstimulation can cause damage and even neuron death. Not surprisingly, high glutamate and consequent toxicity is associated with mental health disorders and neurodegenerative conditions.

Conditions Associated with High-Glutamate Toxicity

Mental health

- Depression

Mood disorder

- Anxiety
- Obsessive-compulsive disorder
- Schizophrenia

Neurodegenerative diseases

- Alzheimer's disease
- Parkinson's disease
- Amyotrophic lateral sclerosis (Lou Gehrig's disease)
- Multiple sclerosis
- Stroke
- Fibromyalgia
- Chronic fatigue syndrome

The connection between high-glutamate damage and ketamine's glutamate antagonism is obvious. Neurons with ketamine treatment show increased blood flow and decreased damage. In the future, ketamine will likely play a role in the management of acute brain damage such as from stroke or hemorrhage. Additionally, with its use in mental health disorders such as depression, already commonplace, treatment of neurodegenerative disease is likely on the horizon.

Finally, inflammation is another risk to the brain. Ketamine decreases systemic inflammation, and thus protects the brain from neuroinflammation that can cause neuron damage and death. Ketamine mitigates these effects in the brain as it does in the rest of the body.

In Practice

With a deeper understanding of how ketamine works and where it's applicable, the next question is how to use it. Medicine can be taken in a variety of ways, and ketamine is no exception. Different problems and patients may need different "routes of administration."

How *Not* to Use Ketamine

First, ground rules on how *not* to take ketamine. The 16th-century physician Paracelsus famously observed, "The dose makes the poison." This means the amount of a substance can determine whether it helps or harms the body. This could be changed to "the route makes the poison." The amount of something taken by mouth should not be taken by injection, and vice versa. In the interest of patient safety, ketamine should only be used as directed by a medical professional and with the purpose of improving physical and mental health.

Commonly, ketamine is recreationally used by *insufflation*, aka snorting a powder. While insufflation can be used for some medications, it is rare and has *never* been used for medicinal ketamine.* Ketamine is also taken as a pill recreationally. This is where our friend Paracelsus returns, the dose of recreationally used oral ketamine is much higher than when taken medicinally. As a rule, concentrations for medical use (other than anesthesia) should not be high enough to cause dissociation.

*Insufflation is not the same as intranasal; see intranasal esketamine spray for depression.

How to Use Ketamine

When used properly, ketamine can be administered orally (swallowed by pill), sublingually (in a lozenge, or *troche*) under the tongue, by intranasal spray, and transmucosal patch. Injections in both muscle and fat and intravenous (IV) are also common. Our clinic prefers IV for its efficiency and level of control. Common doses for each route are listed below.[2] Doses will range depending on the route, patient demographic, medical history, and disease being treated.

Common routes and dosages

- Intravenous (IV) 0.1–0.5 mg/kg
- Intramuscular 0.1–0.5 mg/kg
- Subcutaneous 0.1–0.5 mg/kg
- Sublingual 0.25 mg/kg
- Intranasal 28 mg per nostril
- Oral 10–50 mg up to 4×/day

Common conditions and doses (IV)

- General anesthesia 1–4.5 mg/kg (average ~2 mg/kg)
- Emergency analgesia 0.2–0.5 mg/kg (average ~0.3 mg/kg)
- Chronic pain 0.5–1 mg/kg/hr.
- Depression*28 mg intranasal spray per nostril

*IV dose, see below.

Doses range for different routes because of how they enter the body. IV or injections are placed directly into the circulation, so the doses are much lower compared to oral or intranasal. The amount the body uses is much higher intravenously than orally, because it bypasses the loss of medication in the gastrointestinal system (termed the *first-pass effect*). This measurement of route efficiency is termed *bioavailability*.

Time

Another important factor in ketamine use is when and how long it's taken. This is applicable to IV administration because the drip rate can be changed in response to how the patient is affected. In the above table, treatment-resistant depression,* a common indication of IV ketamine, is not listed with its normal dose. This is because practitioners don't generally agree on the ideal dose and infusion length.

Many practices offer ketamine infusions over thirty to sixty minutes. While common, it's not the most efficacious. Studies and clinical practice show that a longer infusion rate leads to better results and fewer side effects.[34] This is how we keep patients from ever experiencing the "k-hole."

Our Protocol

Ketamine infusions should be a part of a comprehensive treatment plan. For patients with depression, we recommend infusions as part of a multidisciplinary plan that includes a healthy diet, a mental-health provider, plenty of physical activity, and psychotherapy. Our protocol entails low-dose ketamine infusions ranging from 0.15–2 mg depending on the patient. Each infusion lasts approximately four hours. During this time, clinic staff carefully monitors patients for any adverse reactions.

Conclusion

The number of individuals in the battle against chronic Lyme and/or tick-borne disease is significant and growing every day. The physical and mental symptoms are fierce, and allies are required to defeat the enemy. Many patients struggling with Lyme disease and mold toxicity will develop limbic and vagal dysfunction and Mast Cell Activation Syndrome.

Current evidence and research places ketamine at the forefront of treatment. Through my clinical experience with patients, I've seen ketamine change people's lives. It's a proven ally in reducing symptoms and hastening full recovery, a concept that some never thought possible. Our educating people on its uses and safety will make ketamine a key to the future of medicine.

A Note on Psychedelics

Only in the past few years has ketamine become more widely known by the public and the medical field. Despite mounting evidence, there are still skeptics of its utility outside the operating room. Psychedelics are even further outside the gaze of traditional medicine. The concept of using these compounds in a professional medical setting is likely to raise the eyebrows of any traditionalist—but that isn't to say the movement isn't growing.

As noted above, psychedelics are serotonergic, interacting with the 5-HT2AR receptor like most anti-depressants. This makes them ideal for the treatment of mood disorders. Similarly, they're known to increase cognitive flexibility and imagination. There is mounting anecdotal and clinical evidence for controlled use of psychedelics in mental health treatment. New procedures, such as micro-dosing, are bringing consistency to research and treatment.

Riding on the coattails of esketamine's FDA approval, psilocybin and MDMA were designated "breakthrough therapies" in the treatment of depression and PTSD respectively. This gives them priority consideration in the approval process. A plethora of research in the last five years backs this therapeutic potential.

LSD has been shown to elicit psychosis-like symptoms but to improve psychological well-being long term.[9] Psilocybin was shown to decrease depression and anxiety in those with terminal cancer.[17] When compared to traditional SSRIs, psilocybin showed greater efficacy in antidepressant effects.[8] Ayahuasca-based DMT reported significant antidepressant effect compared with placebo.[32]

Despite these advances, research remains difficult. Most psychedelics are on the DEA's list of Schedule 1 controlled substances. This defines them as having no accepted medical use and a high potential for abuse. This is unlikely to remain, however, with increased research and regulation to maintain safe use in the medical field. Ketamine, and CBD before it, pushed through the prejudice of recreational use into acceptance by modern medicine. Psychedelics are treading a similar path. I hope this note helps raise awareness of the future of these promising treatments.

References

1. Abby Pribish, Nicole Wood, Arun Kalava, "A Review of Nonanesthetic Uses of Ketamine," Anesthesiology Research and Practice, vol. 2020, Article ID 5798285, 15 pages, 2020. https://doi.org/10.1155/2020/5798285.
2. Andrade, C. (2017, July). Ketamine for Depression, 4: In What Dose, at What Rate, by What Route, for How Long, and at What Frequency? Pyschiatrist.com. Retrieved August 11, 2022, from https://www-psychiatrist-com.lecomlrc.lecom.edu/jcp/depression/ketamine-for-depression-dosing-administration-and-duration/.
3. Bathina S, Das UN. Brain-derived neurotrophic factor and its clinical implications. Arch Med Sci. 2015 Dec 10;11(6):1164-78. doi: 10.5114/aoms.2015.56342. Epub 2015 Dec 11. PMID: 26788077; PMCID: PMC4697050.

4. Begec, Z., Yucel, A., Yakupogulları, Y., Erdogan, M. A., Duman, Y., Durmus, M., & Ersoy, M. O. (2013). Efectos antimicrobianos de la Cetamina en combinación con el propofol: UN Estudio in vitro. Brazilian Journal of Anesthesiology (Edicion En Espanol), 63(6), 461–465. https://doi.org/10.1016/j.bjanes.2012.09.004.

5. Bell, Josh D. MD, PhD. In Vogue: Ketamine for Neuroprotection in Acute Neurologic Injury. Anesthesia & Analgesia: April 2017 - Volume 124 - Issue 4 - p 1237-1243. doi: 10.1213/ANE.0000000000001856.

6. Berman RM, Cappiello A, Anand A, Oren DA, Heninger GR, Charney DS, Krystal JH. Antidepressant effects of ketamine in depressed patients. Biol Psychiatry. 2000 Feb 15;47(4):351-4. doi: 10.1016/s0006-3223(99)00230-9. PMID: 10686270.

7. Bollen J, Trick L, Llewellyn D, Dickens C. The effects of acute inflammation on cognitive functioning and emotional processing in humans: a systematic review of experimental studies. J Psychos Res 2017; 94: 47–55.

8. Carhart-Harris R, Giribaldi B, Watts R, Baker-Jones M, Murphy-Beiner A, Murphy R, Martell J, Blemings A, Erritzoe D, Nutt DJ. Trial of Psilocybin versus Escitalopram for Depression. N Engl J Med. 2021 Apr 15;384(15):1402-1411. doi: 10.1056/NEJMoa2032994. PMID: 33852780.

9. Carhart-Harris RL, Muthukumaraswamy S, Roseman L, Kaelen M, Droog W, Murphy K, Tagliazucchi E, Schenberg EE, Nest T, Orban C, Leech R, Williams LT, Williams TM, Bolstridge M, Sessa B, McGonigle J, Sereno MI, Nichols D, Hellyer PJ, Hobden P, Evans J, Singh KD, Wise RG, Curran HV, Feilding A, Nutt DJ. Neural correlates of the LSD experience revealed by multimodal neuroimaging. Proc Natl Acad Sci U S A. 2016 Apr 26;113(17):4853-8. doi: 10.1073/pnas.1518377113. Epub 2016 Apr 11. PMID: 27071089; PMCID: PMC4855588.

10. Chen, J. (2022, March 9). How ketamine drug helps with depression. Yale Medicine. Retrieved August 10, 2022, from https://www.yalemedicine.org/news/ketamine-depression.

11. de Andrade Neto JB, da Silva CR, Barroso FD, do Amaral Valente Sá LG, de Sousa Campos R, S Aires do Nascimento FB, Sampaio LS, da Silva AR, da Silva LJ, de Sá Carneiro I, Queiroz HA, de Mesquita JRL, Cavalcanti BC, de Moraes MO, Nobre Júnior HV. Synergistic effects of ketamine and azole derivatives on Candida spp. resistance to fluconazole. Future Microbiol. 2020 Feb;15:177-188. doi: 10.2217/fmb-2019-0082. Epub 2020 Feb 20. PMID: 32077323.

12. Drug scheduling. DEA. (n.d.). Retrieved August 17, 2022, from https://www.dea.gov/drug-information/drug-scheduling.

13. FDA approves new nasal spray medication for treatment-resistant depression; available only at a Certified Doctor's Office or clinic. U.S. Food and Drug Administration. Retrieved August 3, 2022, from https://www.fda.gov/news-events/press-announcements/fda-approves-new-nasal-spray-medication-treatment-resistant-depression-available-only-certified.

14. Ferreira, S.R., Machado, A.R.T., Furtado, L.F. et al. Ketamine can be produced by Pochonia chlamydosporia: an old molecule and a new anthelmintic?. Parasites Vectors 13, 527 (2020). https://doi.org/10.1186/s13071-020-04402-w.

15. Fujimoto T, Nishiyama T, Hanaoka K. Inhibitory effects of intravenous anesthetics on mast cell function. Anesth Analg. 2005 Oct;101(4):1054-1059. doi: 10.1213/01.ane.0000166955.97368.80. PMID: 16192519.

16. Glutamate: What it is & function. Cleveland Clinic. (n.d.). Retrieved August 9, 2022, from https://my.clevelandclinic.org/health/articles/22839-glutamate.

17. Griffiths RR, Johnson MW, Carducci MA, Umbricht A, Richards WA, Richards BD, Cosimano MP, Klinedinst MA. Psilocybin produces substantial and sustained decreases in depression and anxiety in patients with life-threatening cancer: A randomized double-blind trial. J Psychopharmacol. 2016 Dec;30(12):1181-1197. doi: 10.1177/0269881116675513. PMID: 27909165; PMCID: PMC5367557.

18. Guidelines for safe administration of low-dose ketamine. (2020, October 7). Retrieved August 12, 2022, from https://www.health.pa.gov/topics/Documents/Opioids/Ketamine%20Guidelines.pdf.

19. Gulyaeva NV. Molecular Mechanisms of Neuroplasticity: An Expanding Universe. Biochemistry (Mosc). 2017 Mar;82(3):237-242. doi: 10.1134/S0006297917030014. PMID: 28320264.

20. Hanna AF, Abraham B, Hanna A, Smith AJ. Effects of intravenous ketamine in a patient with post-treatment Lyme disease syndrome. Int Med Case Rep J. 2017 Aug 18;10:305-308. doi: 10.2147/IMCRJ.S137975. PMID: 28860873; PMCID: PMC5571854.

21. Hartney, E. (2022, June 20). Taking ketamine can mean experiencing a K-hole. Verywell Mind. Retrieved August 16, 2022, from https://www.verywellmind.com/what-is-a-k-hole-21861#:~:text=A%20k%2Dhole%20is%20when,state%20between%20intoxication%20and%20coma.

22. Holz RW, Fisher SK. Synaptic Transmission. In: Siegel GJ, Agranoff BW, Albers RW, et al., editors. Basic Neurochemistry: Molecular, Cellular and Medical Aspects. 6th edition. Philadelphia: Lippincott-Raven; 1999. Available from: https://www.ncbi.nlm.nih.gov/books/NBK27911/.

23. Hudetz JA, Pagel PS. Neuroprotection by ketamine: a review of the experimental and clinical evidence. J Cardiothorac Vasc Anesth. 2010 Feb;24(1):131-42. doi: 10.1053/j.jvca.2009.05.008. Epub 2009 Jul 29. PMID: 19640746.

24. Johnstone M. The cardiovascular effects of ketamine in man. Anaesthesia. 1976 Sep;31(7):873-82. doi: 10.1111/j.1365-2044.1976.tb11898.x. PMID: 970587.

25. Lois F, De Kock M. Something new about ketamine for pediatric anesthesia? Curr Opin Anaesthesiol. 2008 Jun;21(3):340-4. doi: 10.1097/ACO.0b013e3282f82bde. PMID: 18458551.

26. Loix, Sébastien, Marc De Kock, and P. J. A. A. Henin. "The anti-inflammatory effects of ketamine: state of the art." Acta Anaesthesiol Belg 62.1 (2011): 47-58.

27. M. Carstensen, A. M. Møller, Adding ketamine to morphine for intravenous patient-controlled analgesia for acute postoperative pain: a qualitative review of randomized trials, BJA: British Journal of Anaesthesia, Volume 104, Issue 4, April 2010, Pages 401–406, https://doi.org/10.1093/bja/aeq041.

28. Mandal S, Sinha VK, Goyal N. Efficacy of ketamine therapy in the treatment of depression. Indian J Psychiatry. 2019 Sep-Oct;61(5):480-485. doi: 10.4103/psychiatry.IndianJPsychiatry_484_18. PMID: 31579184; PMCID: PMC6767816.

29. Maxwell SP, Brooks C, McNeely CL, Thomas KC. Neurological Pain, Psychological Symptoms, and Diagnostic Struggles among Patients with Tick-Borne Diseases. Healthcare (Basel). 2022 Jun 23;10(7):1178. doi: 10.3390/healthcare10071178. PMID: 35885705; PMCID: PMC9323096.

30. Molderings GJ, Haenisch B, Brettner S, Homann J, Menzen M, Dumoulin FL, Panse J, Butterfield J, Afrin LB. Pharmacological treatment options for mast cell activation disease. Naunyn Schmiedebergs Arch Pharmacol. 2016 Jul;389(7):671-94. doi: 10.1007/s00210-016-1247-1. Epub 2016 Apr 30. PMID: 27132234; PMCID: PMC4903110.

31. Nma. (2022, January 22). Navigating Ketamine Doses. Peak. Retrieved August 14, 2022, from https://www.withpeak.com/blog/navigating-ketamine-doses.

32. Palhano-Fontes F, Barreto D, Onias H, Andrade KC, Novaes MM, Pessoa JA, Mota-Rolim SA, Osório FL, Sanches R, Dos Santos RG, Tófoli LF, de Oliveira Silveira G, Yonamine M, Riba J, Santos FR, Silva-Junior AA, Alchieri JC, Galvão-Coelho NL, Lobão-Soares B, Hallak JEC, Arcoverde E, Maia-de-Oliveira JP, Araújo DB. Rapid antidepressant effects of the psychedelic ayahuasca in treatment-resistant depression: a randomized placebo-controlled trial. Psychol Med. 2019 Mar;49(4):655-663. doi: 10.1017/S0033291718001356. Epub 2018 Jun 15. PMID: 29903051; PMCID: PMC6378413.

33. Puderbaugh M, Emmady PD. Neuroplasticity. [Updated 2022 May 8]. In: StatPearls [Internet]. Treasure Island (FL): StatPearls Publishing; 2022 Jan-. Available from: https://www.ncbi.nlm.nih.gov/books/NBK557811/.

34. Rasmussen KG, Lineberry TW, Galardy CW, et al. Serial infusions of low-dose ketamine for major depression. Journal of Psychopharmacology. 2013;27(5):444-450. doi:10.1177/0269881113478283.

35. Reiff CM, Richman EE, Nemeroff CB, Carpenter LL, Widge AS, Rodriguez CI, Kalin NH, McDonald WM; the Work Group on Biomarkers and Novel Treatments, a Division of the American Psychiatric Association Council of Research. Psychedelics and Psychedelic-Assisted Psychotherapy. Am J Psychiatry. 2020 May 1;177(5):391-410. doi: 10.1176/appi.ajp.2019.19010035. Epub 2020 Feb 26. PMID: 32098487.

36. Rodriguez, C., Kegeles, L., Levinson, A. et al. Randomized Controlled Crossover Trial of Ketamine in Obsessive-Compulsive Disorder: Proof-of-Concept. Neuropsychopharmacol 38, 2475–2483 (2013). https://doi.org/10.1038/npp.2013.150.

37. Schwenk ES, Viscusi ER, Buvanendran A, Hurley RW, Wasan AD, Narouze S, Bhatia A, Davis FN, Hooten WM, Cohen SP. Consensus Guidelines on the Use of Intravenous Ketamine Infusions for Acute Pain Management From the American Society of Regional Anesthesia and Pain Medicine, the American Academy of Pain Medicine, and the American Society of Anesthesiologists. Reg Anesth Pain Med. 2018 Jul;43(5):456-466. doi: 10.1097/AAP.0000000000000806. PMID: 29870457; PMCID: PMC6023582.

38. Sedef Gocmen, Unase Buyukkocak & Osman Caglayan (2008) In Vitro Investigation of the Antibacterial Effect of Ketamine, Upsala Journal of Medical Sciences, 113:1, 39-46, DOI: 10.3109/2000-1967-211.

39. Sheehy KA, Muller EA, Lippold C, Nouraie M, Finkel JC, Quezado ZM. Subanesthetic ketamine infusions for the treatment of children and adolescents with chronic pain: a longitudinal study. BMC Pediatr. 2015 Dec 1;15:198. doi: 10.1186/s12887-015-0515-4. PMID: 26620833; PMCID: PMC4665913.

40. Titulaer, J., Björkholm, C., Feltmann, K., Malmlöf, T., Mishra, D., Bengtsson Gonzales, C., Schilström, B., & Konradsson-Geuken, Å. (2021). The importance of ventral hippocampal dopamine and norepinephrine in recognition memory. Frontiers in Behavioral Neuroscience, 15. https://doi.org/10.3389/fnbeh.2021.667244.

41. Torres G, Hoehmann CL, Cuoco JA, Hitscherich K, Pavia C, Hadjiargyrou M, Leheste JR. Ketamine intervention limits pathogen expansion in vitro. Pathog Dis. 2018 Mar 1;76(2). doi: 10.1093/femspd/fty006. PMID: 29365093.

42. Visser E, Schug SA. The role of ketamine in pain management. Biomed Pharmacother. 2006 Aug;60(7):341-8. doi: 10.1016/j.biopha.2006.06.021. Epub 2006 Jul 5. PMID: 16854557.

43. Ward, A. (2021, December 29). A cure for the common—and not so common—blues? Psychedelia. Retrieved August 17, 2022, from https://psychedelia.live/content/a-cure-for-the-common-and-not-so-common-blues/.

44. Wernersson S, Pejler G. Mast cell secretory granules: armed for battle. Nat Rev Immunol. 2014 Jul;14(7):478-94. doi: 10.1038/nri3690. Epub 2014 Jun 6. PMID: 24903914.

45. YouTube. (2021). Jeffrey Becker, M.D. The Science of Ketamine: What's Really Going on in Your Brain? YouTube. Retrieved August 3, 2022, from https://www.youtube.com/watch?v=MgBXD7Px4zg.

46. Zunszain, P., Horowitz, M., Cattaneo, A. et al. Ketamine: synaptogenesis, immunomodulation and glycogen synthase kinase-3 as underlying mechanisms of its antidepressant properties. Mol Psychiatry 18, 1236–1241 (2013). https://doi.org/10.1038/mp.2013.87.

DR. ANDREAS GROSSGOLD graduated from the New Granada Military School of Medicine in Bogota, Colombia, at age twenty-four, and completed his internship and residency at several hospitals in Houston, Texas, including MD Anderson, Memorial Hermann, Lyndon B. Johnson, and Texas Children's Hospital. He then dedicated himself to the field of Integrative Medicine, graduating with a doctorate at Capital University in Washington, D.C. He went on to complete a postdoctoral fellowship in cellular regeneration and gene therapy at Baylor College of Medicine. He is currently a commander with the U.S. Navy Reserves.

Dr. Grossgold practices as an integrative internist and pediatrician and treats myriad complex cases, including Lyme and associated diseases, myalgic encephalomyelitis, mold, petrochemicals, heavy-metal toxicity, neurological disorders, and genetic and autoimmune conditions. He is currently completing another fellowship in Integrative Psychiatry with the University of Colorado School of Medicine and the Integrative Psychiatric Institute. He practices at The Grossgold Clinic in Clearwater, Florida—www.thegclinic.org.

Acknowledgments

Dr. Grossgold appreciates the assistance of Joseph Johnson, a third-year medical student at Lake Erie College of Osteopathic Medicine in Bradenton, Florida, in the preparation of this chapter. Joseph graduated with honors from University of South Florida in 2020 and plans a career in primary care.

Part V

Putting It All Together

Chapter 27: Guide to Evaluation and Treatment of the Sensitive Patient

Neil Nathan, MD

If you've read this far, you now likely have an excellent grasp of what conditions can contribute to the evolution of extreme sensitivity and how to approach it from many different perspectives. To put all this information together in a practical form, I'll lay out how to evaluate a sensitive patient, and how to decide which treatments you'd want to receive or provide, and in what order.

Evaluation

Questions to Ask

Learn the details of the sensitivity.

Exactly what are you sensitive to? Light? Sound? Touch? Chemicals? Smells? Foods? EMF? We need to know whether sensitivity is global, suggesting the possibility of carbon monoxide exposure, or, later (to decide on potential treatments), whether exposure to light or sound can trigger a negative reaction.

When you *do* react to a chemical or smell, how *quickly* do you react and what is that reaction? Is this true MCS, in which the reaction is immediate, or merely aversion? In the case of food sensitivities, is it immediate (MCAS) and does it fit with histamine release, or is it delayed, suggesting another etiology?

How severe is your reaction? This provides an important clue as to the intensity of limbic and/or vagal involvement.

History of Exposures

Have you ever lived in a moldy home or gone to a school where mold was known to be present? Has there ever been water damage to a home you lived in? If so, was it promptly remediated, and how was it remediated? (Was the water dried up quickly, or did the landlord just paint over the mold?)

Have you ever been bitten by a tick or lived in a Lyme-endemic area?

Have you ever been bitten or scratched by a cat or had exposure to fleas?

Did you ever live near a chemical plant or any type of toxic dump?

Did you ever live on a farm or near a farm where pesticides were used?

Does your drinking water come from a well or from a city system?

What electronic devices do you use, and how often do you use them?

Have you lived near a cell tower or power line?

Does your home have a smart meter? If you live in an apartment, where are the smart meters in relationship to your home?

Does your home use propane or natural gas in any way? Do you have a carbon monoxide meter?

Diet and Nutrition

What's your diet like? A food diary covering several days can be helpful, Do you eat a lot of fast foods, carbohydrates, sugar, gluten, or milk products?

Do you mostly eat organically grown food?

Do you consume smoothies regularly? (Looking for excessive kale or spinach as possible sources of oxalates or perhaps thallium toxicity).

History of Trauma or Stress

Surgical history: Have you had any surgical procedures that had complications?

Obstetric history: Have you had any difficult birthing experiences, including postpartum? Any difficulties with lactation?

Have you been in any motor vehicle accidents? How severe were they?

Have you had concussions or injuries to your neck or back?

Have you had broken bones or other injuries that led to hospitalization or disability?

Early childhood stressors: Did you experience any verbal, physical, or sexual abuse? Were your parents emotionally distant? Were your needs met as a child or teenager?

Have you experienced any jaw dysfunction? Have you had any jaw or dental surgery? Have you been told about TMJ (*temporomandibular joint disorder*)? Did you have braces or wear a dental appliance?

Have you ever fallen onto your tailbone or low back?

Have you had any recent vaccinations?

Did you have COVID? If so, how did it affect you?

Medication History

Have you taken antidepressants or anti-anxiety medication?

Have you needed any medication for sleep?

Are you taking, or have you taken, metformin?

Please provide a list of all the supplements you currently take. Also, please list any supplements you were unable to take, and why.

Are you allergic to any medications or supplements? Please provide details.

Evaluation and Testing

Every patient is unique, especially from a genetic and biochemical perspective. The specific evaluation and treatment you choose should be based on your own comprehensive approach and shouldn't follow any sort of rigid algorithm. The information below is a suggestion for the kinds of approaches that might be useful. Some might not apply to you at all; others could be very important.

Physical Examination

- General appearance: look for state of nourishment, weight gain or loss, signs of metabolic syndrome.
- Hair and nails: look for signs of nutrient deficiencies.
- Tongue and pharynx: look for thrush or inflammation. Check the gag reflex.
- Heart and lungs: look for breath sounds and heart sounds.
- Abdominal exam: look for distention, bowel sounds, tenderness.
- Reflexes of upper and lower extremities: look for possible cervical trauma, fibromyalgia.
- Nervous system: evaluate for cognitive impairment, visual impairment, hearing impairment, peripheral neuropathy.
- Musculoskeletal system: evaluate areas of pain, spasm, or fasciculation (muscle twitch).
- Lymph nodes: look for any areas of adenopathy (swollen lymph nodes).
- Skin: look for dehydration or rashes.

For Mast Cell Activation Syndrome

Given the transitory presence of the mediators released by mast cells when they're active, measurement is inherently difficult. For most of our patients, observing the effects of empirical treatment, without testing, is sufficient. Check for dermatographia.

A number of tests can suggest the presence of MCAS:

- If a tissue biopsy has been performed, looking at the tissue using a CD 117 stain can be diagnostic. You might need to specifically request this, even on biopsies done previously, as the usual staining is insufficient to make the diagnosis.
- Total serum tryptase
- Plasma heparin and/or histamine
- Chromogranin A
- Urinary N-methyl histamine
- Urinary PG D2
- Leukotriene E4

For Mold Toxicity

- Measure urine mycotoxins
- Measure visual contrast
- OAT testing
- Stool testing for yeast/Candida

Using mold plates or ERMI testing, check your home, workplace, and car for possible mold exposure. Consult an environmental engineer for a more comprehensive evaluation.

Dr. Jill Crista's questionnaire (see chapter 7) might help point in the direction of mold toxicity.

For Lyme Disease and Coinfections

At a minimum, Igenix IgM and IgG Immunoblot or Infectolabs for Lyme disease; for a more comprehensive evaluation, a complete Igenix panel and/or Infectolab panel.

Dr. Richard Horowitz's Assessment Test might help point in the direction of Lyme disease.

For Environmental Toxins

Great Plains Environmental Toxin Panel, including glyphosate

Test the patient's drinking water for heavy metals and PFAs.

For EMF Evaluation

Get a meter that can measure what you're being exposed to at home or at work or in other situations.

Check your home for dirty electricity.

It might help to work with an environmental engineer for a more comprehensive evaluation.

For Structural Evaluation

Consult with an osteopathic or chiropractic physician to learn whether there are any structural limitations preventing healing.

Consult with a dentist and/or osteopathic physician to evaluate jaw function for its possible role in sensitization.

For Evaluation of Thiamine Deficiency

Consider an erythrocyte transketolase test followed by a thiamine pyrophosphate effect.

A therapeutic trial with thiamine should always be considered.

For Evaluation of Oxalates

An organic acid test (OAT) from Great Plains has three measurements of oxalate, all of which can suggest that this is another component of sensitization. It's often connected to mold toxicity, since several mold species, notably *Aspergillus*, contribute to the formation of oxalates in the body.

For Evaluation of Sulfation

An unusually low homocysteine level (<7) might suggest difficulties here, and any genomic issues involving the genes SUOX, CBS, CTH, CDO, Hs3St1, or PAPPS suggest that we might need to look here for clues.

Genetic/Genomic Evaluation

Look at a patient's SNPs to provide guidance to prioritize which areas you might want to focus on from a biochemical perspective.

Associated Hormonal Dysregulation

- Sensitivity worsens premenstrually
- Early menopause or estrogen dominance
- Decreased libido
- Adrenal and thyroid deficiencies

Treatment

Treatment Plans

A comprehensive treatment plan needs to start with "root cause." We need to focus on the components of the illness that are the primary triggers for it. I've found that mold toxicity, Lyme disease and its coinfections, environmental toxins, and EMFs are the most common primary issues in triggering a sensitive patient. In turn, those commonly trigger limbic- and vagal-nerve dysfunction and mast-cell activation, which often limit a patient's ability to progress until they are addressed.

I emphasize once again that each patient has a unique biochemical, genetic, and stress history, which requires us to formulate a treatment plan that will be specific to that individual. This discussion can therefore only be general and not specific to any case, but I hope it serves as a template that the patient's information can be put into to create their own healing plan.

Start with the most limiting condition(s) (if present): The three most common conditions that limit our sensitive patients' ability to heal and to tolerate the treatments that would otherwise address the root cause(s) of their illness are limbic dysregulation, vagal dysfunction, and mast-cell activation.

Limbic Dysregulation

The two programs I've used most (I estimate that over 1,000 of my patients have used each of these) that I know to be effective in the majority of patients are the Annie Hopper DNRS program (see chapter 1 for a detailed discussion) and the Ashok Gupta Amygdala retraining program (see chapter 2 for a detailed discussion). By reading these chapters, patients or physicians who are interested in working with these systems can get a feel for the differences and for which programs might best fit your specific needs. I've occasionally encouraged very sensitive patients to do a bit of both programs to get started, and this has been effective. Also, I've observed that for unusually sensitive patients, it might be necessary to start with just 10–15 minutes a day, as longer usage can be a bit overwhelming for them. As they respond and improve, longer sessions become possible.

I know of several other programs that have evolved from the pioneering work of Annie and Ashok, but have only had a few patients use them, so my inexperience limits additional comment. Still, I wanted patients and physicians to be aware that other approaches are being developed. These include David Hanscom's DOC (Direct your Own Care) Program, which is especially designed for, and helpful for, sensitive patients who are coping with severe pain. Cathleen King has created her Primal Trust program, which address both limbic and vagal issues.

Vagal Dysfunction

To make it a bit more cohesive, I added some of this information at the end of Stephen Porges's chapter on polyvagal theory. It bears repeating here, to provide you an overview of treatments we've found effective in essentially rebooting vagal dysfunction.

In addition to the Safe and Sound program developed and described by Dr. Porges, other treatments that have proven especially helpful include:

The exercises described by Stanley Rosenberg in his book *Accessing the Healing Power of the Vagus Nerve*, 2020.

Osteopathic Cranial Manipulation (see chapter 16).

Frequency Specific Microcurrent (FSM), a unique medical device capable of not only treating the vagus nerve but other nerve and brain contributing effects as well.

Brain Tap, a medical device developed by Patrick Porter, PhD, that uses frequencies of sound and light, delivered through the eyes and ears simultaneously, to treat vagal-nerve dysfunction.

Dr. Porges also recommends a vagal-nerve stimulator, developed by Dr. Peter Staats, called gammaCore, available from electroCore, Inc. Another vagal stimulator that has been effective is the Apollo Neuro device, worn on the wrist for brief periods of time to start (for our sensitive patients 3–5 minutes, once daily, and slowly increasing to 10 minutes twice daily, as tolerated).

Emotional Freedom Technique is a method for tapping specific areas (acupuncture points) over the face and shoulders to reduce vagal dysfunction. EMDR is an equivalent procedure.

Singing, humming, gargling, and gagging have been used for many years, as described by Dr. Datis Kharrazian in his publications and YouTube presentation ("The Gut/Brain Axis"). While they're helpful, I've found the other modalities more specific for our purpose.

Mast Cell Activation Syndrome (MCAS)

As discussed in chapter 4, it's only recently been recognized that mast-cell activation is far more common than previously appreciated. Estimates range widely, but a reasonable starting point is to allow that 10–15% of all people are at risk for developing this condition. In patients with mold toxicity and Lyme disease, the estimate goes up markedly: over 70% of those patients who've become sensitive will, over time, develop Mast Cell Activation Syndrome. Many patients with MCAS respond better to either pharmaceuticals or to natural supplements, and occasionally to both, so I often start treatment with H1 and H2 blockers and quercetin to see whether my patient has a preference, so I can focus on what's most likely to be effective.

The more different materials and approaches one can bring to MCAS the more effective treatment becomes. A single substance is unlikely to work very well; the combinations work far better.

To organize possible treatment options in this way, I'll list the pharmaceutical and botanical options and their main mechanism of action so you can work to optimize treatment.

Pharmaceuticals

H1 histamine-receptor blockers include Claritin (loratadine), Allegra (fexofenadine), Zyrtec (cetirizine), Benadryl and Xyzal (levocetirizine). Sensitive patients should start with a single dose at bedtime and, if tolerated, a second dose, midday. If these are not tolerated, having them made by a compounding pharmacy, in lower-than-usual doses, is a good place to start.

H2 receptor blockers include Pepcid (famotidine), often starting at bedtime and then adding a second dose midday; the same suggestions for treatment (compounded and in lower doses) apply here as well.

Ketotifen, made by compounding pharmacies, is one of the most effective treatments, since it has multiple modes of action: it's an H1 receptor blocker, but also a mast-cell stabilizer and leukotriene inhibitor. For especially sensitive patients, I start at 0.1mg at bedtime and slowly increase to 0.5mg 30 minutes before a meal and slowly increase to 0.5mg 30 minutes before each meal. Patients who are less sensitive can start at 0.25 or 0.5mg, and the dosage can be increased as tolerated. Remember, it's always best to start with a lower dose, because if you start with too strong a dose, you'll only get the limbic system to fear this medication and subsequent efforts to take it might fail.

Singular (montelukast), a leukotriene inhibitor, is often helpful, with the usual dose of 10mg daily. It too might need to be compounded and taken at lower doses for sensitive patients.

At times, Vistaril (hydroxyzine) and Sinequan (doxepin) can be helpful as well. This discussion is intended to just get you started, not to be a comprehensive review of all possible medications.

Cromolyn sodium is an excellent mast-cell stabilizer, and one can take 100mg (one vial) 30 minutes before a meal, working up to 30 minutes before each meal. Very sensitive patients can start with lower initial doses.

Herbal/Botanical Supplements

Quercetin is an excellent mast-cell stabilizer, if tolerated. I have found that about 20% of sensitive patients can't, for various reasons, tolerate it at any dose, but it's worth a try. For the most sensitive patients I suggest starting with Neuroprotek LP, one capsule 30 minutes before a meal, working up to one capsule 30 minutes before each meal and at bedtime, and if this is well tolerated, doubling the dose. For patients who are less sensitive, starting at 250mg or 500mg of quercetin taken the same way is effective, and that can be increased, if tolerated, to 1000mg before each meal and at bedtime.

Perimine appears to be well tolerated by sensitive patients, and is another effective mast-cell stabilizer. One tablet (which can be cut in half or into quarters for sensitive patients) before each meal is the target dose.

Allqlear is a tryptase inhibitor made from quail eggs, and can be taken as a chewable, one before a meal, working up to one before each meal. It can be doubled if well tolerated

Supplements such as Mirica, which contain PEA (palmitoylethanolamide), are mast-cell stabilizers and also help reduce inflammation in the nervous system. Starting slowly at one capsule a day, working up to 2-3 capsules twice daily is the target dose.

DAO (diamine oxide) supplements provide an enzyme that the body makes to metabolize excess histamine, and is often an excellent addition. Starting with one capsule 30 minutes before a meal and working up to 2–3 capsules before each meal is the target dose.

Again, this discussion includes an assortment of substances that do best combined. It is not an exhaustive list, but it's a good start.

Next Step: Treat the Root Cause(s)

Once a patient has become noticeably less sensitive and reactive, which may take a few weeks or sometimes many months, then you can move on to treating the root cause(s), which will ultimately make it likely that the mast-cell activation and vagal and limbic dysfunction will be much improved.

There are a few physicians who treat mast-cell activation and vagal and limbic dysfunction as a primary diagnosis. Yes, this will help, but it will rarely get the patient well until the root cause is addressed. Some of those physicians, who do not look for or treat the root cause, believe strongly that these conditions will need to be addressed for a patient's entire life.

The majority of my patients, however, when their mold toxicity or Lyme disease or other factors are properly addressed, get completely well. They don't need to take the supplements that helped them when they had MCAS, and neither do they need to continue their limbic/vagal training. They are, as far as I and they can tell, completely well. I can then, with a clear conscience, tell my patients that if we provide a comprehensive program, there's an excellent chance that they can recover completely. As you might imagine, merely hearing that is an excellent start at helping their limbic and vagal systems recover. With this in mind, let me review, in the order that I find these conditions causative, the root causes of sensitivity that need to be looked for and treated.

Both Annie Hopper and Ashok Gupta have shared with me that they've each had quite a few sensitive clients improve completely with limbic retraining alone. That I only occasionally see this underscores the individuality of each patient. I've taught and mentored hundreds of physicians, and comparing notes with them I've realized that we medical-care providers attract patients to us in our own unique ways. This means that it's hard to compare any practitioner's practice with another's—we're literally seeing different kinds of patients. Thus, comparing our results, and noting which treatments benefit which patients, varies greatly from practitioner to practitioner. However you choose someone to work with, be aware of this, because it works best if you can match your own style and needs and belief system to your physician's. This might not be easy to do, but it reflects the ideal of what we hope will happen.

Mold Toxicity

Anyone who's become unusually sensitive should be tested for the possibility that they've acquired mold toxicity, which is the most common trigger for such sensitization. With a strong suspicion of mold toxicity, confirmed by history, mold tests of the patient's environment, symptoms, and urine mycotoxin testing, mold toxicity is the single most important thing to treat to reverse sensitivity (and cure the mold toxicity). While it's central to treatment for many patients, we must always try to ascertain just how sensitive our patient is so as to clarify our treatment plan. This means deciding at an early visit whether our patient needs to start by working on limbic or vagal dysfunction and/or mast-cell activation first. A tricky question that often arises here is whether they can start to treat mold toxicity concurrently with the other strategies or whether they need to wait until their sensitivities are under better control. I don't know any scientific way to figure this out, so I often allow my patients to begin by taking tiny doses of mast-cell materials first, and if those are tolerated, tiny amounts of clay, charcoal, and *Saccharomyces boulardii* next. How they handle these supplements gives me immediate feedback as to how to proceed with treatment.

If they handle these tiny amounts well, we can slowly increase the doses of supplements to tolerance. If they don't, we know that this is a very sensitive system, which must be honored, and we'll focus instead on just limbic and vagal approaches for several months.

Given this as an outline, I always remind patients that there are four essential components to treatment (see chapter 6 for details):

Evaluate the home, office, or car for the presence of toxic mold. A patient cannot get well if they continue to be exposed.

Take the appropriate binders that match the mycotoxins that show up in their urine testing.

If necessary (which will be true for most patients), add antifungal and biofilm treatments for the two main reservoirs of colonized mold in the body—the sinuses and gastrointestinal tract.

Improve the patient's ability to detoxify. Look at table #1 in chapter 7 ("Mold Toxicity") to see details on which foods and supplements are specifically useful in improving detoxification of the toxins found on urine-mycotoxin testing. Look below for the general description of improving detoxification for other environmental toxins.

Remember that we also need to be mindful of our patients' ability to detoxify and to support that throughout treatment. Our patients might also be allergic to mold, which is especially problematic if it has colonized and is growing inside their bodies. Immunotherapy for mold allergy can be helpful for many patients. Mold toxins often produce hormonal dysregulation, and treatment of adrenal, thyroid, and sex hormones will be helpful for both immediate improvement and long-term benefit.

I remind patients that treatment is best continued until the urine-mycotoxin testing has normalized. The symptoms might resolve sooner, but there's a significant chance of relapse if the mold isn't adequately removed from their bodies. It usually takes a year or more to fully treat the mold toxicity, and it's important that a patient start with realistic expectations that the process will take quite a bit of time and effort, but that it's is likely to reward them with a return to health.

Lyme Disease and Coinfections

Right behind mold toxicity as a major cause of sensitization is Lyme disease (see chapter 8 for details). While I believe that the mold toxicity, if present, should be treated first, some Lyme experts believe the opposite. Either way, Lyme disease, and particularly the coinfection *Bartonella*, should also be looked for in most patients who've become sensitive, especially if they've gotten better but not completely well, through their treatment of mold toxicity. The opposite is also true: if a patient has gotten better, but not completely well, with the treatment of Lyme disease and its coinfections, then looking for mold toxicity (which produces similar symptoms) should be the next step.

As with mold toxicity, the treatment of Lyme disease and its coinfections is a long and sometimes arduous process that could take several years, but sticking with treatment is usually rewarded by getting well. Experts argue about whether Lyme disease and *Bartonella* can be completely "cured." I've had thousands of patients get well, meaning that they've been off antibiotics, are receiving no treatment, and have had no symptoms for years after treatment was completed. We can argue whether they are "cured," meaning there is not a single pathological organism left in their body, or whether their immune systems have recovered sufficiently to keep the infections under control, but this might be a moot point. From the perspective of healing the limbic and vagal systems, I find it more helpful to allow these patients to feel like they're cured, rather than strain the limbic system by having them constantly look over their shoulders, worried, with every symptom they've experienced previously, that their Lyme is "coming back."

It's important to understand the complexity of Lyme disease, and Dr. Horowitz's aptly-named 16-point program emphasizes this. We've learned that it's not enough to treat the infecting organisms; we must also deal with the toxicity they create, the hormonal dysregulation they engender, and the biochemical distresses they produce. Protecting the gut with adequate probiotics throughout treatment is paramount.

Other Environmental Toxins

When a patient gives a history for exposure to environmental toxins, testing for it is important. Depending on which substance is toxic, different treatments apply (see chapter 11 for more details). Often central to treatment is working on the body's ability to detoxify, by doing some basic interventions:

- Drink pure water
- Eat organic as much as possible
- Evaluate skin care products for safety
- Dietary approaches, such as those detailed in Dr. Joseph Pizzorno's book *The Toxin Solution*, have been helpful.
- Saunas, 20–30 minutes 2–3 times a week. Sensitive patients might need to start with 5 minutes, using lower temperatures.
- Dry brushing
- Oil pulling. Sensitive patients might need to start at just 2–3 minutes a day and slowly work up to 20 minutes daily.

Glutathione

Using liposomal glutathione can help improve the body's ability to detoxify, but many of our sensitive patients can't take it in any quantity without mobilizing toxins faster than they can excrete them, and thus glutathione is contraindicated for them. A trial of glutathione, and the patient's ability to tolerate it, is helpful, but if poorly tolerated, put glutathione on a back burner until the patient is much better and much less sensitive.

It's important to improve the function of the organs of elimination. This brief list of materials is intended only as a starting point:

Liver

Milk thistle, alpha-lipoic acid, Apo-HEPAT. Sensitive patients often benefit from small doses of ToxEase GL, starting at one drop a day and slowly increasing to 2 drops twice daily, with a target of 5–10 drops twice daily if tolerated.

Gall Bladder

Improving the body's ability to make bile by using phosphatidyl choline or ox bile can help, as can using bitters to improve the gall bladder's ability to empty.

Skin

Sweating in any form is helpful. In addition to saunas, hot baths, hot tubs, foot baths, ionic salts or Epsom salts are helpful.

Lymphatics

Lymphatic massage is often of great value. The homeopathic Itires, starting with 1 drop once daily and working up to 5–10 drops twice daily has been of value.

Kidneys

Drinking an adequate amount of water daily is important. Some authorities recommend eight 8-oz. glasses of water, but this would be far too much for some patients. Each patient needs to experiment to find their optimal amount of hydration. The use of the homeopathic Renelix, in the same dosing as ToxEase GL and Itires, can help.

If heavy metals, especially mercury and lead, are noted on testing, specific treatments are indicated. Your physician will help guide you in using the most effective treatments. Sensitive patients, as always, need to consider using smaller-than-usual doses in order to tolerate and benefit from treatment.

For mercury: The use of intravenous DMPS is very effective. If that's not readily available, oral DMSA can help. Sensitive patients might be able to start at 50–100mg twice a week, and gradually increase to 200mg twice a week. The IMD protocol from Quicksilver is often well tolerated and effective.

For lead: The use of intravenous EDTA is very effective. If that's not readily available, oral DMSA can help.

Other heavy metals: See chapter 11 for a more detailed discussion on this subject.

EMFs

We are increasingly realizing that EMFs are adding another level of disability to our sensitive patients. The switch from 4G to 5G might play a role here. I encourage all patients to purchase a hand-held meter that can measure the exposure they get from each of their home devices and appliances. An excellent resource to find a good meter and exactly how to shield those devices can be found in Nicolas Pineault's book *The Non-Tinfoil Guide to EMFs*. In addition, it might be necessary to check your home for dirty electricity, using a Stetzerizer Microsurge Meter. Many of our patients have found that an environmental engineer has been very helpful in defining the problems and limiting exposure. Once shielded, many of our patients report immediate improvement.

Thiamine Deficiency

The important role of thiamine in helping heal the autonomic nervous system is described in detail in chapter 18. While testing for thiamine deficiency is possible, accurate testing isn't readily available. It's easiest to just supplement with thiamine and see how your patient responds.

Most sensitive patients can start with 100mg of thiamine hydrochloride daily, but a few need to start at lower doses (10–25mg) and slowly work up from there. Once 100mg is tolerated, increasing to twice daily, then doubling that, can be helpful. If thiamine hydrochloride is tolerated, switching to benfotiamine or TTFD may provide a form of thiamine that can move more easily through the blood-brain barrier into the brain and hence be more effective.

Oxalates

Several tipoffs suggest that oxalates are contributing to a patient's sensitivities. A history of kidney stones, especially if they're recurrent, or a history of chronic pelvic pain, interstitial cystitis (IC), recurrent vaginitis, or pain with intercourse, could point in this direction.

See chapter 12 for a detailed discussion of oxalates. A brief review of possible treatments includes:

Magnesium and/or calcium citrate. These can bind to oxalates to help remove them from the body.

Low-oxalate diet: While potentially very helpful, one must go slowly on instituting this diet because of the possibility of oxalate dumping; it can make the patient worse if they decrease their body content of oxalates too abruptly.

Sulfation

See chapter 13 for a detailed discussion of this issue. An overview of treatment options includes:

Low-sulfate diet: Common sources of sulfate include garlic, onions, animal protein, dairy, broccoli, eggs, cauliflower, brussels sprouts, asparagus, cabbage, kale, and spinach. It would be best to work with a dietician to slowly introduce this, or any, dietary change.

Molybdenum as a supplement to improve the process of sulfation; also hydroxocobalamin, CoQ10, and butyrate.

Epsom salt baths, nightly at first, starting with 1 cup, and working up to 4 cups of Epsom salts per bath, eventually cutting back to 2–3 times a week. Especially sensitive patients might need to start treatment with ¼ or ½ cup and work up from there.

Structural Issues

Any part of our anatomy that's unable to move properly might put a strain on the body that can show itself as pain, stiffness, or restricted motion. These in turn can compress or restrict the function of arteries, veins, nerves, or lymphatics, decreasing the flow of blood, fluids, or energy to parts of the body that need it. The most obvious example would be a decreased flow of oxygen, vital to all organs and tissues, if arteries or veins are compressed.

Previous injuries, surgery, or childbirth can create these structural issues, and an assessment and treatment can be very helpful in promoting healing and decreasing the strains on a body that add to the process of sensitization. Evaluation by a trained osteopathic physician, chiropractor, or physiatrist may be needed (see chapter 16 for more details).

A particularly important area to be aware of is dental/facial structural imbalance, which can play a unique and important role in either initiating sensitization or worsening it. If a sensitive patient has a history of TMJ or jaw misalignment, and perhaps oral surgery, addressing this might be a starting point of treatment before other treatments can be tolerated (see chapter 15 for more details).

Ketamine and Micro-dosing of Psychedelics: See chapter 26.
Salicylates: See chapter 14.
LDI/LDA: See chapter 25.
Carbon Monoxide Poisoning: See chapter 22.
Secondary Porphyrias: See chapter 23.
Genetic/Genomic Considerations: See chapter 19.

Prevention and Treatment of Long-Haul COVID

Many authors have written about a variety of supplements that have, in their extensive experience, helped prevent the onset of Long COVID after an episode of infection.

These include taking an adequate amount of vitamin D (check blood levels—they should be at least 60–80 nmol/L), N-acetyl cysteine, glutathione, alpha lipoic acid, lysine, vitamin C, and zinc, among others. See Dr. Horowitz's published paper "Three novel prevention, diagnostic and treatment options for COVID-19, urgently necessitating controlled, randomized trials" in *Medical Hypotheses*, October 2020, 143: 109851.

Treatment of Long-Haul COVID

Recent research by Bruce Patterson, MD, has shown that patients with Long-Haul COVID show a predictable pattern of cytokines that can be measured by a blood test from InCellDx laboratories. Using a combination of maraviroc and pravastatin, Dr. Patterson has found remarkable effectiveness in healing Long-Haul COVID. Further research into cytokine panels on blood testing gives promise that we'll find other patterns that can help clarify the diagnostics of our patients who have chronic inflammatory illness, one of the major triggers for sensitivity.

Oxygen As Therapy

I'm not certain about exactly how this works, but I'll share with you the benefits of low-dose oxygen therapy, found to be of great benefit by William Rea, MD, who pioneered the treatment of environmental sensitivity. We have found that sensitive patients often respond well to 2 liters of oxygen per minute, delivered by nasal canula for 2 hours a day. Many sensitive patients will react to the plastic in the nasal mask or tubing that connects with the oxygen tank, so a ceramic mask and hypoallergenic tubing might be necessary. It's possible that this might help those with carbon monoxide poisoning, but the benefits seem to be so generalized that I suspect another mechanism is in play here. The bottom line is that the regular use of oxygen will help many sensitive patients.

A Simplified Approach to Treatment

Given the complexity of what I've laid out here, it might be helpful if I simplified by emphasizing what I consider the basics of treatment. These suggestions are all contingent on the proposed treatment being relevant to the patient, based on their symptoms; i.e., if a patient has no symptoms that suggest mast-cell activation, it might not be necessary to try treatments for it unless the patient isn't responding well to what they've been trying. Similarly, if the patient has no known exposure to Lyme disease and their Lyme testing is negative, treating Lyme or its coinfections might be unnecessary and inappropriate.

Each patient must be treated according to their own individual presentation, symptoms, biochemistry, and genetics. Given this as our starting point, a simplified approach to treatment for a sensitive patient might include:

Starting with limbic/vagal and/or mast-cell activation treatments and being assured that EMF exposure has been minimized and the home or work environment has been evaluated, additional treatments can then be used. I encourage starting with mold toxicity, which will be present in the majority of patients. Thiamine replacement should be considered as an early intervention. When this has been adequately addressed, move on to Lyme and coinfection treatment if they're present.

If patients aren't responding to these basics, look into oxalates, salicylates, dental and structural issues, secondary porphyrias, carbon monoxide exposure, and other environmental exposures or toxicities.

Hopefully this will help keep our focus on what we need to do, and in what order, for most patients. This approach has been effective in helping thousands of my patients recover their health, so please keep your hopes up that you'll respond too!

Acknowledgments

This book was a wonderful collaborative effort. From the inception of the idea that we could bring this information to the attention of the public and the medical world, I was touched by the willingness of the twenty authors who readily agreed to volunteer their time and expertise to bring this volume to life.

What we've produced is a cutting-edge discussion of a medical condition that hasn't received the recognition it merits. We anticipate that this information will help countless individuals who are struggling with their health. It will also provide a road map for physicians to understand and effectively treat these patients with precision.

It takes a fabulous team to be able to pull all this together, so first, let me thank the authors of these chapters, in the order that we present them. I am forever grateful to Jill Crista, Annie Hopper, Ashok Gupta, Frances Goodall, Stephen Porges, Beth O'Hara, Andrew Maxwell, Deborah Wardly, Kurt Woeller, Richard Horowitz, Riina Bray, Magda Havas, Martin Pall, Lyn Patrick, Emily Givler, Greg Nigh, Tasha Turzo, Carmine Van Deven, James Greenblatt, Chandler Marrs, Bob Miller, Ty Vincent, and Andreas Grossgold for their contributions. Just by that list, you can see how much effort went into putting this together.

There are so many others who have contributed to this effort by teaching me and helping me understand these complicated concepts. While I can't possibly name all of them, I want to single out Robert Naviaux, whose Cell Danger Response model of chronic illness is central to these understandings. I would also like to thank Stephanie Seneff, who wrote a chapter and then connected me with Greg Nigh to make that chapter even better.

This book could not have come into being without the vision and dedication of our publishing team at Cypress House. With gratitude to my publisher, Cynthia Frank, and my editor, Joe Shaw, for their help in uniting all of this information, in its diverse forms, into a cohesive volume.

This book could not have come into being without the support of my wonderful family, most especially Cheryl, my muse and the love of my life, who inspires me daily to be the best version of myself. And always, my children, Aviva, Jules, and David, and my grandchildren, Avinash, Anjali (I did spell it right this time!), and Wilder. And my two providers of unconditional puppy love, Sasha and Eddie.

Thank you all, always, for everything!

Index

twitching in muscle, 86–87
type I and II primary hyperoxaluria, 238
tyrosine, 317

ulcerative colitis, 110, 392, 400
underactive *vs.* overactive enzymes, 338–340
upper airway resistance syndrome (UARS), 79–80
uridine, 383
urine mycotoxin testing, 124

vaccination-induced autonomic dysregulation
    lithium orotate, low dose, 386
      Monolaurin, 386
      vagus nerve therapies, 386–387
vagal anti-inflammatory reflex, 38
vagal compression syndrome, 280–281
vagal dysfunctions, 38, 281, 434–435
vagal inflammatory reflex, 41, 118
vagal nerve dysfunction, 5, 103–104
vagal nerve-entrapment syndrome, 275
vagal nerve system, 1, 38
vagal parasympathetic activity, suppression of, 384
vagal-system dysfunction, 38
vagus-nerve function, 17–18
vagus nerve therapies, 386–387
Valium, 307
Valsalva maneuver, 79–80
venous and lymphatic circulation, 297
ventral vagal complex, 36–37
vertebrobasilar insufficiency, 78
VGCC calcium-channel blockers for treatment
    of EHS, 184–185

Vincent, T., 391, 401–402
viscerosomatic reflex, 291
Vistaril (hydroxyzine), 436
vitamin B-1, *see* thiamine
vitamin B6, 238–239, 241–242, 314–315
vitamin B12, 257, 313–314
vitamin C, 236
vitamin D, 249–250, 315
    activation, 97
    deficiencies, 182
vocalizations, acoustic features of, 36
Voice Dialogue, 368
volatile organic compounds (VOCs), 196, 199
voltage-gated calcium channel (VGCC), 151

Wardly, Deborah, 84
Wardly Phenomenon, 81–82
Welchol (colesevalam), 124
Wernicke's encephalopathy, 325
Wilson, D., 358
Wilson's syndrome, 358
Winkelman, S., 368
Woeller, Kurt N., 100
Wolff Parkinson White syndrome, 153

Xanax, 307
Xyzal (levocetirizine), 436

zearalenone, 111, 124
zirconium dioxide, 160
Zyrtec (cetirizine), 436

About the Author

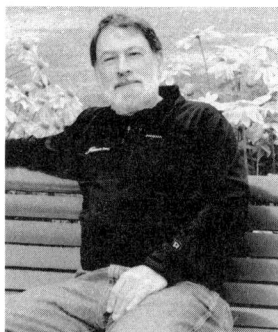

Neil Nathan, MD, has practiced medicine for over five decades. Board certified in Family Practice and Pain Management, he is a Founding Diplomate of the American Board of Integrative Holistic Medicine, and served as a board member of the International Society for Environmentally Acquired Illness (ISEAI). For many years, he has worked primarily with patients whom conventional medical sources could not diagnose, and especially with those whose illness has made them unusually sensitive and hence difficult to treat.

An internationally recognized speaker, Dr. Nathan has lectured to medical audiences both nationally and internationally. The books he has written include *Healing is Possible: New Hope for Chronic Fatigue, Fibromyalgia, Persistent Pain, and Other Chronic Illnesses; On Hope and Healing: For Those Who Have Fallen Through the Medical Cracks; and Toxic: Heal Your Body from Mold Toxicity, Lyme Disease, Multiple Chemical Sensitivities and Chronic Environmental Illness.* He also authored *Energetic Diagnosis: Groundbreaking Thesis on Diagnosing Disease and Chronic Illness,* and the e-book *Mold and Mycotoxins: Current Evaluation and Treatment 2022.* A researcher as well, he is a coauthor, with Dr. Robert Naviaux, of the groundbreaking medical paper "Metabolic Features of Chronic Fatigue Syndrome," published in *Mitochondrion* (https://doi.org/10.1073/pnas.1607571113).

Dr. Nathan has hosted an internationally syndicated radio program/podcast on VoiceAmerica called *The Cutting Edge of Health and Wellness Today.* He has also mentored nearly 200 physicians, teaching them the principles of treatment for chronic inflammatory illnesses that trigger increased sensitivity. Learn more about his mentoring program (with Dr. Jill Crista) at www.neilnathanmd.com. Dr. Nathan is available for consultations with patients and to coordinate his suggestions for healing with their primary treating physicians; contact him at askdrnathan@gmail.com.